Cognitive Therapy for Depressed Adolescents

MENTAL HEALTH AND PSYCHOPATHOLOGY
A MacArthur Foundation Research Network Series

DAVID J. KUPFER, Series Editor

COGNITIVE THERAPY FOR
DEPRESSED ADOLESCENTS
T. C. R. Wilkes, Gayle Belsher, A. John Rush,
Ellen Frank, and Associates

PERSONALITY AND DEPRESSION:
A CURRENT VIEW
Marjorie H. Klein, David J. Kupfer, and M. Tracie Shea, *Editors*

Cognitive Therapy for Depressed Adolescents

T. C. R. WILKES
GAYLE BELSHER
A. JOHN RUSH
ELLEN FRANK
and Associates

Foreword by Aaron T. Beck

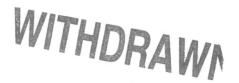

THE GUILFORD PRESS
New York   London

Printed in the United States of America

This book is printed on acid-free paper.

Last digit is print number: 9 8 7 6 5 4 3 2 1

Library of Congress Cataloging-in-Publication Data
Cognitive therapy for depressed adolescents / T. C. R. Wilkes . . . [et
al.] and associates; foreword by Aaron T. Beck.
    p.   cm.—(Mental health and psychopathology)
    Includes bibliographical references and index.
    ISBN 0-89862-119-4
    1. Depression in adolescence—Treatment.   2. Cognitive therapy for
teenagers.   I. Wilkes, T. C. R. (Thomas C. R.)   II. Series.
    [DNLM: 1. Depressive Disorder—in adolescence.   2. Depressive
Disorder—therapy.   3. Cognitive Therapy—in adolescence.
4. Cognitive Therapy—methods.   WM 171 C67595 1994]
RJ506.D4C64   1994
616.85′27′00835—dc20
DNLM/DLC
for Library of Congress   94-13340
                                              CIP

Contributing Authors

Aaron T. Beck, M.D., Center for Cognitive Therapy, University of Pennsylvania, Philadelphia, Pennsylvnia

Gayle Belsher, Ph.D., Department of Psychiatry, University of Calgary, Calgary, Alberta, Canada; present address: Department of Psychology, Calgary District Hospital Group, Calgary, Alberta, Canada

David A. Brent, M.D., Department of Psychiatry, University of Pittsburgh Medical Center, Western Psychiatric Institute and Clinic, Pittsburgh, Pennsylvania

Graham J. Emslie, M.D., Department of Psychiatry, University of Texas Southwestern Medical Center at Dallas, and Children's Medical Center of Dallas, Dallas, Texas

Ellen Frank, Ph.D., Department of Psychiatry, University of Pittsburgh Medical Center, Western Psychiatric Institute and Clinic, Pittsburgh, Pennsylvania

Miriam S. Lerner, Ph.D., Department of Psychiatry, University of Pittsburgh Medical Center, Western Psychiatric Institute and Clinic, Pittsburgh, Pennsylvania; present address: Allegheny General Hospital, Wexford, Pennsylvania

Anthony Nowels, M.D., Grant Center Hospital and University of Miami School of Medicine, Miami, Florida

A. John Rush, M.D., Department of Psychiatry, University of Texas Southwestern Medical Center at Dallas, Dallas, Texas

Warren A. Weinberg, M.D., Department of Pediatrics and Neurology, University of Texas Southwestern Medical Center at Dallas, and Children's Medical Center of Dallas, Dallas, Texas

T. C. R. Wilkes, M.D., Department of Psychiatry, University of Calgary, Foothills Hospital, Calgary, Alberta, Canada

Acknowledgments

This work owes much to the support of David J. Kupfer, M.D., Director of the John D. and Catherine T. MacArthur Foundation Research Network on the Psychobiology of Depression and Other Affective Disorders.

This book represents a combination of many years of clinical practice and research interest in the field of adolescent depression. Indeed, many people have contributed to this book—clinicians, researchers, and patients. In particular, we would like to thank our colleagues who made suggestions and comments regarding the revision of the manual when we organized an open pilot study at the Dallas, Calgary, Hamilton, and Toronto child and adolescent divisions. These include, from Dallas, Denise McCallon, Ph.D., Sunita Stewart, Ph.D., and Betsy Kinnard, Ph.D; from Calgary, Brian Cram, M.D., and Allan Donsky, M.D.; from Hamilton, the child and adolescent assessment team members Ted Ridley and Tom Alexander, together with Linda Archer, Ph.D.; and, from Toronto, Robert Stein, M.D., and George Papatheordorow, M.D.

T. C. R. Wilkes
Gayle Belsher
A. John Rush
Ellen Frank

Foreword

Among the exciting developments in cognitive therapy has been its application to disorders and populations not originally envisioned in my early writings. The initial approach to the common garden variety of disorders such as depression, anxiety, and phobias has now been modified and extended to a wide variety of disorders ranging from hypochondrias to schizophrenia. With the passage of time, therapists involved in treating specific disorders not described in earlier publications have found that they are able to adapt cognitive therapy to almost any clinical problem that they encounter. Empirical work continues at a high rate to validate these newer applications.

Therapists working with a broad range of populations also have found that they can utilize cognitive approaches in dealing with patients of both genders, children, adolescents, adults, and elderly individuals. It has not been necessary to devise a whole new armamentarium in treating these population groups. Using their own experience and ingenuity, therapists have been able to integrate the cognitive approach within the framework that they have already been utilizing. The essence of cognitive therapy is not so much the specific technology that is used but rather the elaboration of an appropriate cognitive model and then its modification to a specific population.

The present authors have succeeded admirably in developing and publishing a cognitive approach to depressed adolescents. Until recently, depression in childhood and adolescence was often questioned as a valid clinical entity on the grounds that the development of a mature superego structure would not as yet have occurred. Depression in adolescence was largely dismissed as a "transient phase" in development. However, epidemiological research has revealed prevalence rates of adolescent depression in the community and in hospital-based clinics ranging from 5 to 40%. Longitudinal investigations have subsequently revealed that the average length of the depressive episode among children could be from 6 to 8 months, whereas dysthymia could last up to 3½ years. In light of all this research, it is not surprising that the National Institute of Mental Health in 1990 published a position paper identifying depression in childhood and adolescence as a high priority.

In the late 1970s, the publication of our volume *Cognitive Therapy of Depression* stimulated much research into the treatment of adult depression. The latter work, together with the relatively disappointing results from the controlled trials of pharmacological treatment for adolescent depression, was the main impetus for adapting cognitive therapy for adults to depressed adolescents. The present volume represents a combination of many years of clinical practice and research interest in the field of adolescent depression.

The first two parts of the book include the first six chapters. Chapter 3 reviews the special issues of diagnosis and assessment of depression in adolescents. The other chapters are devoted to demonstrating the differences between cognitive therapy with adolescents and with adults. Special attention needs to be given to the formation of a therapeutic alliance. Since adolescents are qualitatively different from adults, any psychotherapy for depression in this younger age group has to tease out the differential contributions of the adolescent phase itself, the unique contribution of learning style and temperament, and, finally, the signs and symptoms of a depressive disorder. Chapter 2 in particular emphasizes 10 key principles that cognitive therapists should take into account when they treat depressed adolescents. A detailed review of cognitive development stages in Chapter 4 illustrates further the differences between adult and adolescent patients in therapy. In Chapter 6, the role of the family in treating adolescents with depression is discussed. The authors have tried to dispel the myth that cognitive therapy is an individual therapy that cannot be applied to groups, couples, or families. They also describe the common therapeutic problems encountered in families of depressed adolescents, mainly hidden agendas and the problem of social control.

Part III is designed to help the reader go through a "how to do" approach to therapy from the initial through the middle and final phases of treatment. Emphasis has been placed on the conceptual macrostages involved in making a cognitive formulation which then dictates the microstages of specific cognitive techniques. Chapter 7 reviews setting goals and priorities. The authors avoid a cookbook approach by including many clinical vignettes that highlight the importance of individualized cognitve formulations. Formulations are changed as new information emerges regarding adolescents' core assumptions and beliefs, the prevalence of their affective states, and their behavior.

The authors have emphasized repeatedly the importance of a trusting, secure relationship with the therapist. This attitude reminds the reader perhaps of Bowlby, who also developed the idea of an internal map of the world, a set of schemas in which self and others and their relationships are represented. This conceptualization clearly integrates well the cognitive model's concepts of core beliefs and primary and secondary assumptions about self and others and the future. As a result of the collaborative approach, the therapist shares the adolescent's perception of loss and pain. Therapist and patient are able to reconstruct narrative, a process that facilitates for patients a more helpful view of their world, themselves, and their future. Chapter 8 pays particular attention to five steps in treatment, especially the monitoring of mood changes and the identifying of automatic thoughts and common cognitive distortions characteristic of this age group. Chapter 9 addresses the importance of setting age-appropriate goals, particularly in view of the fact that the developmental matrix the therapist finds himself in will frequently merge issues of depression with issues of separation and individuation, and therefore identity formation.

Part IV describes what all child and adolescent psychiatrists are only too well aware of—the ubiquitous comorbidity that occurs with adolescent depression, particularly substance abuse and sexual abuse. Chapter 10 shows how cognitive therapy and recovery, especially the 12-step program, can be combined in a hospital-based program. Chapter 12 describes the role of cognitive therapy with depressed adolescents who are hopeless and suicidal.

Parts V and VI acknowledge that outpatient cognitive therapy is but one of many paradigms for the treatment of depressed adolescents. Chapters 13 and 14 review the role of hospital inpatient settings with depressed adolescents, and Chapter 14 considers the role of multimodal therapy for depressed adolescents as well. The authors recognize that the therapist's reality will often be determined by the context in which he is working. Nevertheless, the authors believe that the cognitive therapy paradigm can be very helpful for the depressed adolescent. Chapter 15 incorporates common obstacles and questions that many therapists have raised during supervision. It also addresses the problem that some adolescents may be a "poor fit" with the cognitive model or that the therapy may be focusing inappropriately on cognitive distortion when there is really a deficit in social skills, such as accurate empathy, consequential thinking, coping strategies, and problem-solving ability. The authors indicate that therapy must be shaped to meet the needs of the adolescent: They avoid the blind approach of applying congitive techniques in a cookbook fashion!

This book will be of value to clinicians of all disciplines dealing with adolescents. Experienced psychologists, psychiatrists, social workers, and psychiatric nurses will find much to enhance their therapeutic skills, and neophytes and students will discover a rich source of information.

AARON T. BECK, M.D.

Preface

This manual provides general guidelines and specific case examples for the use of cognitive therapy in treating depressed adolescents. It borrows heavily from and provides adaptations to the use of Aaron T. Beck's cognitive therapy for depression in adults (Beck et al., 1979).

We developed this manual for trained psychotherapists—physicians, psychologists, mental health nurses, social workers, and child-care workers—who are dealing with depressed or dysthymic adolescents. It is not intended for the treatment of adolescents with bipolar or psychotic depression, although it does attempt to address adolescents who are depressed with significant comorbidity from posttraumatic stress disorder or alcohol and drug abuse. The emphasis of the manual is on outpatient treatment, since this is the setting in which cognitive therapy has typically been provided. However, since brief periods of hospitalization are fairly regularly part of the management of depressed adolescents, we have devoted one chapter to the use of cognitive techniques in the inpatient setting. The reader of this manual who wishes to use it in practice should (1) have previous basic psychotherapy training with adults and adolescents, and (2) have read and had experience in using cognitive or behavioral methods with depressed adults.

As is the case with all therapy, and with adolescent therapy in particular, treatment manuals cannot be used as recipe books. Rather, the general approach of therapy (problem definition, designation of alternative strategies, selection of a specific strategy, implementation, assessment of the effect of the implementation, revision in problem definition, and so on) is an interactive, educational, but still trial-and-error process. Thus, the reader should note that both the principal strategies, as well as particular tactics, described here are provided as examples without intending to cover all possibilities. Creative therapists will blend what is provided herein with their previous experience and a "feel" for the particular patient at a particular moment to develop new tactics and strategies and to adapt our recommendations to their own practices and environments.

The other word of caution we wish to offer is that the efficacy of the cognitive approach with depressed adolescents has not been established empirically. We have used it in our own work with this population and, with adaptations, have found it useful enough to prepare this manual. However, the therapist should be aware that the cognitive approach to depressed adolescents may be useful for only a subset of such patients and, in some cases, may be ineffective. Thus, repeated assessment of the patients' signs and symptoms and, indeed, follow-up of those who appear to have responded, are strongly recommended, since a failure to respond after a reasonable period of time should alert the clinician to the need for a diagnostic reappraisal and potential changes in the treatment plan. Conversely, for those patients who respond, careful longitudinal follow-up is essential, since many patients may suffer a relapse or recurrence.

We hope readers find our limited experience to be a useful guide in their own practice, and we welcome their feedback in order to add to the body of experience in using cognitive techniques in treating an adolescent population.

REFERENCE

Beck AT, Rush AJ, Shaw BF, Emery G: *Cognitive Therapy of Depression.* New York, Guilford Press, 1979.

Contents

Cognitive Therapy for
Depressed Adolescents

PART I

Introduction and Overview

CHAPTER ONE

Adaptation of Cognitive Therapy for Depressed Adolescents

A. JOHN RUSH

ANTHONY NOWELS

INTRODUCTION

Cognitive therapy of various psychiatric disorders has been the subject of several recent reviews (Beck, 1976; Rush, 1982; Jarrett and Rush, 1986; Beck and Rush, 1989; Jarrett, 1990). For syndromal disorders as outlined in Axis I of the *Diagnostic and Statistical Manual of Mental Disorders*, third edition, revised (DSM-III-R; American Psychiatric Association, 1987),[1] cognitive therapy is a short-term, time-limited psychotherapy aimed at specific target conditions. Cognitive theory suggests that negative thinking plays a pivotal role in the development and/or maintenance of depression. In applying cognitive therapy, symptoms of the depressive syndrome are used as clues to define specific negative automatic thoughts (verbal thoughts or pictorial images) that contribute to the symptomatic state and to identify assumptions, core beliefs, or schemas that account for psychological vulnerability.

---

[1]This manual refers to diagnoses by DSM-III-R categories since DSM-III-R is currently the most widely used psychiatric nosological system and is, therefore, likely to be familiar to most readers. When the authors refer to "depression," they typically mean major depressive disorder as defined in DSM-III-R terms. However, the cognitive techniques described in this volume are also likely to be appropriate for milder forms of depression such as dysthymic disorder or for less well-defined forms, such as depressive disorder not otherwise specified. DSM-IV is expected in May 1994. The symptom criteria for major depressive disorder and dysthymic disorder were unchanged from DSM-III-R.

The initial phase of treatment aims at symptom reduction. The therapist tries to teach patients to recognize and record their negative automatic thoughts. Thereafter, patients use objective evaluation and experimentation to learn how these negative automatic thoughts modify their thinking patterns.

The second half of therapy aims at the identification and modification of specific assumptions (schemas or dysfunctional attitudes) that are inferred from the patient's stereotyped thinking and behavioral patterns. These schemas are values or notions that derive from previous personal experiences that support the negatively biased moment-to-moment automatic thinking, culminating in the symptomatic state. The schemas are viewed as vulnerability factors for future recurrence. Cognitive therapy thus aims at both acute symptom reduction and subsequent prophylaxis.

HISTORICAL BACKGROUND

Cognitive therapy derives from the so-called "phenomenological" school of psychology, the philosophical basis for which is described elsewhere (Spielberg, 1971, 1972). The phenomenologists assign a central role to an individual's view of himself[2] and the world as determinants of behavior—a notion initially proposed by the Stoic philosophers of Greece.

Alfred Adler emphasized the idea that each of us lives in a personal conceptualization or representation of the objective world (Ansbacher and Ansbacher, 1956). According to Adler, the profusion of stimuli that bombard us is immediately organized, conceptualized, and given meaning based on our personal, unique prior experiences. He coined the term "phenomenal field" to denote this constructed representation of objective reality. The phenomenal field of subjective reality explains why different people respond differently to the same event or series of events. For example, moving to a new city may be seen as a loss by some and as an adventure by others. Thus, it is not events in themselves but the views we take of them that please or upset us. The phenomenological emphasis apparently arose in the 20th century, in part from dissatisfaction with unconscious motivation as a sufficient explanation for various behaviors. In general, unconscious motivations are inferred

---

[2]For ease of reading and to avoid awkward sentence construction, the authors follow the standard English convention of using the masculine pronoun form to include both genders.

from a behavioral pattern by examining the results of the behavioral sequence. The clinician assumes that the consequences of the behavioral pattern make apparent one's unconscious wishes and desires. Thus, if the person denies that he actually desires the end products of a behavioral sequence, this denial may be discounted.

However, if the consequences of a behavior constitute the sole basis for inferring unconscious motivations, diagnostic errors may result. For instance, one may erroneously infer an unconscious desire from a behavioral consequence that the individual neither desired nor foresaw. Motivational inferences based exclusively on the consequences of a behavior assume (1) that the patient can make anything happen that he wants, (2) that nothing happens that he does not want, and (3) that he can consciously or unconsciously foresee all the consequences of any particular behavioral sequence before undertaking it. Obviously, these assumptions are rarely applicable to everyday situations.

On the other hand, cognitive theory assumes that a person chooses those options that are in his own best interest, based on his particular, albeit idiosyncratic, view of things. However, these views are rarely objective and are often highly biased in a stereotyped fashion. Cognitive therapy views self-defeating behaviors not as a desire to lose, for example, but as a result of the patient's inability either to conceive of or to carry out more constructive alternatives.

Initially, the cognitive therapist clarifies how patients view things (i.e., how they conceptualize and give meaning to particular events): What are the bases of these views? Are they accurate? To what behaviors and feelings do these views lead? For instance, depressed persons often fail to undertake common-sense measures that might relieve their depression, not because they want to suffer (one of several possible unconscious motivational assumptions), but because (1) they cannot conceive of the particular steps needed to reduce the depression, (2) they do not believe that any actions will result in relief, or (3) they may not believe that they can successfully complete the needed steps. If patients are convinced that corrective actions are unavailable or doomed to failure, this conviction logically leads to a decision not to try.

Beck (1963, 1976) has emphasized the critical role that automatic thoughts (conscious verbal or pictorial mental activity) and assumptions or beliefs play in stereotyped, repetitive, "neurotic" behavior. In recent decades, ego-psychoanalytic (Klein, 1970), neobehavioral (Mahoney, 1974; Meichenbaum, 1977), and cognitive-psychological (Kelly, 1955; Ellis, 1962) movements have also emphasized the importance of moment-to-moment thinking patterns on behavior.

A cognitive explanatory system allows for a significant degree of direct empirical testing of many of the presumed determinants of behavior. If patients' views of events lead to particular responses, and if their views are written, then their awareness and consciousness are available to them, and the relationship between their views and observed behaviors can be evaluated. Thus, a cognitive perspective allows for greater empirical testing than does a strictly unconscious motivational explanation of behavior. Indeed, key elements of Beck's theory are supported by a range of empirical data (for a review see Beck and Rush, 1978).

COGNITIVE THEORY OF DEPRESSION

The cognitive theory of depression is a formulation that grew out of careful clinical observation and experimental testing. This interplay of clinical and experimental information has fostered the careful evolution of this model and of the psychotherapy it has spawned. The cognitive model postulates three specific notions to explain depression: the cognitive triad, schemas, and cognitive errors.

The Cognitive Triad

The cognitive triad consists of the patient's view of himself, his world or day-to-day experiences, and his future. The negative view of the self is apparent in depressed patients' beliefs that they are defective, inadequate, or unworthy and in their attribution of their unpleasant experiences to physical, mental, or moral defects in themselves. Such patients believe they are undesirable and worthless because of their presumed defects. They underestimate or criticize themselves because of these defects. Finally, they believe they lack the attributes deemed essential to the attainment of happiness and contentment.

Second, depressed persons interpret their ongoing experiences in negative ways. They see the world as making exorbitant demands on them and/or presenting insurmountable obstacles to their reaching their life goals. They misinterpret their interactions with those around them as evidence for defeat and deprivation. Depressed patients negatively construe situations even when less negative, more plausible alternative interpretations are available. However, depressed persons are often able to revise their initial negative interpretations if they can learn to employ more objective, less negative explanations. In this way, they come to realize that they automatically tailor facts to fit their preconceived negative conclusions.

The third component of the cognitive model, negative view of the future, is evident as depressed persons look ahead. They anticipate that current difficulties or suffering will continue indefinitely. They expect unremitting hardship, frustration, and deprivation. When they consider undertaking specific tasks, they believe they will fail.

Cognitive theory suggests that many associated signs and symptoms of depression are maintained by or may follow from the activation of the negative cognitive triad. For example, if patients incorrectly think they are being rejected, they react with the same negative emotion (e.g., sadness, anger) that occurs with actual rejection. If they erroneously believe they are social outcasts, they feel lonely.

The depressed person's relationships to others (e.g., increased dependency) can also be explained cognitively. Because depressed people see themselves as inept and undesirable, they unrealistically overestimate the difficulty involved in normal tasks and expect things to turn out badly. Patients seek help and reassurance from others whom they consider more competent and capable.

If depressed individuals expect negative outcomes, they will not commit themselves to a goal or specific undertaking. Suicidal wishes are understood as extreme expressions of desires to escape from what appear to be insoluble problems or unbearable situations. Depressed persons often see themselves as both worthless and as burdens on others, thereby concluding that they are better off dead.

Finally, negatively biased thinking may also exacerbate the physical symptoms of depression. Apathy and low energy may result from the patients' view that they are doomed to failure in all their efforts. A negative view of the future leads to or supports a sense of futility, which may exacerbate "psychomotor inhibition."

Schemas

Schemas are the second major ingredient in the cognitive model. They explain why depressed patients continue to believe in painful attitudes despite objective evidence of positive factors in their lives.

Each situation is composed of a plethora of stimuli, to which individuals attend selectively. They combine these elements into patterns by which they conceptualize situations. Although different persons conceptualize the same situation in different ways, a particular person tends to be consistent in his responses to similar events. Relatively stable patterns of conceptualization explain the regularity of interpretations of a particular set of situations. The term "schema" designates these stable thinking or conceptualizing patterns.

When a person faces a particular circumstance, a schema related to the circumstance is activated. The schema is the basis for molding raw sensory information into automatic thoughts (defined as any mental activity with verbal or pictorial content). Schemas provide the rules for screening out, differentiating, and encoding these raw sensory stimuli into ideas. They help us to categorize and evaluate our experiences in a consistent way. Schemas, however, are inferred from the patterns of automatic thoughts (mental events that are available to the consciousness).

Schemas determine how individuals structure different experiences. A schema that is inactive at one time can be activated by specific environmental events. The schemas activated by specific situations directly determine how persons cognitively conceptualize and affectively respond to those situations. For example, if a person is concerned about whether he is competent and adequate, he may be assuming the validity of the schema "Unless I do everything perfectly, I'm a failure." In this case, he will evaluate various situations in terms of personal adequacy, even when this question is not obviously related to the situation. For instance, while swimming at the beach (an apparently enjoyable activity not related to personal competence), this person may think, "Is my swimming good enough? Do I look as good as others?"

The depressed patient's conceptualizations of specific situations are distorted to fit particular schemas. The orderly matching of the objective stimulus and appropriate schema is upset by the intrusion of overly active, idiosyncratic schemas that displace more appropriate ones. As these idiosyncratic schemas become more active, they are evoked by a wider range of stimuli that are less and less logically related to the schemas. The patient's growing inability to invoke other, more appropriate schemas causes him to lose control of his thinking processes.

In milder depressions, patients may be able to view their negative thoughts with some objectivity. However, as the depression worsens, their thinking is increasingly dominated by negative ideas, although there may be no logical connection between actual situations and negative interpretations. Patients become increasingly less able to entertain the notion that their negative interpretations are erroneous, possibly because the stronger idiosyncratic schemas interfere with reality testing and reasoning. These hypervalent schemas lead to distortions of reality and, consequently, to systematic errors in the depressed person's thinking.

Cognitive Errors

As schemas become more pronounced, systematic errors in the logic of the depressed person's thinking become more apparent. These errors include arbitrary inference, selective abstraction, overgeneralization, magnification or minimization, and personalization. *Arbitrary inference* refers to the process of drawing a conclusion that either is contrary to the data or is not supported by the evidence. *Selective abstraction* consists of focusing on a detail taken out of context, ignoring other more salient features of the situation and conceptualizing the whole experience based on this element. *Overgeneralization* refers to drawing a general conclusion on the basis of a single incident. *Magnification and minimization* are errors in evaluation based on over- or underemphasizing either the entire or selected aspects of the situation(s). *Personalization* is inappropriately relating external events to oneself without an obvious basis for making such connections.

Cognitive theory hypothesizes that an individual's predisposition to depression is based on his early experiences, which may constitute the basis for forming a negative view about himself, the future, and the world around him. These schemas may generally be latent but become activated by specific circumstances that are analogous to the experiences that were initially responsible for embedding the negative attitude.

For example, disruption of a marital situation may activate the concept of irreversible loss associated with the death of a parent in childhood. Alternatively, depression may be triggered by the development of an illness that activates the notion that one is destined to prolonged suffering. While these and other events might be painful to most people, they do not necessarily produce a depression unless the person is particularly sensitive to the situation because of previous experience and consequent predepressive cognitive organization or schemas. In response to current trauma or stressful events, the average person will still maintain interest in and realistically appraise other nontraumatic aspects of his life. However, the thinking of depression-prone persons becomes markedly constricted, and they develop negative ideas about many aspects of their lives.

There is substantial empirical support for the cognitive theory of depression from naturalistic, clinical, and experimental studies that have documented the presence and intercorrelation of the constituents of the "cognitive triad" in association with depression. Several studies have demonstrated the presence of specific thinking deficits, such as impaired abstract reasoning and selective attention, in depressed or suicidal persons. Dysfunctional attitudes or schemas have been found to be present in depressed patients. Although more experimental investigations are needed, cognitive theory has led to a specific psychotherapy for depression and other forms of psychopathology.

AN OVERVIEW OF THE PROCEDURE OF COGNITIVE THERAPY

Cognitive theory forms the basis for cognitive therapeutic methods. The therapy consists of a number of specific techniques for treating depressed patients, as well as a theoretical perspective by which to organize the clinical data, to conceptualize the treatment plan, and to proceed in the conduct of therapy. These techniques and procedures for adults have been detailed elsewhere (Beck et al., 1979). This section illustrates a few of these techniques to provide a flavor for how treatment is conducted.

Cognitive therapy is a short-term, time-limited psychotherapy usually involving a maximum of 20 sessions over a period of 10 to 15 weeks. Although more sessions may be needed with adolescents, the time limits should be retained. The therapist actively directs the discussion to focus on selected problem areas or target symptoms presented by the patient. Questioning is frequently used to elicit specific thoughts, images, definitions, and meanings. For example, the therapist may say, "What did the phone call mean to you?" or "What were you thinking just as you hung up the telephone?" In addition, questioning is used to expose inner contradictions, inconsistencies, and logical flaws in the patient's thinking or conclusions. However, skill and tact are required, especially with adolescents, to assure that this questioning is not construed as an interrogation or cross-examination. Such a view might lead depressed persons to conclude that their reasoning powers are defective.

The therapist and patient collaborate, using empirical methods to identify and resolve specific problems. The therapist must clearly understand the patient's conceptualizations of himself and the world around him. In essence, the therapist must be able to see the world "through the patient's eyes." If the patient's conceptualizations differ from the therapist's view of reality, the patient and therapist reconcile these differences with a logical-empirical approach.

In essence, the patient's thoughts are regarded as hypotheses that require validation. During this validation process (often conducted as homework), the patient needs to understand clearly what beliefs or ideas (hypotheses) are being tested; therefore, he must understand the purpose of each homework assignment. Technically, cognitive therapy is comparable to scientific investigation in that it follows a procedural sequence: (1) collecting data that are as reliable and valid as possible; (2) formulating hypotheses based on these data; and (3) testing and, if indicated, revising these hypotheses (i.e., thinking patterns) based on new information.

The data consist of the patient's "automatic thoughts," which are collected as oral or written reports from the patient. The therapist accepts these thoughts as truthful (although not necessarily accurate) representations of reality, since a basic premise of cognitive theory is that depressed persons negatively misconstrue their day-to-day experiences. The automatic thoughts of adolescents may be obvious in emotional outbursts within the session itself, or they may be sought through more projective techniques, such as writing poetry, telling stories, or discussing movies or television programs.

The therapist first tries to elicit the automatic thoughts surrounding each upsetting event. Once these thoughts are identified, the therapist tries to obtain specific evidence for or against the patient's potentially distorted or dysfunctional thinking by questioning him about the total circumstances and specific details of a particular upsetting event. Often this process reveals a pattern of distorted thinking that occurs across a range of events. For adolescents it is important not to prematurely counter their particular thoughts, since such questions may produce patient attrition. Sometimes, in working with adolescents, a metaphor such as the good coach or bad coach may animate the concept of automatic thoughts: The good coach thinks of options; the bad coach is overly critical and demanding.

Then, the cognitive therapist teaches the patient to identify specific errors of logic in his thinking (e.g., arbitrary inference or overgeneralization). Learning to recognize and correct these errors helps the patient to repeatedly assess the degree to which his thinking mirrors reality.

Next, the therapist helps the patient to identify or infer the assumed attitudes that underpin these recurrent negative automatic thinking patterns. For example, such a thesis might be "expecting to fail" or "reading rejection into personal situations." The therapist helps the patient to see that such beliefs may not necessarily reflect reality. For example, the therapist would use logic, persuasion, and evidence from the patient's current and past functioning to get the patient to view a belief (e.g., "I am unable to learn") as an idea or hypothesis requiring validation, rather than as a fact.

The patient and therapist collaborate to identify basic attitudes, beliefs, and assumptions that (according to the model) shape moment-to-moment thinking. Sometimes an attitude may be so dominant or pervasive that, despite changes in environmental events, the conclusion never varies (i.e., "I can't be happy unless I'm loved"). By articulating these attitudes, the therapist helps the patient not only to develop a basis for empirical validation but also to recognize subsequent cognitions based on these attitudes.

Cognitive techniques are designed to facilitate changes in specific target symptoms found in depression (e.g., inactivity, self-criticism, lack of gratification, suicidal wishes). In general, a therapy session begins with a discussion of the previously assigned homework, which typically focuses on the patient's thinking. The latter part of each session is spent developing and planning the next homework assignment.

In the initial sessions, therapy tends to emphasize increased activity and environmental interaction (i.e., behavioral changes). In the course of such changes, patients learn to recognize, report, and/or record their thinking associated with particular behaviors, activities, or changes in mood. This early emphasis on behavioral objectives is based on our recognition that severely depressed patients are often unable to engage in cognitive tasks because of difficulty in abstract reasoning.

As the depression lessens, concentration improves, and the intensity of the mood decreases. Patients learn to collect, examine, and empirically test their negative automatic thinking. In subsequent sessions, the assumptions supporting these automatic negative thoughts are identified and subjected to empirical validation through homework assignments. These cognitive-change techniques require an ability to abstract and use logic and, therefore, can be employed only after the depression lessens in severity. However, if the patient is less severely depressed, the therapist may employ these cognitive-change techniques from the outset. In addition, a task designed mainly to alter behavior will also influence the patient's thinking. Similarly, a change in thinking patterns may result in a behavioral change as well.

Table 1.1 lists several behaviorally oriented techniques as well as some techniques aimed more particularly at changing cognitions or be-

TABLE 1.1. Behavioral and Cognitive Techniques

Behavioral techniques
    Activity scheduling
    Mastery and pleasure ratings
    Graded-task assignments
    Cognitive rehearsal
    Assertiveness training/role playing
    Mood graph

Cognitive techniques
    Recording automatic thoughts (cognitions)
    Reattribution techniques
    Responding to negative cognitions
    Counting automatic thoughts
    Identifying assumptions
    Modifying shoulds
    Pro–con refutation of assumptions
    Homework to test old assumptions
    Homework to test new assumptions

liefs. These lists of techniques are not exhaustive but are meant to provide examples of the application of the cognitive model, as discussed in detail in Chapter 8 (Beck et al., 1979). In fact, an experienced cognitive therapist will design homework assignments for each individual patient in each session, depending on the cognitive and behavioral targets to be addressed.

Homework assignments (sometimes called "experiments" with adolescents who eschew the term "homework") are critical to treatment. They are designed to help patients (1) develop objectivity about situations that otherwise are stereotypically misconstrued, (2) identify underlying assumptions, and (3) develop and test alternative conceptualizations and guiding assumptions.

The therapist selects specific techniques, depending on the degree and type of psychopathology that is present. For example, the therapist provides greater structure, direction, and guidance to more severely depressed patients who are less able to think objectively. Typically, therapy begins with techniques that focus on behavioral monitoring and change. These techniques are often simple; they are designed to provide patients with success experiences. Subsequently, task assignments are given to provide stimuli for the collection and later correction of cognitions.

CONTRAINDICATIONS

Although Beck et al. (1979) caution that many depressed patients may require medication or may not respond to cognitive therapy, specific contraindications to this treatment are yet to be identified. Clinical experience suggests that patients with impaired reality testing (e.g., hallucinations, delusions), impaired reasoning abilities or memory function (e.g., organic brain syndromes), borderline personality structures, and schizoaffective disorder will not respond to this treatment, at least not in its short-term, time-limited format. Whether patients with antisocial personality with major depression or other forms of secondary depression will respond to cognitive therapy is yet to be empirically established. However, clinical experience suggests that many secondary depressions will respond.

The reasons for a poor outcome with cognitive therapy have recently been reviewed by Rush and Shaw (1983), and it has been suggested that cognitive therapy may be contraindicated for patients suffering from endogenous depression with associated dexamethasone nonsuppression. However, such recommendations are as yet based on anecdotal information. Perhaps, in the future, specific biological measures will help to identify responders and nonresponders to cognitive or other psychotherapies.

Most adult patients who ultimately respond well to cognitive therapy will do so within 5 to 7 weeks of twice-a-week treatment with cognitive therapy alone. If a 50% symptom reduction assessed by the Hamilton Rating Scale for Depression (HRS-D; Hamilton, 1960) or the Beck Depression Inventory (BDI; Beck et al., 1961) is not achieved within 14 sessions, the treatment plan should be revised. Whether this recommendation is applicable to depressed adolescents as well remains unclear to date.

It is surprising that no reports of adverse reactions to cognitive therapy have yet emerged, although adverse reactions may be difficult to differentiate from lack of efficacy. For instance, suicide attempts, as well as premature terminations, may be evidence of either adverse reactions or lack of efficacy.

Some—but not all—adult studies suggest that cognitive methods are associated with a significantly lower premature dropout rate than antidepressant pharmacotherapy alone. One might suspect that the structured, planned, directive nature of this approach helps retain depressed outpatients in treatment. If so, cognitive therapy might be particularly useful for those who are psychologically less sophisticated (e.g., adolescents, patients from lower socioeconomic classes).

RATIONALE FOR COGNITIVE THERAPY
WITH ADOLESCENTS

Over the past few decades, there has been a "significant revolution" in the identification and treatment of depression in adolescents. Previously thought by many to be a rare condition that was distinctly different from adult depression, adolescent depressive disorders are now viewed as being on a continuum with adult major depression and responsive to many of the same treatments (although the role of medication is yet to be established significantly in adolescents). Unfortunately, research evidence is lacking in many areas of adolescent evaluation and treatment; yet, clinicians proceed with psychotherapeutic and pharmacological interventions and ancedotally report good results. Teenagers are often described as being "more difficult to treat" or "less likely to respond to antidepressant medication," but evidence in support of these statements is scanty.

The extension of cognitive techniques to the treatment of adolescent depression is a natural extension of the success obtained with adult patients. Many practitioners have simply taken the techniques and strategies designed for adults and used them with teenagers (apparently with some success). This result is consistent with the view of adolescent depression as being on a continuum with adult major depressive illness.

Anecdotally, others have reported success with cognitive methods while acknowledging that there are "differences," especially the need for the therapist to adapt the techniques to the special developmental issues relevant to teenage patients. As we await the scientific evidence supporting the efficacy of cognitive therapy with teenagers, an expanding number of therapists are already using these methods to treat adolescents with depressive illness, both alone and in combination with antidepressant medication. This manual is an attempt to describe the special problems that arise in using cognitive techniques with depressed teenagers, calling on the experience of a number of "experts" and providing clinical case material to enable therapists to "imagine" how these techniques can be applied with their own patients.

DEVELOPMENTAL ISSUES

Clearly, teenagers are in a different developmental stage than adults. For example, it is therapeutically useful to actually see the family myths still in action, since they serve as a framework for the adolescent's self-assumptions. There are even markedly different developmental needs and processes occurring at the beginning of adolescence than at the end. Such changes can be as confusing for the therapist as for the patient, yet the success of treatment depends on the therapist's awareness of these changing biological, social, and psychological developments. Interventions that may be effective during early stages of adolescence become too simple or direct later when developmental maturation occurs.

As an example, let us consider a youngster who is trying to deal with the negative, joking remarks of an older sister and her girlfriends, who daily appear to assault the patient's self-esteem. With a 17-year-old, an "inventory" can be suggested, with logical processing of alternative understandings of the sister's actions and why these so affect the patient. But a 13-year-old in the same situation might require acknowledgment of the pain, with little effort to dissect the specific events logically. Later, attempts at concrete descriptions of the feelings might be tried, but the important issue is how an early adolescent would be treated differently from an older teenager.

Cognitively, teenagers are working through the development of formal operations. Whether one accepts Piagetian theory or not, the changes in thinking style and complexity from early to late adolescence for many (but clearly not all) youngsters is an extremely dramatic process for therapists working with these patients. Clearly, both the selection and application of cognitive techniques must take this metamorphosis into account. Yet, whatever disadvantage the early or even preformal operations patient may present for a cognitive therapist, it may be far outweighed by the advantage of conducting therapy with patients with the more fluid cognitive structures characteristic of the cognitive development process. Indeed, it may turn out (as some feel) that early adolescence is the (theoretically) most powerful time for application of cognitive techniques. The excitement that many teenagers feel as they experience "thinking about thinking" can easily carry over into the therapy process. It is then fun to work on these issues, and resistance to change is sometimes markedly less than with adults, as this example illustrates:

A 17-year-old girl was experiencing a severe, painful depressive episode that was triggered by her breakup with a boyfriend while simultaneously seeing her school grades fall. Although on one level an intellectualization, she enjoyed the process of self-exploration, and particularly of being able to understand the interrelationships of her feelings, her losses at school and with her boyfriend, and how her self-esteem was artificially tied to her mother's views. This self-pleasure greatly supported her self-esteem during this difficult time, even leading to her taking an honors psychology course the next year in school. She wrote: "I think about how I think about things, and now I know why these things happen to me. I wish I could have understood this before; I don't think I would even have felt so badly."

Because teenagers are often "reluctant" patients who reject treatment and mobilize enormous defensive denial in the face of both major depressive symptoms and the experience of seeing a therapist, therapists have sought the means to engage teenagers, keep them in treatment, and have them participate meaningfully in the overall therapeutic process. The literature on teenage-targeted interventions is replete with caveats concerning the difficulties of "engagement" and the problems of rebellious, therapy-rejecting patients. Most texts on the subject reject, or at least modify, a distant or "silent" therapeutic stance in favor of greater therapist participation and revelation. Cognitive techniques are ideal in their promotion of a therapeutic process that minimizes the "powerful therapist–poor patient" dichotomy and also allows for the establishment of mutual goals in a "cotherapy" environment. Objective "change" measures in the form of behavior logs, essays, and other strategies that are "owned" by the teenager himself are used to assist the teenager to view the process as helpful. Many therapists, working long before cognitive techniques were specifically identified, reported that the processes inherent in this system are very "comfortable" and similar to those developed over years of working with difficult teenage patients.

A 14-year-old ninth-grade boy came to the evaluation session alternating between angry rejection and near-mute responses. Several previous therapists had "failed" in the eyes of the family, and the private school was now pressuring the family to get help for this very bright but failing youngster, or it would expel him for a series of provocative behavioral events. "You don't understand me, you just want my parents' money," was followed with occasional curses and then silent refusal to answer any personal questions. "You'll just listen to my parents anyways, so ask them," led to a joint family session where the "rules" for treatment were laid down. While the parents were identified as the payers for the treatment, the treatment was identified as belonging to the patient. Anything the parents told the therapist was subject to being revealed to the patient; there would be no secrets from the patient. But the reverse was not true—the patient could decide what his family would be told. The family was asked not to telephone the therapist without the patient available to be part of the call. The patient was also responsible for getting a check from the family to pay for treatment and for bringing it to each therapy session.

The next session began with a specific listing of the patient's goals, which, although similar to those of his parents, he insisted must be kept separate. He delighted in the process of paying for the session himself and kept detailed logs, never again rejecting therapy.

SEXUAL ISSUES

Teenagers are intensely sexual creatures, and many therapists underestimate the power of sexual urges and teenage fantasies. Caution must be used to ensure that the cotherapy, working-together environment is not misconstrued as sexually provocative. Therapists must also take care not to dismiss these intense feelings as teenage "puppy love" or something the adolescent will somehow "grow out of." Although the reality and intensity of these feelings can be overwhelming, they are also highly pleasurable. They can also be the source of great fear and embarrassment. A depressed teenager's greatest worry may be the loss of these intense experiences. He thus becomes a potential "victim" of another who would abuse that need to be loved, liked, or included. An important part of therapy may be to acknowledge these intense feelings without giving permission for acting out the accompanying impulses.

For example, Melissa was a 16-year-old 11th grader whose referral for treatment of a significant bulimic eating disorder did not address the intense recurrent depressive episodes with which she was also struggling. Her parents minimized her growing up, her attractiveness, and her relationships with boyfriends.

M: No one realizes how important he [her current boyfriend] is to me. He's the reason I'm alive! Everyone wants me to stop seeing him because he's 21.

T: (*after many attempts at exploration made her angry*) Why don't you help me understand by writing an essay about your feelings?

M: You want me to stop seeing him just like [my stepfather]. You don't understand.

T: Maybe writing about it will help everyone understand.

Two sessions later Melissa talked about her essay: "Some of what I wrote sounded so stupid—but I did show it to my mother, and she seemed to understand—we talked a lot. But I'm still not going to break up with him."

It was important for the therapist to allow Melissa her feelings, to identify with their importance, yet to have her explore the feelings without her believing they were being ridiculed or rejected. An essay proved to be the best neutral device—making sex a safe, but important, subject. The sexualized nature of her relationship with her father, the therapist, and, to some extent, all men was left to a later, more appropriate time.

IDENTITY ISSUES

As teenagers seek to develop their own separate sense of self—different from the child who was so attached to the family—the pressure of significant depressive problems tends to inhibit their developing self-esteem. Cognitive methods can powerfully assist in reversing self-condemning internalized statements, help the teenager question any negative assumptions about the future and the world around him, and help him stop using overgeneralizations and illogical interpretations of life events. Since these personality constructs are being laid down during adolescence, the teenager is perhaps more vulnerable to depression or at least to its effects on identity development. Treatment becomes all the more important to prevent these deficits from becoming more permanent.

Perhaps, treatment can be particularly effective because the psychological machinery for the self-assessment, self-exploration, and development of a physical self-image and self-concept is already extremely active or at least (with the younger adolescent) easily moved into an active, cognitive role. It becomes the therapist's role to use this developing self-concern as an integral part of the treatment, not to dismiss it as an adolescent narcissistic problem.

For example, Brian was a 15-year-old gifted 10th grader whose depression with prominent low self-esteem centered around his feelings of loneliness and isolation from peers. Sessions often became a long series of "mind reading" episodes, where Brian would talk of how he *knew* others did not like him or was sure others would reject him—often with his choosing to reject them first. Early on, these "mind reading" episodes were logically explored, with Brian intellectually accepting the maladaptive nature of his assumptions about others but never changing the process. He reported:

B: Why don't you just give up? there's no way to fix this. That's just the way [these people] want me to be.

T: You want me to give up?

B: I wish my parents would. I can't take all this therapy shit.

T: Help me understand.

B: I'm failing this—you—like everyone. (*tearful*)

T: If treatment doesn't seem to be fixing everything, that's your fault! (*silence*)

B: You know what I mean. It's what everyone else thinks.

T: What you think is what you need to think about—you keep telling me about what others think.

B: What I think keeps changing. I don't know what I think.

Brian was asked to log his self-opinions and self-thoughts on a nightly basis. He gradually became much more comfortable with his own ideas and thoughts and, finally, was able to share them.

When adolescents are unable to discuss their feelings, or when contradictory statements emerge, this inconsistency is often not merely resistance but a reflection of the uncertain and changing self-concept that is a natural part of adolescence. The therapist should probably help the patient become comfortable with his uncertainty and then discuss specifics as they arise, especially when depression may begin assaulting identity formation. With Brian, the logs gradually became the method for this self-exploration process. But this could happen only when he became aware of and could separate out his own feelings and thoughts. Early adolescents often have problems doing this.

Teenagers are attempting to deal simultaneously with a number of complex developmental sequences, often simplified in some texts as their need to "move away from the family toward independence," to seek the end of "role confusion and move toward identity development," to achieve the "capacity for intimacy," and to learn to cope with enormous biological changes and the sexual and aggressive impulses that accompany them. The therapist working with a teenager must be aware of the "developmental soup" in which he is immersed with his patient. Cognitive-behavioral interventions appear to be particularly adaptable to this changing, difficult therapeutic environment.

Many significant problems must be addressed in applying cognitive therapy to adolescents. This manual describes those problems and how some experienced therapists have successfully dealt with their teenage patients.

SELECTED READINGS

American Psychiatric Association: *Diagnostic and Statistical Manual of Mental Disorders*, third edition, revised. Washington, DC, American Psychiatric Association, 1987.

Ansbacher HL, Ansbacher RR: *The Individual Psychology of Alfred Adler: A Systematic Presentation in Selections from His Writings*. New York, Basic Books, 1956.

Beck AT: Thinking and depression: I. Idiosyncratic content and cognitive distortion. *Archives of General Psychiatry* 1963; 9:324–333.

Beck AT: *Cognitive Therapy and the Emotional Disorders*. New York, International Universities Press, 1976.

Beck AT, Rush AJ: Cognitive approaches to depression and suicide, in *Cognitive Defects in Development of Mental Illness*. Edited by Serban G. New York, Brunner/Mazel, 1978.

Beck AT, Rush AJ: Cognitive therapy, in *Comprehensive Textbook of Psychiatry/V*. Edited by Kaplan HI, Sadock BJ. Baltimore, Williams & Wilkins, 1989.

Beck AT, Rush AJ, Shaw BF, Emery G: *Cognitive Therapy of Depression*. New York, Guilford Press, 1979.

Beck AT, Ward CH, Mendelson M, Mock JE, Erbaugh JK: An inventory for measuring depression. *Archives of General Psychiatry* 1961; 4:561–571.

Ellis A: *Reason and Emotion in Psychotherapy*. New York, Lyle Stuart, 1962.

Hamilton M: A rating scale for depression. *Journal of Neurology, Neurosurgery and Psychiatry* 1960; 12:56–62

Jarrett RB: Psychosocial aspects of depression and the role of psychotherapy. *Journal of Clinical Psychiatry* 1990; 51 (Suppl. 6): 26–35

Jarrett RB, Rush AJ: Psychotherapeutic approaches to depression, in *Psychiatry*, Vol. 1. Edited by Cavenar JO. Philadelphia, Lippincott, and New York, Basic Books, 1986.

Kelly GA: *The Psychology of Personal Constructs*. New York, Norton, 1955.

Klein GS: *Perception, Motives and Personality*. New York, Knopf, 1970.

Mahoney MJ: *Cognition and Behavior Modification*. Cambridge, MA, Ballinger, 1974.

Meichenbaum D: *Cognitive-Behavior Modification: An Integrated Approach*. New York, Plenum Press, 1977.

Rush AJ (ed): *Short-Term Psychotherapies for Depression*. New York, Guilford Press, 1982.

Rush AJ, Shaw BF: Failures in treating depression by cognitive behavior therapy, in *Failures in Behavior Therapy*. Edited by Foa EB, Emmelkamp PMG. New York, Wiley, 1983.

Speilberg H: *The Phenomenological Movement*, Vols. 1 and 2. The Hague, Nijhoff, 1971.

Spielberg H: *Phenomenology in Psychology and Psychiatry*. Evanston, IL, Northwestern University Press, 1972.

CHAPTER TWO

Ten Key Principles of Adolescent Cognitive Therapy

GAYLE BELSHER

T. C. R. WILKES

INTRODUCTION

Principles of cognitive therapy are the "ground rules" that must be observed throughout therapy. Principles do not refer to specific techniques of intervention, rather, they represent more general practices or "attitudes" adopted throughout the course of therapy. Novice cognitive therapists are sometimes tempted to employ specific techniques too readily, but more important than any cognitive therapy technique is the consistent application of therapeutic principles. In fact, therapists who are thoroughly familiar with cognitive theory and observe key principles when working with adolescents will be in a prime position to exercise their own creativity in developing therapeutic techniques.

Many of the principles discussed below would certainly apply to models of intervention other than cognitive therapy. However, the discussion that follows focuses on how the principles are specifically manifest within the context of adolescent cognitive therapy. The principles are not mutually exclusive nor are they exhaustive; more or fewer could have been identified and their use illustrated within a cognitive therapy context. The list of 10 is intended to give therapists one way of conceptualizing the basic guidelines for cognitive therapy with depressed adolescents.

1. ACKNOWLEDGE THE ADOLESCENT'S NARCISSISM

"Narcissism" refers to the tendency of adolescent patients to be somewhat egocentric in their interests and goals, often with little regard for the wishes of others and little ability to take others' points of view. No pejorative tone is intended in using the term "narcissism"; in fact, the adolescent's greater tendency to focus on "self" relative to many adult patients is viewed as developmentally appropriate. As such, both the adolescent and his parents need to understand that the therapist accepts this greater relative egocentrism and will not insist that the adolescent give this up entirely. If the adolescent's narcissistic position is not acknowledged, the therapist risks promoting an oppositional stance, wherein the adolescent may feel obliged to defend his views strongly and thereby prematurely veto discussion on various issues.

Communication of the therapist's understanding of an adolescent's greater concern with himself is not achieved with use of the terms "narcissism" or "egocentricity," which patients or their parents may interpret inappropriately. Instead, the therapist communicates this message indirectly, for example, by asking numerous questions about the adolescent's view of himself, his "world" or current circumstances, and his "future" or goals, fantasies, and predictions. Questions are used to elicit information about how the adolescent patient sees things beyond what he volunteers. In other words, the therapist tries to enhance the information initially volunteered by asking questions about how the patient perceives relationships among problems, people, and events, for example. Questions indicate that the therapist is interested in the details of the adolescent's life and "feed" the narcissism in a way that is useful both for understanding the depression and for designing appropriate interventions.

Adolescents generally want to be understood as individuals, so it is important for therapists to reflect back their understanding more frequently than might be the case with adult patients. Rather than using statements, questions are often the best way of reflecting to adolescents. For example, the question "Would it be correct to say that you think...?" formally acknowledges the adolescent as the best judge of his own views. Because adolescents generally want to feel special or unique, the therapist must normally avoid use of "leveling" comments such as "All teenagers feel that way," or "I've heard this before," or "When I was a teenager. . . ." There are some exceptions to this guideline, so the therapist should be aware of these special circumstances and use such comments only with foresight and specific purpose. For example, the therapist may wish to "normalize" something that the adolescent feels is abnormal or wrong by indicating that other adolescents have similar concerns. Alternatively, the therapist may wish to instill hope about the resolution of a particular problem or recovery from depression by indicating that other adolescents have overcome similar difficulties.

The adolescent's sense of importance may also be acknowledged and enhanced by offering choice. As such, the cognitive therapist should make a special effort to provide the adolescent patient with a menu of choices catering to his therapeutic needs. For example, when designing homework tasks, the therapist can offer the adolescent various alternatives. Although the therapist may have a particular technique in mind, two or three "versions" of it, differing in detail, can be presented to the patient. For example, one use of record keeping is to make patients aware of the relationship between environmental stimulus events, their own emotions, and their own thoughts at the time of the events. Adolescents could be asked to keep a three-column record of events, emotions, and thoughts in the usual "adult" way. Alternatively, they may be more inclined to keep a personal diary that records a narrative story from which the therapist can (in session) identify the components of the three columns with the adolescent. For some adolescents, the format of a calendar with large empty squares in which to record daily events, feelings, and thoughts is appealing. Homework designed to accomplish the same therapeutic ends could be handwritten in various formats; alternatively, some adolescents we have seen would only do the homework on their computers; others might like to dictate the information on a small tape recorder. The important point is that adolescents will probably respond better to a choice, and the therapist will usually have to take the major responsibility for generating the menu of choices. The purpose of generating choice, as is the purpose of various other suggestions above, is to acknowledge and use the adolescent's narcissism in the service of treating the depression.

2. ADOPT A MODE OF COLLABORATIVE EMPIRICISM

The term "collaborative" means cooperating with the adolescent, joining with him to treat the depression. The term "empiricism" means that factual data are the basis for changing cognitions or behaviors that maintain or exacerbate the depression. Although the principle of collaborative empiricism is central to cognitive therapy with any age group, observation of this principle with adolescents requires that the therapist make some adjustments relative to what might be the case in using cognitive therapy to treat adult patients.

By virtue of age, life experience, education, and social norms, among other things, adolescents will usually enter therapy with the perception that they are in a "one-down" position relative to the therapist. Therapists and adolescent patients are less "equal" in many objective ways than are therapists and adult patients. This is especially the case when the adolescent has been brought to therapy against his own wishes by concerned adults. Because of the hierarchical status difference between therapists and their adolescent patients, it is particularly important that the therapist consciously work to build and maintain a collaborative relationship. The goal of the therapist is to convey a willingness to cooperate in finding ways to ameliorate the depression.

Working in collaboration with the adolescent means that the therapist is not a "dictator" who knows best and prescribes solutions to problems. Neither is the adolescent given free rein to control the therapy by avoiding issues or focusing on tangential problems of his own choosing. The therapist must develop the skill of simultaneously "being in the room with the patient" and "adopting a metaposition" whereby the therapist guides the interaction, carefully titrating therapist and patient control of each session. Generally speaking, adolescents are acutely aware of interpersonal alliances and will react to perceived allegiances of therapists to parents or to themselves. Adopting a mode of collaboration with an adolescent does not mean that the therapist becomes a "co-conspirator" of the patient. Implied threats or blackmail by the adolescent are not condoned, and it is important early in therapy for the adolescent to understand boundaries and limitations about such issues as confidentiality.

Collaboration is enhanced by being a voice for the adolescent with significant others. It is often the case that the therapist must raise difficult issues or questions with authority figures such as parents. The therapist may have to speak the adolescent's fears for him in the presence of others. This goal can be achieved without reporting directly to significant others exactly what the adolescent has revealed in individual therapy sessions. For example, the therapist could take the responsibility in a family session for voicing a concern about family stability that was central to an adolescent girl's depression by using an introduction such as "I wonder if your daughter is fearful that you [her parents] are going to divorce."

Collaboration is continuously demonstrated throughout all interactions with the adolescent patient. Setting the agenda at the beginning of a therapy session is always a joint exercise of the therapist and patient. The difference between adult and adolescent patients is that the willingness and ability to participate in agenda setting will be more variable with the younger population. Some adolescents will readily demonstrate their agenda by initiating a one-sided narrative as soon as they enter the therapy room. Others will politely state something of concern when invited to do so, whereas still others initially will deny that there is anything of consequence to discuss in the session. Even when adolescent patients have been socialized into the cognitive therapy model, it is less likely that they will respond well to the direct question "What should we put on our agenda for today?" Instead, the therapist should be prepared to take a quick survey of various "life spheres" or "known problem areas" in order to identify relevant agenda topics. When this approach to identify agenda items is employed, the adolescent may launch into a long and detailed monologue about a particular event. Fortunately, adolescents generally seem quite accepting of the therapist's interruption in this presentation if the therapist identifies the issue as something to list on the agenda for further discussion later in the session. As always, the therapist also participates in setting an agenda by stating his own topics; but with adolescents, as compared to adults, the importance of modeling is exaggerated. This means that the cognitive therapist working with adolescents should enter each therapy session mindful of the cognitive formulation regarding the adolescent's depression so that an appropriate amount of leadership can be demonstrated in constructing an agenda that addresses issues central to the depression.

Not only is setting the agenda with adolescents a shared venture; throughout the session, therapists demonstrate collaboration with respect to time spent talking, consideration of points of view, designing homework, and scheduling future therapy sessions, for example. Relative to adult therapy, adolescent therapy may require the therapist to encourage cooperation (either more patient participation or more therapist participation) more often and to model cooperation more explicitly.

A collaborative relationship can also be encouraged indirectly. For example, adolescents seem to live in a verbal world rich with slang, which is often specific to a particular geographical location or subgroup with which the patient identifies. The adolescent does not necessarily expect the therapist to know or use this idiosyncratic jargon without being educated as to its meaning but will usually appreciate being asked what some expression means and will often enjoy the therapist's incorporation of the jargon into his own language during the session. This is not to suggest that the therapist "becomes the adolescent patient" by mimicking slang but, rather, that the therapist acknowledges the patient's creative use of English, sometimes in a humorous way. For example, a therapist can parenthetically insert such comments a ". . . or as you would say . . ." into his own speech. Other indirect means of encouraging a collaborative relationship include mirroring the adolescent's style with use of humor, varied tones of voice, varied rates of speech, or varied pace in the session.

It is important that the message of collaboration be conveyed to the adolescent in a way that suggests that the therapist is cooperating to achieve what is best for the adolescent in the long run or in the big scope of things rather than to achieve short-term egocentric demands that are not central to the adolescent's depression. For example, although a particular adolescent may be focused on reconciliation with a boyfriend or girlfriend, the therapist may need to forgo cooperating on this specific goal in favor of a more general goal such as working with the adolescent to correct a habitual cognitive distortion about the meaning of disagreements between people who purportedly like each other (e.g., boyfriends or girlfriends).

With respect to "empiricism," cognitive therapists working with adolescents will usually need to adopt a somewhat less "academic" approach than would be the case with adults. Adolescents will generally be less interested in discovery of maladaptive thinking patterns unless the discovery can be directly related to some issue of central importance to them at the current point in time. Since the issues of greatest concern to adolescents are apt to change quickly, even from week to week, therapists may more quickly need to introduce the "label" for a particular cognitive distortion that seems operative in the adolescent's depression. Related to adolescents' sense of urgency and their relative impatience with taking a global view of themselves and their lives, therapists should be prepared to work in the "here and now" to a greater extent than might be the case with adult patients. Some of the best empirical data that can be presented to adolescents will be generated in the therapy session in the form or words or behaviors demonstrated by the patients themselves. Some therapists have found it very effective to read verbatim statements back to adolescent patients and inquire about the "problematic word" or the "pattern" that might be contributing to depression.

In general, adolescents will require more assistance to generalize from specific examples of maladaptive thinking. It is incumbent on the therapist to remember previous examples, complete with names of relevant people and places specific to the adolescent's life. To assist with the process of generalization, it is useful to interject brief "summaries" throughout a therapy session as well as at the end of the session so that the "take-home points" are emphasized frequently for adolescents in brief but potent doses.

With adolescents, empirical data may often be more behavioral than cognitive, especially in the beginning stages of therapy. As behavioral data are more concrete, they often have more impact, particularly with younger adolescents or those with comorbid diagnoses such as attention deficit hyperactivity disorder. Thus, for example, homework that directs an adolescent to do some novel activity rather than to think something different may more rapidly achieve the desired cognitive change. With respect to homework, specific techniques of empirical data collection must be tailored to the patient's level of cognitive development as well as to the patient's immediate concerns. In general, adolescents are less inclined to do homework out-of-session than are adults, so it is particularly important to exercise ingenuity in defining homework that the adolescent is highly motivated to complete. Of course, the term "homework" is seldom used because of its possible negative association with school experiences.

Finally, the therapist must use empirical data to "adjust" the maladaptive cognitions of the adolescent rather than directly challenge them as "wrong." If the therapist attempts to "shift" cognitive style on a continuum of adaptivity rather than to "change" it, the goal usually will be met with less resistance by the adolescent.

3. ADOPT AN OBJECTIVE STANCE

A therapist who has adopted an "objective stance" is one whose position is somewhat removed from the intricacies of the adolescent's life. This does not mean that the therapist is disinterested or uncommitted but, rather, able to stand back and look at the entire global picture without getting caught up in side issues or special agendas of the adolescent or his parents. Although an objective stance is crucial to cognitive therapy regardless of the patient's age, it is sometimes harder to maintain with adolescents because they themselves are less able to suspend their narcissistic tendencies in order to consider themselves and their lives from any perspective other than the one to which they currently subscribe. Because adolescents generally adhere so strongly to their views, the therapist may feel an inordinate amount of covert pressure to agree with the patient's highly subjective point of view. Maintaining an objective stance with adolescent patients may be more difficult in some cases because the parents present a particularly one-sided view and consider themselves "unavowed experts" on their own children. Since parents are necessary participants in most adolescents' therapy for instrumental (e.g., driving to sessions) as well as therapeutic reasons, the therapist may be tempted to give more weight to parents' points of view than a more objective stance would support.

By definition, maintaining an objective stance requires that the therapist avoid overidentification with either the adolescent's or his parents' point of view. Objectivity need not be sacrificed by acknowledging the narcissistic nature of adolescents. Knowing in detail how the adolescent views things does not mean that the therapist agrees that this is the only way to view them. One of the most effective ways of avoiding overidentification and of communicating the goal of objectivity to the adolescent is to involve the patient's parents in therapy from time to time. By so doing, information is gathered from a variety of sources, and the therapist gains greater perspective. The necessity of involving family members in the adolescent's therapy cannot be overemphasized. This position is in contrast to that of cognitive therapy with adults, where more commonly, therapists see only the identified patients and work with their points of view regardless of what these are.

Objectivity is enhanced by avoiding the adoption of a "problem-solver" role where the therapist prescribes solutions. Rather, the therapist focuses on teaching adolescents how to develop skills for coping or resolving problems themselves. In this way, the therapist does not get entangled in the details of any particular problem but takes a more "removed" position, helping the adolescent identify and address skill deficiencies or maladaptive cognitions that are common to a variety of situations.

The maintenance of an objective stance is also enhanced by the principle of collaborative empiricism. If the therapist and patient use empirical data to support or challenge particular points of view, then they probably will be less invested in upholding any one position and more willing to be influenced by relevant factual evidence. The act of "collecting data" itself reinforces the patient's and therapist's view of therapy as objective.

Apart from overt demonstrations of therapist objectivity by collecting points of view from various information sources or gathering empirical data through observations and record-keeping, the therapist can covertly enhance his own objectivity by developing the skill of "parallel processing" or "multilevel analysis" of content and process in therapy sessions. While actively participating in the therapy session with such activities as asking questions, introducing topics, and directing conversation, the therapist must also listen for evidence of cognitive distortions and maladaptive beliefs inadvertently expressed in the speech of the adolescent or other family members. Whether or not identification of the distortions or beliefs is the stated goal of the ongoing interactions in the therapy session, it is crucial that the therapist listen with a "third ear" for patterns in cognitive style that may be related to the depression. For example, an adolescent reviewing his previous week's activities might report objective evidence of many positive occurrences (e.g., a skiing trip, passing a difficult exam, buying new clothes) but sound depressed and indicate that "nothing really good is happening in [his] life, which continues to be as bad as ever." Further questioning about the activities may lead the observant therapist to note a disproportionate amount of time spent describing small details of things that were not "perfect" in the adolescent's eyes, and lead the therapist to form (silently) the hypothesis that the adolescent upholds the same perfectionistic standards that have been noted in the patient's high-achieving parents. Furthermore, the therapist might suspect that the adolescent habitually disqualifies the positive, magnifies the negative, and tends to personalize serendipitous events, thereby maintaining a depressogenic view of his life and himself. The practice of listening with a third ear helps the therapist maintain an objective stance (avoiding premature commiseration with the adolescent) by raising the possibility, at least in the therapist's mind, that there is another way of interpreting the same events. Many adolescents are experts at giving passionate presentations of depressing points of view, which, if adopted by the therapist, would make amelioration of the depression extremely difficult. The therapist accepts the narrative as the true current perspective of the depressed adolescent but does not agree that another perspective is not possible. It should be noted that, in some cases, the adolescent's complaints are entirely accurate as stated, in which case the therapist collaborates to solve a problem or instruct the patient in coping or skill acquisition, rather than identifying and changing cognitive distortions. In any case, the therapist's goal of objectivity is enhanced by actively, consciously, and constantly using information provided by the patient to formulate and test hypotheses about the cognitions that may be related to the adolescent's depression.

4. INCLUDE MEMBERS OF THE SOCIAL SYSTEM

The social system of adolescents comprises not only their immediate family members but also extended family, school personnel, friends, and sometimes other professionals such as child welfare workers or nonparental guardians. When others are invited to participate in therapy, sessions will most often include family members or guardians, less often include other professionals, and rarely but sometimes include friends or school personnel.

Because the adolescent is not independent of parental figures and is often not in a position to make decisions or changes that affect him, the therapist sometimes must act as a mediator or provider of information to these members of the social system. Family members with whom the adolescent patient lives or interacts play a central role in the development of the adolescent's beliefs about himself, his world, and his future. As such, it will usually be advantageous to know the prevailing attitudes of family members about the adolescent's depression and various factors contributing to it. Often, adolescent patients will hold depressogenic views of themselves, their lives, or their futures that are reinforced by interactions with their family members. Unless the therapist includes these influential others in some therapy sessions, the risk is great that therapeutic gains made by the adolescent in individual sessions will be inadvertently undone by members of the social system who have not been involved in the same processes of cognitive restructuring as has the adolescent patient. For example, when depressed adolescents hold particularly unrealistic views of themselves as inadequate, unskilled, unintelligent, or inferior members of their families, it is often the case that a family session will uncover the family belief that the patient in question does not live up to family standards. But these family standards may be overly demanding or "perfectionistic." Parents themselves may hold depressogenic beliefs about success or accomplishment, for example, which they unwittingly teach their children through the demands they make for performance, either overtly or covertly, through such mechanisms as the reinforcement contingencies operative in the family. To make headway with the depressed adolescent in question, it will be necessary to identify and adjust the family's beliefs about performance so that expectations are more realistic. It is not always the case that family members hold the same depressogenic beliefs as the depressed adolescent, so another reason for involving the family in therapy is to highlight for the adolescent pertinent information that will challenge beliefs that are supporting the depression. In addition, family members are often helpful in the task of problem-solving, thereby addressing the adolescent's deficient self efficacy or sense of helplessness that may accompany depression.

Less commonly, it may be necessary to involve other professionals such as child welfare caseworkers in therapy sessions. The goal of the therapist may be to achieve the environmental change (e.g., temporary placement) necessary for the safety of the adolescent. In such cases, it is obvious that the helplessness accompanying depression and cognitions about self, circumstances, or future could not be successfully addressed in therapy without first addressing the issue of safety.

When people other than the depressed adolescent are invited to a therapy session, their involvement should be framed as participation in treating the adolescent's depression. The therapist continues to work in a cognitive model by maintaining uppermost in mind a cognitive formulation about the adolescent's depression. In other words, the therapist involves other people to the extent that their participation is necessary to alter the depressed adolescent's maladaptive beliefs about himself, circumstances, or the future that are thought to be maintaining the depression. Regardless of who is invited to participate in therapy sessions, the focus of the therapist remains on the depressed adolescent, and the therapist's first obligation is to this individual patient. Even though other family members might benefit from therapeutic intervention or even though the family as a whole might benefit from what would traditionally be considered "family therapy," the purpose of family involvement is to ameliorate the adolescent patient's depression by addressing maladaptive cognitions. With families who are reluctant to become involved in "family therapy," it is often the focus on the depressed adolescent that convinces them to participate in the therapy process. When framed as "participating in therapy to help their child/sibling overcome the depression," reluctant family members often become useful therapist's allies who do, in fact, undergo change themselves, albeit indirectly and in the service of helping a family member other than themselves. When members of the adolescent's social system are involved in therapy, therapists must withstand the temptation to adopt primarily a "case manager" or "problem-solver" role. Also, therapists experienced in other models of therapy may have to contain their inclinations to become "prescriptive" in any way that defeats the cognitive therapy principle of collaborative empiricism.

Just as the therapist listens with a "third ear" for evidence of possible cognitive distortions or maladaptive beliefs in the adolescent's individual sessions, so he must do in sessions that involve other people from the depressed adolescent's social system. In fact, the importance of active listening and silent generation of hypotheses is probably even more important in these sessions as a way of maintaining a cognitive therapy orientation focused on the individual adolescent patient.

5. CHASE THE AFFECT

To "chase the affect" is to investigate signs of emotion exhibited by the adolescent during therapy sessions. Regardless of the patient's age, most models of psychotherapy and all cognitive therapists will be concerned with displays of emotion. The rationale for attending closely to affect is that it is often the window to cognition. Relative to their adult counterparts, adolescent patients generally have less ability to "think about thinking" and will need more help to engage in observation of their own thought processes. Fortunately for therapy, adolescents often are also less emotionally controlled than their adult counterparts and, as such, give the therapist clues to cognitive domains that are particularly relevant to the depression.

Chasing the affect requires investigation of changes in emotion as well as demonstrations of high emotion. Behavioral indicators of change in emotion may include shifts such as from talkativeness to silence, or from argumentative behavior to cooperative participation (or the respective reverses). A particular indicator of affect, such as tears, may be associated with various emotions such as sadness or anger, for example. Also, different adolescents will display the same emotion in different ways. For example, sadness may be expressed through tears by one depressed patient and with a silent downward glance by another. The cognitive therapist must be vigilant for all signs and changes of emotion and must guard against assuming the meaning of the affect shown.

Since the relationship between affect and cognition is central to cognitive therapy, it is essential that the therapist investigate affect with questions such as "What were you frowning about?" or by making investigatory comments such as "You seem to be thinking about something that made you sad." Adolescents often will have more difficulty than adults in responding to such open-ended inquiries about their thoughts. When this is the case, the therapist may need to probe with statements such as "I wonder if your tears mean you are are sad about your parents' divorce?" or "Do you suppose your angry tone of voice has anything to do with thinking that people are being unfair to you?"

Although adolescents will seldom endorse exactly what is offered to them in this manner, they often can be encouraged to correct the therapist's hypothesis, thereby providing their own understanding of the relationship between their affect and cognitions. Sometimes, the therapist may have to offer several variations of a hypothesis before the adolescent can identify an association between his affect and cognitions. Consistent with adolescents' relative difficulty generalizing from a particular example, hypotheses about their displays of emotion will often need to be quite specific to the people and events in their lives.

In addition to the difficulty of making associations between emotions and thoughts, some adolescents will be unable to label their affect. Therapists may need to provide educational remediation in this regard by providing adolescent patients with a set of affective labels and instructing them in the recognition of emotional states. With particularly young adolescents, such instruction may require the use of pictorial facial stimuli or vignettes.

One of the benefits of including family members in sessions with the depressed adolescent is the opportunity to observe the powerful influence of family members on the patient's affect. Therapists sometimes feel as if they are working with two "different" adolescents, who behave and respond emotionally differently in the presence of family members than when seen individually. Sudden and dramatic shifts in the patient's affect are often observed during family sessions when particularly potent topics central to the adolescent's depression are raised. These are prime opportunities for the therapist to investigate the adolescent's cognitions directly or to ask family members about their hypotheses concerning the adolescent's depressogenic cognitions.

The therapist working with depressed adolescents must tolerate greater extremes in affective display than would normally be acceptable with adult patients. It is not uncommon for adolescents to scream unreasonably, to use derogatory language directed at the family or therapist, to rip at their clothes, or even to leave the therapy room. Tolerance of emotional extremes does not mean that the therapist is nonresponsive to them. It is often most useful if the extreme affect is framed as an indicator of something about which the adolescent believes strongly. In this way, emotional outbursts, which family members may view as intolerable, or which the adolescent himself views as reprehensible, can be discussed as opportunities to gain greater understanding of the thinking that underlies the emotional demonstrations.

When depressed adolescents seem particularly defeated, displaying deep sadness or hurt, for example, it is sometimes tempting for the therapist to offer comfort by quickly suggesting reasons for optimism or solutions to problems, or by changing the topic to one less affectively "potent." However, because of the crucial relationship between affect and cognition, progress in therapy is slowed by succumbing to such temptation. In rushing to the adolescent's rescue, the therapist forgoes the opportunity to work collaboratively with the patient to understand the distortions or maladaptive beliefs that may be contributing to the extreme emotional pain. At such times, it is particularly important for the therapist to listen carefully to the spontaneously offered, uncensored flow of thoughts that may emerge. At such times, the adolescent frequently issues a string of depressogenic beliefs in rapid succession.

6. USE SOCRATIC QUESTIONING

"Socratic questioning" refers to the process of asking a series of questions intended to lead the patient to challenge his own adherence to assumptions, beliefs, or behaviors that are contributing to the depression. The use of direct questions or interrogative statements is central to all cognitive therapy. Questions are used not only to collect information, but also to convey information, to raise topics, or even to offer suggestions.

More than is usually the case with their adult counterparts, adolescent patients will be unfamiliar with the role of participating in focused discussion or meaningful inquiry. Adolescents more often come to therapy in the position of being told what to do or with the belief that their opinions are unimportant or unwelcome. As such, although the practice of Socratic questioning may be liberating to some adolescents, for others it may initially be threatening. Furthermore, adolescent patients, more often than their adult counterparts, will assume that there is a "correct" answer to questions being asked and generally will have had less experience in exploring a variety of responses, all of which might be quite tenable. Cognitive therapists working with adolescents can do much to dispel the misconception of therapist as "prosecutor" and patient as "witness" by asking questions of themselves, leaving questions unanswered, or even prefacing questions with comments such as "I'm not sure there is an answer to this question . . ." or "Different people probably will have different answers to this question. . . ." Also effective in disarming the initial defensiveness about questioning is the adoption of a "Columbo" style of "innocent" questioning or "playing dumb." This style of "being confused" about something is particularly useful when the therapist wants to draw attention to some discrepancy in factual information or some inconsistency in logic. For example, suppose a therapist wants to draw a depressed girl's attention to the cognitive distortion "disqualifying the positive" that seems to be operative whenever she evaluates her own achievements. Rather than stating that her thinking about the issue is in error, a Socratic questioning process would be exemplified by asking, "Will you help me understand how your parents can tell me you are a very capable daughter, your sister tells me she wishes she could do all the things you can, you tell me yourself that your friends admire your abilities, but somehow you think you're stupid, to the point of being nearly worthless? How does all that fit together?" (asked confusedly).

Although some adolescents will welcome the invitation to participate actively in therapy sessions guided by the therapist's use of questions, other, more reluctant patients, perhaps forced to attend sessions by parents, will resist the invitation to participate either with silence or the ubiquitous "I don't know" response. Therapists need not be deterred by such initial reluctance, which can usually be addressed by wondering aloud about potential answers the adolescent could have offered, or in family sessions, by asking other family members to guess what the silent adolescent would say if he did respond. Especially with adolescents who seem reluctant to answer questions, the therapist must be careful not to use seemingly "rapid-fire" questions in sequence in order to avoid unintentionally activating a "cross-examination" schema. Most adolescents are extremely sensitive filters of innuendo in content or tone of speech, and therapists should remember that questions can be asked in a wide variety of tones of voice. For example, tone can indicate surprise, disbelief, curiosity, uncertainty, or wonder, as well as lack of factual knowledge.

Many adolescents are more concrete in their thinking than adults. If the Socratic questioning process is to lead to the desired ends, therapists must pose specific questions rather than make vague general inquiries. Extra effort will be required to communicate to the adolescent patient what point is being made or what question is being asked. For example, it usually is not sufficient to ask, "How did you feel?" or to give the directive "Tell me more about that," because the adolescent is likely to respond about something tangential to the therapy or ask for further instruction like "Feel about what, when?" or "What do you want to know about?" Adult cognitive therapy patients may understand better exactly what the therapist is asking, but an adolescent patient will respond to the intended question more appropriately if the therapist is specific, for example, "When you were sent to your room after hitting your sister, what words would you use to describe your emotions at that exact moment?"

Responses to questions often indicate that the adolescent missed the point the first time the question was asked. Repetition of the same manifest content in a question will often be necessary. It is not uncommon, especially with younger adolescents, to ask the same question in three or four different ways. When repeating questions, the repetition can be disguised to avoid offending the adolescent, for example, by responding to the first answer in some acknowledging way such as "OK, that's one possibility and in addition . . ." (repeat the question using different words). Additionally, the therapist should usually take the responsibility for obvious misunderstanding with such statements as "I'm not asking that question very well. Let me try to do a better job . . ." (then rephrase the question).

7. CHALLENGE THE BINARY MOTIF

The "binary motif" of adolescents refers to their proclivity to think in "all–none" or "black–white" terms. Although depressed adults, as well as adolescents, will often engage in dichotomous thinking that contributes to their depression, the pervasiveness of this thinking style may be greater with younger patients. Binary categories simplify the world, so this way of conceptualizing things would seem to be developmentally appropriate, at least initially in life. For very young children, the oversimplification is probably adaptive and contributes to learning. Furthermore, adults may protect young children from potentially confusing exceptions to their largely binary world view. But adolescents begin to experience problems with the oversimplification engendered by dichotomous thought because they increasingly become victims of an unrealistic world view that clashes with reality, causing cognitive dissonance or emotional upheaval.

Adolescents' tendencies to think in a binary motif are often evident in their descriptions of affective states. For example, one week an adolescent may describe himself as "depressed" and identify a variety of presumed causal agents. The next week, the same adolescent may report some positive occurrences and describe himself as "happy." The rapid substitution of a new emotional state for the former one is not viewed as anything unusual by the adolescent patient, who may describe his emotional life as a roller coaster between these two extremes.

But since such a description of emotional experience suggests a binary motif and likely portends continued vacillating between two polar extremes, the therapist must work actively to challenge this style of dichotomous categorization. Especially with younger adolescents, it may be necessary to provide some form of an "emotional thermometer" with gradations for both the "happy" and "depressed" affective states. Some patients may even need to work with the therapist to generate numbered divisions and "anchors" from experiences in their own lives to convey the concept of graded emotional response. For example, the therapist could ask for an event that would correspond to a "1," "5," and "9" on a "0-to-10" scale of "sadness." Alternatively, the therapist could provide examples of upsetting events from the patient's life and ask the adolescent to rate them on a "0-to-10" scale. For example, the therapist could ask, "What would losing your favorite baseball be?" or "What was the rating when your cat died?" The binary motif of affective experience also may be effectively challenged by developing a vocabulary of emotional terminology to correspond to numbered points on the continuum. For example, an event rated as "1" might be "annoying," whereas one rated a "5" might be "maddening," and one rated a "9" might be "infuriating."

Not only in describing their emotional experience, but in many other areas as well, adolescents will tend to adopt an all-or-none view. Questions such as "What proportion of responsibility would you estimate to be yours?" or "What part of the depression is related to your boyfriend?" are often useful. Visual representations such as a line continuum, proportional pie diagram, or balance scales can also be effective in challenging the binary motif.

In addition to labeling and correcting black-and-white thinking overtly, the cognitive therapist must challenge the binary motif covertly throughout all therapy sessions. Of particular importance is the language of the therapist whose choice of words implies a dichotomous or a continuous frame of reference. Rather than asking if some event were categorically "good" or "bad," for example, the therapist should attempt to ask questions that imply an underlying continuum of judgment by offering choices such as "better" or "worse" as response alternatives.

8. AVOID BLAME

"Blaming" refers to the view, either stated or unstated, that the patient is a "bad or defective person," a view that indicates a "global" judgment of character rather than a focus on a particular behavior or problem. Because a negative self-view is a central component of depression for many patients when they enter therapy, and because a depressogenic attributional style reflects the increased tendency of depressed patients to postulate internal, stable, and global causal explanations for negative events, it is especially important for the therapist to guard against inadvertently reinforcing such maladaptive cognitions. Although a negative self-image and a depressogenic attributional style may be components of the depression for both adults and adolescents, the increased tendency for younger patients to think in dichotomous black-and-white terms may make them more susceptible to selfblame. For some depressed adolescents, the cognitive formulation might focus less on a negative self-view and more on an unrealistically negative "world" or "future" view. Nonetheless, the therapist should guard against holding or portraying a blaming stance because narcissistic injury is easily inflicted on many adolescents who appear exquisitely sensitive to any information that can be construed as criticism of their character.

When discussing the adolescent's depression, avoiding blame means the therapist avoids implying that the depression is some kind of basic "character flaw." Reference to the adolescent's depression as a psychiatric disorder that can be treated will be especially important when there is a family history of depression or when the adolescent has had recurrent depressive episodes. These events in the adolescent's history will often lead families to formulate hypotheses about the "innate nature" of the depressed adolescent that suggest that little can be done to ameliorate the psychiatric condition. Therapists often find it useful to talk about "beating" or "controlling" the depression in order to shift the locus of control and address a potential sense of helplessness. Even when discussing behaviors that may alleviate or exacerbate the depression, the emphasis is on choice of behaviors and their consequences rather than on "fault" for being depressed.

Most therapists who work with adolescents will encounter a proportion of their patients whose behaviors are clearly unacceptable in some respect. A 14-year-old boy who does not hold a driver's license but who is involved in stealing his parents' car would be one such example. The cognitive therapist would avoid blame by refusing to construe the act of stealing the car as evidence of the adolescent's "bad character" or "rotten core," as his parents may see the situation. Instead, the therapist must attempt to engage the adolescent in a discussion of responsibility for one's actions, and review the potential consequences of such behavior. Through discussion of this type, the depressed adolescent must come to understand that acting badly or doing something wrong is behavior for which he is responsible and for which consequences may be levied. Such an interpretation is quite different from believing that one is "all bad" or flawed in some major way that is sure to affect all other spheres of life with little or no hope of change for the better. Because adolescents often interpret comments or questions as accusations of blame when they are not intended as such, cognitive therapists should use consequential reasoning with the depressed and misbehaving adolescent judiciously and with sensitivity. Adolescents may be less likely to misinterpret discussion of action–consequence associations if the therapist begins the discussion with review of the potential advantages and disadvantages of a particular misbehavior, perhaps allowing the adolescent to "justify" his actions by verbalizing the perceived advantages before being asked to evaluate the disadvantages. Often it is helpful to examine a variety of alternatives and their respective pros and cons, rather than to challenge any particular action or intention directly.

Avoiding blame must remain uppermost in the therapist's mind when family members are invited to participate in the depressed adolescent's therapy. As mentioned previously, family members may blame the adolescent for being depressed. Alternatively, parents or siblings may think the adolescent's depression is the family's fault. The exploration of the family's maladaptive attitudes or beliefs in relation to those of the depressed adolescent need not leave parents feeling blamed for their child's depression. Rather, such a discussion can promote a greater awareness of the existence and perpetuation of maladaptive beliefs in general. Discussion often leads to therapeutic reattribution for family members, who may come to understand that their own attitudes and beliefs were shaped by their respective families of origin (external genesis), do not apply without exception to all areas of their lives (specific rather than global application), and are not unchangeable (unstable rather than stable prognosis). The therapist must strive to convey the message that no one is to blame for depression and that family members as well as the adolescent have choices regarding behaviors or beliefs relevant to the alleviation or exacerbation of the depression.

9. OPERATIONALIZE THE ABSTRACT

To "operationalize" means to define in observable, specific, exact terms what can be "measured." The specification of what is meant by abstract terms such as "depression" or "happiness" or "caring," for example, is necessary in all cognitive therapy, but especially so with depressed adolescents because the connotative meaning of abstract concepts is often highly idiosyncratic to members of this younger age group. Adolescents are not "little adults" who use language in the same way with the same intent as their adult counterparts. A common error of less experienced cognitive therapists is to assume what adolescents mean. Therapists working with this younger population must ask their patients constantly about the meaning of abstract terminology. Questions such as "How would you know . . . ?" or "How would you notice . . . ?" or "How would someone else be able to tell . . . ?" or "What would be going on differently . . . ?" help to convey to patients the therapist's request for operationalization of the abstract.

More so than is the case with depressed adult patients, depressed adolescents may have difficulty specifying in observable terms what something means. The therapist often will need to assist them by offering a list of alternatives or a menu from which to choose the appropriate interpretation. For example, a therapist wanting to know what "wanting dad's love" means to an adolescent girl might ask, "When you say you want your dad to love you, do you mean that he should give you an allowance, or that he should look at your report card, or that you should get the car whenever you want? Or do you mean something else?" Parents, too, must be encouraged with similar questions to operationalize their wishes for change. For example, a father complaining that his son is not "more responsible" could be asked, "How would your son behave differently if he were a more responsible teenager?" or "What changes would you notice if your son were to become more responsible?"

Once the abstract has been operationalized, the therapist is in a position to collaborate with the adolescent to examine empirical data relevant to the depression. Once the abstract has been made more specific, cognitive distortions often become apparent and unfounded assumptions are more easily changed. In the previous example of the depressed girl whose negative self-view as an "unlovable" person was founded on the belief that "her father didn't love her," operationalization of the concept "father's love" could lead to a list of behaviors that fathers who love their children exhibit, and it could allow observation of her own father with regard to his demonstration of these behaviors with her and her siblings at home. Through the process of collaborative empiricism, the therapist might help the depressed girl to identify her tendency to "disqualify the positive" and "personalize" the financial difficulties of the family. Sometimes operationalization of the abstract does not lead to cognitive change in the depressed adolescent directly but is preceded by behavioral change in the adolescent or his family members.

Once an abstract concept has been clearly defined so that everyone involved in the therapy knows what is meant by it, therapists often find it useful to label the concept using some "tag" that is meaningful to both the adolescent and the therapist. This "tag" might be the abstract jargon originally used by the adolescent or some other metaphor introduced by the therapist. In the previous example of the adolescent whose negative view of himself was founded on the belief that he was "lazy and would never amount to anything," exploration of what his father meant by "being more responsible" could lead to enumeration of behavioral indices of responsibility that could then be subjected to empirical analysis. Subsequent reference to "the responsibility thing" by the adolescent would then carry with it an understanding of the fullness of meaning previously explored and become a shorthand way of encapsulating a complicated concept. When such abbreviating is done, the therapist should check with the adolescent from time to time to be certain he still remembers what the "tag" means.

10. MODEL FOR THE ADOLESCENT

Therapists who "model" for their patients will demonstrate, nearly continuously, the behaviors and thinking styles they wish to teach. Such demonstrations can occur even without drawing the patient's conscious attention to the fact that a skill from the repertoire associated with cognitive therapy is being modeled. Modeling is an important part of cognitive therapy with both depressed adults and adolescents. However, in light of their developmental stage, which is characterized by rapid learning and change, modeling may have relatively more impact on the younger patient population. Furthermore, modeling allows several "messages" to be conveyed simultaneously by the therapist. For example, while asking a series of questions about why a particular adolescent dislikes attending therapy sessions, the therapist will be collecting information about the stated issue (dislike of therapy) but will also be modeling how not to jump to conclusions or catastrophize or personalize (all cognitive distortions to which the depressed adolescent will be susceptible). The therapist could also use this situation to model cognitive techniques, for example, by thinking aloud about the relationships between the situation (patient complaining about therapy), the therapist's possible emotional response (e.g., some degree of depression), and the therapist's possible automatic thoughts that might be associated with this emotion (e.g., "I've failed with this patient," or "I'm no good at being a therapist"). The ability to convey several different messages at once may be particularly important in the case of adolescent patients who require a lot of repetition and who may require generally shorter therapy sessions than is the case with adult depressed patients.

Modeling can be undertaken at various levels of patient awareness. At one end of the continuum, the patient's attention may be drawn to a particular technique, which is labeled and practiced by the therapist and patient in purposeful role play of some hypothetical situation relevant to the patient's depression. For example, a therapist who wishes to teach the cognitive skill of "generating alternative explanations" to help a depressed adolescent counter the cognitive distortions of "jumping to conclusions" and "mind reading" might design a role play in which the therapist takes the patient role and the adolescent takes the role of a friend. Each would consciously attempt to think like the assigned character, but, in addition, the therapist would "think aloud" in the voice of the adolescent patient whose character he is playing to demonstrate how to stop jumping to conclusions and mind reading and how to replace the maladaptive cognitions that exemplified these distortions with more adaptive thoughts. Alternatively, a therapist may teach skills covertly, without ever drawing the adolescent's attention to what might be of note about the therapist's behavior. For example, by asking questions with words that imply an underlying "continuum" rather than a two-category forced choice, the therapist can covertly model how to avoid the cognitive error of dichotomous thinking.

Not only the "cognitive" skills of therapy can be modeled for the adolescent, but all of the listening, negotiating, problem-solving, assertiveness, and other behavioral skills that a therapist wishes to teach can also be modeled in the therapy session. Sometimes the therapist will demonstrate behaviors without ever directly indicating that modeling is ongoing. For example, a therapist might model assertive behavior with an overbearing father during a session in which a depressed girl's parents are participating. Sometimes it is useful to draw attention to some aspect of the therapist's behavior immediately after its occurrence during the session. Thus, modeling would be immediately followed by identifying for the depressed adolescent what the therapist was doing that the patient might also try. Adolescents seem to enjoy the role of "watch dog" in which they are asked to be vigilant for and notify the therapist when they observe a particular cognitive distortion or cognitive skill being demonstrated during the session. On some occasions, adolescent patients have appeared to take great pleasure in spontaneously identifying cognitive distortions in the speech of family members who are participating in therapy sessions. Family sessions are particularly good opportunities for the therapist to see whether or not the adolescent can generalize to different people and situations some of the cognitive therapy concepts they have been discussing in individual sessions.

Modeling may be at least as important for the parents of depressed adolescents as for the patient, since severe family problems are often related to an inadequate repertoire of parenting skills.

In addition to modeling the cognitive or behavioral skills specific to cognitive therapy, therapists are advised to model the more general behaviors or attitudes requisite to good interpersonal relationships. With adolescents, tolerance (e.g., of forgetfulness, inattention, extreme displays of emotion or behavior) and flexibility (e.g., in scheduling appointments, agenda-setting, pace in therapy, homework tasks) are paramount.

CHAPTER THREE

Diagnosis and Assessment of Depression in Adolescents

GRAHAM J. EMSLIE
WARREN A. WEINBERG

INTRODUCTION

Depression and suicide are major health problems in the adolescent age group. In addition, depression is a major cause of school failure and school dropout in normally intelligent adolescents. Decreasing performance leads to less participation in previously enjoyed activities. Depressed adolescents often abandon their peer groups in favor of new peers who are also doing poorly. Thus, there is no longer debate about whether mood disorders are manifest in children and adolescents. The answer is a clear yes. What is less clear is whether the major depression seen in adolescents is the same disorder seen in adults (with the same phenomenology, genetics, pathophysiology, and treatment responsiveness). There have been large discrepancies in the reported frequencies of child and adolescent depression because of differences in the ages studied, the different measures used (interview vs. self-report), and different criteria for depression. In addition, reports of different rates of depression can be explained by whether the investigators were looking at depressive symptoms or diagnoses. The prevalence of adolescent depression ranges from 2–6% in the general population to 50–60% in psychiatric inpatient populations. Several studies have demonstrated the continuation of this disease into adult life.

In a recent study of a large ($n = 3,294$) representative sample of nonreferred high school students (Emslie et al., 1990) in a large, urban metropolitan school district, we administered two self-report measures of depressive symptoms, the Weinberg Screening Affective Scale (WSAS) and the 21-item Beck Depression Inventory (BDI; Beck et al., 1961). The WSAS consists of 55 statements that require yes or no responses and a fourth-grade reading level. Fifty of the 55 questions relate directly to the Weinberg Criteria for Depression (Weinberg et al., 1973) and assess whether, by self-report, the adolescent fulfills established criteria for depression. The BDI consists of 21 questions with four choices of answers, giving scores of 0–3 for each item and a total score of 0–63.

The sample included 1,825 (55.4%) black, 783 (22.8%) white, 598 (18.2%) Hispanic, and 86 (2.6%) other (Native American and Asian) students, of whom 50.7% were male. The mean age was 15.7 years (range 14–20 years); the median and modal grade was the 10th grade.

On the BDI, 597 (18.1%) of the students scored in the moderate–severe range (score of 16+); this group included 368 (22.7%) girls as compared to 229 (13%) boys. Of the three major ethnic groups, Hispanic girls had the highest proportion in the moderate–severe range (96 of 308, or 31.2%), and white boys had the lowest (36 of 418, or 8.6%). On the WSAS, 440 of 3,294 (13.4%) students met criteria for depression by self-report. Hispanic girls again had the highest percentage of depression (69 of 308, or 22.4%), whereas the white boys had the lowest (33/418 or 7.9%).

With regard to suicidal ideation on the BDI, 101 out of 3,236 students (3.1%) responded positively to "I would like to kill myself," or "I would kill myself if I had the chance." Interestingly, 847 of 3,283 (25.8%) students answered "Yes" on the WSAS item "Sometimes I wish I were dead," and 752 of 3,236 (23.2%) answered positively to the BDI question "I have thoughts of killing myself, but I would not carry them out."

In summary, adolescents in a large metropolitan school district reported a significant amount of depressive symptomatology. Thirteen to 18% showed evidence of depression by self-report. In addition, at a specific point in time, 3% of the population was experiencing significant suicidal ideation. It would appear that depressive symptoms are common in this age group and that a significant number of adolescents are at risk for suicidal behavior.

As mentioned above, only by conducting a clinical interview is it possible to ascertain the number of adolescents with significant depressive symptoms by self-report who actually meet criteria for major depression. Having the disorder requires not only having the symptoms necessary to meet the criteria but also sufficient duration of symptoms and, importantly, dysfunction in daily life (in the family, school, or free time) as a result of the symptoms.

DIAGNOSIS

In adults and adolescents, the development of specific criteria for depression has increased diagnostic reliability. Further, structured and semistructured interviews reduce information variance and improve interrater reliability in clinical and epidemiological research. This section reviews each DSM-IV criterion for major depressive disorder (Table 3.1), with an emphasis on what we feel are unique aspects of the symptoms in adolescents. In addition, criteria for specific use in children and adolescents are presented.

1. *Depressed mood.* This is required to be present objectively or subjectively most of the day and nearly every day. In adolescents, depressed mood may be listed as nonspecifically feeling bad, moody, and irritable (not necessarily sad). Mood and affect appear to be more environmentally influenced in adolescents than in adults. Younger adolescents may report that their sad or dysphoric mood is less persistent over time than adults.

2. *Anhedonia.* This is defined as diminished interest or pleasure in all or almost all activities almost all the time. In adolescents, anhedonia is manifest by dropping out of usual activities such as sports and recreational activities and changing peer relationships. Often adolescents are able to say that they used to enjoy specific activities but do not now. Total anhedonia appears to be rare in this age group, but a marked change in interest or pleasure in activities is often reported. This symptom is often made more difficult to interpret because of secondary rationalization of the changes; in other words, the adolescent attempts to justify or explain why a certain activity is dropped because of age, social group, or a similar excuse. With regard to social interaction, depressed adolescents may not socially withdraw but may instead shift peer groups to a group less acceptable to their parents (i.e., less well functioning) with a justification of seeking more autonomy or self-expression.

3. *Weight loss/gain.* Appetite and weight change in adolescents are less commonly reported than in adults, a factor that may be confounded by developmental changes around puberty. Some adolescents and their parents have little idea of what their weight is and whether it has changed, particularly since, at this age, most adolescents' weight should be increasing along with height. Obtaining regular weights and heights is useful in the ongoing assessment of adolescents.

4. *Insomnia/hypersomnia.* In understanding sleep changes in adolescents, it is important to know about normal adolescent sleep patterns. Normal adolescents tend to sleep less than they need to during the week and sleep longer on the weekends. Studies have shown that such

TABLE 3.1. DSM-IV Criteria for Major Depressive Episode

At least five of the following symptoms have been present during the same two-week period and represent a change from previous functioning; at least one of the symptoms is either (1) depressed mood, or (2) loss of interest or pleasure. . . .

(1) depressed mood (can be irritable mood in children and adolescents) most of the day, nearly every day, as indicated either by subjective account or observation by others

(2) markedly diminished interest or pleasure in all, or almost all, activities most of the day, nearly every day (as indicated either by subjective account or observation by others of apathy most of the time)

(3) significant weight loss or weight gain when not dieting (e.g., more than 5% of body weight in a month), or decrease or increase in appetite nearly every day (in children, consider failure to make expected weight gains)

(4) insomnia or hypersomnia nearly every day

(5) psychomotor agitation or retardation nearly every day (observable by others, not merely subjective feelings of restlessness or being slowed down)

(6) fatigue or loss of energy nearly every day

(7) feelings of worthlessness or excessive or inappropriate guilt (which may be delusional) nearly every day (not merely self-reproach or guilt about being sick)

(8) diminished ability to think or concentrate, or indecisiveness, nearly every day (either by subjective account or as observed by others)

(9) recurrent thoughts of death (not just fear of dying), recurrent suicidal ideation without a specific plan, or a suicide attempt or a specific plan for committing suicide

Note. From American Psychiatric Association (1994). Copyright 1994 by the American Psychiatric Association. Reprinted by permission.

a sleep pattern can result in decreased cognitive performance. Middle and terminal insomnia are relatively uncommon in depressed adolescents, although initial insomnia and trouble awakening are often reported. Again, the trouble falling asleep may be rationalized as staying up late for other reasons; but, after close questioning, the adolescent may admit that he could not fall asleep earlier even if he had tried.

5. *Psychomotor agitation/retardation.* This symptom is required to be observable by others, not just a subjective feeling by the adolescent of being restless or slowed down. In adolescents, this information is difficult to elicit if one has not seen the adolescent in a nondepressed state and if the parents have difficulty attributing the changes to something other than normal adolescence.

6. *Fatigue/loss of energy.* In interviewing adolescents, fatigue and loss of energy can often be confused with other symptoms of depression and with sleepiness. It is important to differentiate not having energy to do

"chores" versus "pleasurable activities" and not to confuse loss of energy with loss of interest. Fatigue is a subjective symptom of feeling tired or having low energy most of the time, even with adequate sleep. A common complaint of adolescents that can cover loss of interest or loss of energy is repeated expressions of being "bored."

7. *Worthlessness/excessive guilt.* It may be hard for an adolescent to admit to feelings of being worthless to an examiner. In addition, adolescents often externalize these feelings with expressions of being picked on. An adolescent may refuse to go to school because other children have called him names. He may deny being worthless, but this reaction to the common occurrence of name calling is often excessive.

8. *Decreased concentration.* This symptom is often one of the more reliable measures of depression in adolescents because of the ability to ask questions about school performance if the patient is unable to report slowed thinking, mind wandering, or similar symptoms. School classes provide a finite period of time in which to do school work. An adolescent who previously has been able to complete the work within the class time allowed, when depressed, may be unable to complete assignments, leading to increased homework because of incomplete work in school. He may then spend long hours doing homework with minimal results. Report cards are obtainable and may show a drop in grades.

9. *Morbid ideation/suicidal thoughts.* As in adults, adolescents will, if questioned, directly admit to wishes of being dead and articulate specific suicidal ideation and plans. The danger in adolescents is that their relatively recent acquisition of abstract thinking tends to lead to more catastrophizing of what adults might consider minor events. Thus, the failure of an adolescent's first relationship may mean to him that he will never have another relationship again. More difficult to assess in adolescents is the preoccupation with death and morbid themes. The parents may report that the adolescent is preoccupied with music and art related to death themes, but this information may not be given spontaneously as the parents may consider such interests to be part of normal adolescence.

The diagnosis of major depression requires at least five of these symptoms to have been present during the same 2-week period, with at least one of the symptoms being depressed mood or loss of interest or pleasure. The primary failure to diagnose depression in adolescents (when present) comes from failure to directly interview the adolescent about the presence or absence of these specific symptoms and the tendency to take at face value superficial rationalizations for the symptoms. Additionally, adolescents vary widely developmentally. Some familiarity with assessing depression in children is necessary in identifying depression in adolescents. Clearly there are significant differences between an immature 14-year-old and a mature 17-year-old.

Specific criteria have been developed for depression in school-aged populations. Although the general consensus is that the same criteria can be used for children, adolescents, and adults, a knowledge of child and adolescent criteria is a useful adjunct to the assessment of an adolescent.

The first criteria developed specifically for children and adolescents from the Feighner et al. (1972) criteria were the Weinberg criteria (Weinberg et al., 1973). As an adjunct to DSM-IV criteria, they have the advantage of clearly defined symptoms and behaviors appropriate for this age group, thus allowing a more structured interview.

The Weinberg criteria have 10 major symptom categories: two essential symptoms and eight auxiliary symptoms. For each symptom category, specific definitions and behaviors relevant to children and adolescents are delineated; these total 40 items. In clinical populations, a criterion of the two essential symptom categories plus four of eight additional symptom categories correlates best with major depression by DSM-IV criteria in children and adolescents. Table 3.2 presents the 10 symptoms and 40 subsymptoms of the Weinberg criteria.

ASSESSMENT

Assessment of depression in adolescents requires systematic evaluation using established criteria for depression. As already mentioned, several criteria sets are available: DSM-IV (American Psychiatric Association, 1994), Research Diagnostic Criteria (RDC; Spitzer et al., 1978), Weinberg (Weinberg et al., 1973), Poznanski (Poznanski et al., 1985), and Feighner (Feighner et al., 1972). The Weinberg and Poznanski criteria have been developed specifically for school-aged populations. The diagnostic assessment is based on clinical interviews of the adolescent, parent historian, and, on occasion, peers and teachers. Self-report measures assessing the range of depressive symptomatolgy are useful adjuncts to clinical interviews. They can also serve as screening measures to assess those needing further evaluation.

The interviewers should use criteria-based structured or semistructured interviews. It is our opinion that, in spite of increased education of professionals about the symptoms of depression in adolescents, the most important factor leading to failure to diagnose appropriately is the

TABLE 3.2. Weinberg Criteria

A. The 10 symptoms and the characteristic behaviors for each symptom. Presence of both symptoms I and II and four or more of the remaining eight symptoms (III through X).

I. Dysphoric Mood

1a. Statements of sadness, loneliness, unhappiness, hopelessness, and/or pessimism
1b. Appearance of sadness, unhappiness, etc.
 2. Mood swings, moodiness
 3. Irritable, easily annoyed
 4. Hypersensitive, cries easily
 5. Negative, difficult to please

II. Self-Deprecatory Ideation

 6. Feelings of being worthless, useless, dumb, stupid, ugly, guilty
 7. Beliefs of persecution
 8. Death wishes
 9. Suicidal thoughts
10. Suicidal attempts

III. Agitation

11. Difficult to get along with
12. Quarrelsome
13. Disrespectful of authority
14. Belligerent, hostile, agitated
15. Excessive fighting or sudden anger

IV. Sleep Disturbance

16. Initial insomnia
17. Restless sleep
18. Terminal insomnia
19. Difficulty awakening in the morning

V. A Change in School Performance

20. Frequent complaints from teachers ("daydreaming," "poor concentration," "poor memory")
21. Loss of usual work effort in school subjects
22. Loss of usual interest in nonacademic school activities
23. Many incomplete classroom assignments
24. Much incomplete homework
25. A drop in usual grades
26. Finds homework difficult

VI. Diminished Socialization

27. Less group participation
28. Less friendly, less outgoing
29. Socially withdrawing
30. Loss of usual social interests

VII. Change in Attitude toward School

31. Does not enjoy school activities
32. Does not want or refuses to attend school

(*continued*)

TABLE 3.2. (*continued*)

VIII. Somatic Complaints
33. Nonmigraine headaches
34. Abdominal pain
35. Muscle aches or pains
36. Other somatic concerns or complaints
IX. Loss of Usual Energy
37. Loss of usual personal interests or pursuits (other than school, e.g., hobbies, sports)
38. Decreased energy; mental and/or physical fatigue
X. Unusual Change in Appetite and/or Weight
39. Anorexia or polyphagia
40. Unusual weight change in past 4 months

B. Interview of patient and historian(s) is conducted using a semistructured, closed-ended technique.
C. A symptom is accepted as positive when at least one of the characteristic behaviors listed for the category is present.
D. Symptoms I and II must be reported by the patient for the symptom to be considered positive. Symptoms III through X can be reported by either patient or historian to be considered positive.
E. Each symptom must be a discrete change in usual self (a new behavior or worsening of an old behavior). The symptom complex must be present for more than one month and associated with a change to maladaption.

Note. Adapted from Weinberg and McLean (1986).

lack of systematic interviewing of the adolescents and parents for the presence or absence of specific criterion signs and symptoms.

Diagnostic interviews and clinician rating scales used specifically with children and adolescents are described briefly below. Adult clinical rating scales have also been used with adolescents, including the Hamilton Rating Scale for Depression (Hamilton, 1960) and the Interview of Depressive Symptoms (IDS-C; Rush et al., 1986).

Diagnostic Inventory for Children and Adolescents (DICA)

The DICA is a structured interview developed by Herjanic and Reich (1982), and the current version is based on DSM-III-R criteria. It consists of two separate interviews with different formats for patients and parents. The instrument's reliability, validity, and parent–child agreement have recently been reviewed and updated (Welner et al., 1987). Studies using this interview schedule show that children/adolescents can provide reliable information as judged by concordance with information given by their mothers (Herjanic et al., 1975), that disturbed children can be distinguished from nondisturbed children (Herjanic and Campbell, 1977), and that adequate interater and intrarater reliability can be obtained (Herjanic and Reich, 1982). In addition, agreement between child and parent on individual symptoms and in diagnostic groups has been assessed (Herjanic and Reich, 1982). Generally, it has been found that children and mothers agree more often about the child's problems when the question concerns concrete, observable, severe symptoms. Mothers report more behavioral symptoms, whereas children report more subjective symptoms relating to their feelings. The interviews with both parents and children take about 2 hours to complete and can be administered by relatively inexperienced interviewers.

Kiddie–Schedule for Affective Disorders and Schizophrenia— Present State (K-SADS-P)

The K-SADS-P (Puig-Antich and Chambers, 1978; Chambers et al., 1985) is an adaptation for children and adolescents of the Schedule for Affective Disorders and Schizophrenia (Endicott and Spitzer, 1978) and has undergone extensive revision and wide use in affective disorder research. The depressive items have been used separately as a severity measure in a double-blind placebo-controlled study of imipramine in children (Puig-Antich et al., 1987). The K-SADS-P also takes 1 to 2 hours to complete and requires an experienced interviewer.

Children's Depression Rating Scale—Revised (CDRS-R)

The CDRS-R is a clinician-rated instrument designed to measure the presence and severity of depression in children and adolescents. Developed by Poznanski (Poznanski et al., 1985), it is modeled on the Hamilton Rating Scale for Depression for adults but also includes questions about school. The CDRS-R consists of 17 items. Fourteen of these are rated on the basis of the subject's response to a series of standardized questions. The remaining three are based on the child's nonverbal behavior. Each item is scored on a 1–5 or 1–7 scale, with a rating of 1 indicating no abnormality. Therefore, the minimum score is 17 and the maximum score is 113. In pharmacotherapy trials using the unrevised version of the CDRS (Geller et al., 1986; Preskorn et al., 1987), a CDRS score of >35 has been used for entry into the study and a score of <25 as an indication of remission. On the revised form, a CDRS-R score of >40 is usually associated with a diagnosis of depression (Poznanski et al., 1985). An equivalent score for remission would be <28. (The unrevised CDRS had fewer items, and most symptoms were rated on a 0–5 or 0–3 scale.) The CDRS has good interrater reliability and correlates highly with global rating of depression. It takes about 30 minutes to obtain sufficient information to score.

Bellevue Index of Depression (BID)

The BID (Petti, 1985), developed by Petti (1978) from the symptoms delineated by Weinberg (Weinberg et al., 1973), can be used as a measure of severity of depressive symptomatology. It is administered in a semistructured interview to both children and parents or other knowledgeable adults and includes 10 major symptom groups and 40 minor symptoms. Each of the minor symptoms is ranked from "absent" to "severe" on a 0–3 scale. The symptoms, to be considered positive, must be of concern to the parent, child, teacher, or referring professional; must be a change from usual self; and must have been present for more than 1 month. The interview is conducted in a semistructured closed-ended format and takes about 30 minutes. There have been no comparisons of the CDRS-R and the BID.

Of the two structured interviews, the choice about which one to use will depend on several factors. The DICA is fully structured and can be completed with the parents and child by a trained technician. It is also available in a computerized version. The DICA is excellent at identifying all possible diagnoses to assist in a differential diagnosis and may be most helpful for clinicians as a supplement to their examination. The K-SADS-P requires more expertise in the field to be utilized. It does a less than effective job with other diagnoses but is probably the best for delineating depressive symptoms, especially for research in affective disorders.

Both the CDRS-R and the BID are good clinical interviews that allow systematic follow- up of depressive symptoms over time; the CDRS-R has more data available regarding cut-off scores and other parameters. However, for the clinician, it is a matter of becoming familiar with one interview so that it can be used regularly.

CONCURRENT DIAGNOSES IN CHILDREN AND ADOLESCENTS WITH DEPRESSION

Initial diagnostic assessment for depression in adolescents requires an evaluation for the presence of other psychiatric disorders as well as depression. In clinical populations, children and adolescents often meet DSM-III, DSM-III-R, or DSM-IV criteria for other psychiatric diagnoses in addition to affective illness. Whether this phenomenon results from the lack of well-developed exclusionary criteria in this age group or represents true comorbid disorders is unclear. Further clarification of this issue is under way from prospective studies. Thus, most children who meet criteria for depression also have symptoms that fulfill criteria for other DSM diagnostic categories.

A recent epidemiological study found concurrent diagnoses in almost 50% of child and adolescent subjects who met criteria for psychiatric disorders (Bird et al., 1988). Using four diagnostic domains of psychopathology from DSM-III (affective, conduct/oppositional, attention deficit disorder [ADD], anxiety), a high rate of comorbidity among the four domains was noted. In those with affective disorder, 24% also manifest conduct/oppositional disorders, 17% ADD, and 17% anxiety disorders.

FAMILY HISTORY

No evaluation of children and adolescents with affective disorders would be complete without a detailed biological family history, including at least first-degree relatives. The offspring of adults with affective illness show a high rate of depression and bipolar disorder. Conversely, children with major depressive disorder have higher familial rates of depression, alcoholism, anxiety, and other psychiatric diagnoses in first- and second-degree relatives. It is expected that adolescents with major depressive disorder will have a positive family history for mood disorders in 50–80% of cases, depending on whether first- or second-degree relatives are evaluated and depending on criteria used (i.e., treated or untreated, definite vs. possible). In evaluating family history, it is necessary to ask more than "Does anyone in your family have psychiatric problems?" Each family member should be asked about individually and screening questions for the major psychiatric disorders asked of each relative. At a minimum, it is preferable to be able to interview both parents of the patient, even if the mother appears at times to know the father's family history better than the father.

MEDICAL EVALUATION

Evaluation of a patient for depression must include a systematic medical evaluation. Depression can be induced by head trauma, viral postencephalitic recovery periods, or medical illnesses such as hyperthyroidism or systemic disseminated lupus. More frequent in adolescents, however, might be induction by various drugs used to treat other medical conditions or select symptoms of depression or mania. The benzodiazepines, stimulants, antihypertensives, and anticonvulsants are notable for heightening the dysphoric symptoms of depression. Additionally, the use of nonprescribed drugs or alcohol should always be assessed. Routine physical examination should include examination for "soft" neurological signs, with appropriate neurological referral as indicated.

BIOLOGICAL CORRELATES

The identification of biological correlates of depression has potential significance for understanding diagnosis, predicting acute treatment and relapse, conducting family and genetic studies, and improving knowledge of the pathophysiology of the disorders. Results from the dexamethasone suppression test (DST)and polysomnography studies seem to be reproducible and offer some potential for further investigation of both diagnosis and prognosis.

The recommended dexamethasone dose for adolescents is 1 mg. Clinically, the DST is not routinely performed for diagnoses, although it may be useful in hard to differentiate populations like the mentally retarded. However, the data suggesting that adolescents with major depressive disorder and a positive DST are less likely to respond to psychosocial treatment alone and less likely to be placebo responders show clinical promise. If these findings are confirmed, then the DST may be useful to assist in treatment planning. Generally, a negative DST is not helpful but a positive DST can be of assistance in management.

Four polysomnographic abnormalities are found in depressed adults: (1) sleep continuity disturbances, (2) reduced delta (slow wave) sleep, (3) increased eye movement density during the early rapid-eye-movement (REM) periods of the night, and (4) shortened REM latency. Polysomnographic studies have also supported a relationship between short REM latencies and major depressive disorder in adolescents.

The question of whether polysomnographic abnormalities are trait or state parameters remains unanswered. However, knowing which variables are persistently abnormal (trait) can, by a process of elimination, give an indication of which variables may be more central to the episode (state). Evidence in adults suggests concordance of reduced REM latency in first-degree relatives of unipolar probands, possibly a genetic (trait) marker. Similarities and differences between adult and child sleep data would contribute to understanding the basic pathophysiology of depression in both groups. Clinically, sleep problems commonly occur in depressed adolescents. A full sleep laboratory assessment (with or without sleep polysomnography) would be indicated in those patients in whom an independent sleep disorder is suspected. The most common problems in adolescence include sleep-phase disorders and excessive daytime sleepiness, secondary to ideopathic hypersomnolence or narcolepsy. Clinically, a common course of action is to treat the depression and see if the sleep difficulties remit.

NEUROPSYCHOLOGICAL/COGNITIVE FUNCTIONING

There is increasing interest in the neuropsychological study of affective disorders in children and adolescents. Several studies have reported findings suggestive of cognitive deficits associated with affective illness in children. Children have been found to have poorer performance on the Wechsler Intelligence Scale for Children—Revised (WISC-R) performance subtests relative to controls. Findings of poorer performance on nonverbal intellectual measures have been interpreted as representing right hemisphere dysfunction. However, it has been suggested that these results may not be indicative of right hemisphere dysfunction but may instead reflect general attention and concentration problems and slower speed on timed measures caused by psychomotor retardation. Conversely, attention, concentration, and psychomotor activity may be right brain functions.

Although no clear evidence for consistent lateralization of deficits currently exists, a pattern of weaknesses has been observed in higher-level cognitive functioning, including problem-solving, abstract reasoning, attention, and concentration. However, comparison of different studies is complicated by whether or not neuropsychological testing (e.g., Halstead–Reitan Neuropsychological Test Battery; Reitan and Davison, 1974) versus general measures of intelligence are used. Additionally, some studies rely on child self-report questionnaires for ascertainment of depression, whereas others require the presence of full-syndrome diagnostic criteria as determined by clinical interviews. These different methods can lead to different study populations and results.

The current literature is significantly deficient in information on the impact of affective illness on the developing brain. Specifically, few longitudinal studies have examined relationships between depressive disorder and the development of cognitive abilities, social competence, and long-term academic achievement.

Whereas no clear pattern of cognitive deficits has specifically been associated with depression, three commonly encountered deficits are clinically important when interviewing an adolescent. They are described in more detail in the next section. First, those adolescents with mild dysphasias (usually trouble recalling words or names in open-ended questions) will respond more cooperatively to questioning involving multiple-choice questions. Second, some adolescents will evidence more right hemisphere dysfunction in spite of intact basic school skills. This symptom is often manifested by adolescents' being disordered, unable to see life as a series of continuous events, and, therefore, unable to give good chronological histories or see natural consequences of actions. The third group tends to have problems with order as described above as well as communication disorders. They are either hyperprosodic or hypoprosodic; in other words, they overexpress or underexpress their internal emotional states in their use of words. In evaluating an adolescent, it is important to separate cognitive deficits from ego defense mechanisms. It may be hard to know whether an oppositional adolescent is purposely being oppositional or is, in fact, unable to answer the questions in the way they are presented.

AFFECTIVE DISORDERS AND LEARNING DISABILITIES

School has been found to be an environment in which children and adolescents can manifest depression either in conjunction with or independent of problems at home and with free time. It is evident that depression and learning disabilities result in poor school performance. However, the resulting interaction between the two remains unknown. Traditionally, studies have focused on classic learning disabilities—dyslexia, dysgraphia, and others—which are thought to be predominantly left brain functions.

Recently, major emphasis on the relationship of the right hemisphere to social competence, nonverbal communication, learning disability, and school failure has developed. Problems with order, prosody, and assessment and processing of nonverbal communication and social cues are believed to be deficits related to right hemisphere dysfunction. This constellation of symptoms has been labeled "nonverbal learning disability." This subtype of learning disability can result in significant problems with adaptation and place the individual at risk for developing depression and suicidal behavior. Rourke and colleagues (1986) found a greater than average frequency of depression and suicide attempts in a population of individuals exhibiting this syndrome. Delong and Dwyer (1988) substantiate the prevalence of affective illness in a group of children and adolescents with right hemisphere dysfunction (Asperger syndrome) and concomitant prevalence of bipolar disease in their biological relatives.

In summary, children who are doing poorly in school, either because of depression or learning disabilities, will frequently manifest both disorders. Three hypotheses have been posed to account for this relationship. The first is that the learning disability leads to increasing frustration and results in depressive symptoms and eventually a depressive syndrome. The second is that depression causes the worsening in school performance and/or the learning disability to become an associated clinical concern. The third hypothesis is the "cerebral dysfunction theory" in which the association between learning problems and depression is explained by their shared etiology. However, an alternative hypothesis is that relationships between learning disorders and depression vary depending on the given individual's genetic predisposition to either depression or learning disability and the environmental stressors he encounters. The "multiple threshold" theory of depression suggests that an individual with high genetic loading may have a depression induced by minimal or no stressors, whereas other individuals with less of a genetic load for depression must experience greater stress before manifesting a depressive episode. Children and adolescents who have affective symptomatology may develop additional symptoms, such as irritability, when stressed by a cognitive or problem-solving task that they are unable to complete successfully. When the task is removed, their mood improves. This scenario is often found in the academic setting, where the depressed child's affective symptoms worsen, contributing to school failure. In classic neurologic thought, a malfunctioning brain, either focal or general (depression), will cause a preexisting neurological deficit (learning disability) to worsen during the acute process.

Clinicians should interview adolescents about school performance, whether they read for fun, have trouble with math, and so on. A mini-mental-status exam, in which the adolescent is asked to read or do some simple math, is also helpful. If a learning difficulty is suspected, then the adolescent can be referred for further systematic psychological testing. However, the clinician should not abrogate the clinical responsibility for knowing how and when to screen for learning disabilities. A semistructured interview for clinician screening has been developed as one possible model (Weinberg and McLean 1986).

CONCLUSION

In summary, the systematic assessment of an adolescent for depression is a complex process requiring careful interviewing of the adolescent and parents. Additionally, an adolescent presenting with problems will also require more general assessment of recent stressors, general coping style, and family interaction as well as an assessment of appropriate developmental issues. The complete assessment of an adolescent is beyond the scope of this chapter. The emphasis on what is only one aspect of assessment is in part an attempt to redress the general failure of professionals to identify a treatable disorder that is often mistakenly identified as a developmental problem, leading to significant morbidity to the adolescent. Additionally, identification of those adolescents with major depressive disorder is the first step in being able to assess treatment response and specificity of treatment as well as to increase our understanding of the basic pathophysiology of this disorder.

SELECTED READINGS

Diagnosis

American Psychiatric Association: *Diagnostic and Statistical Manual of Mental Disorders,* third edition, revised. Washington, DC, American Psychiatric Association, 1987.

American Psychiatric Association: *Diagnostic and Statistical Manual of Mental Disorders,* fourth edition. Washington, DC, American Psychiatric Association, 1994.

Bird HR, Canino G, Rubio-Stipec M, Gould MS, Ribera J, Sesman M, Woodbury M, Huertas-Goldman S, Pagan A, Sanchez-Lacay A, Moscoso M: Estimates of the prevalence of childhood maladjustment in a community survey in Puerto Rico: The use of combined measures. *Archives of General Psychiatry* 1988; 45:1120–1126.

Carlson GA, Cantwell DP: Diagnosis of childhood depression: A comparison of the Weinberg and DSM-III criteria. *Journal of the American Academy of Child Psychiatry* 1982; 21:247–250.

Cytryn L, McKnew DH, Bunney WE: Diagnosis of depression in children: A reassessment. *American Journal of Psychiatry* 1980; 137:22–25.

Geller B, Cooper TB, Chestnut EC, Ankes JA, Schluter MD: Preliminary data on the relationship between nortriptyline plasma level and response in depressed children. *American Journal of Psychiatry* 1986; 143:1283–1286.

Kaplan SL, Hong GK, Weinhold C: Epidemiology of depressive symptomatology in adolescents. *Journal of the American Academy of Child Psychiatry* 1984; 23:91–98.

Kashani JH, Carlson GA, Beck NC, Hooper EW, Corcoran CM, McAllister JA, Fallalin C, Rosenbert TK, Reid JC: Depression, depressive symptoms and depressed mood among a community sample of adolescents. *American Journal of Psychiatry* 1987; 144:931–934.

Kovacs M, Feinberg TL, Crouse-Novak MA, Paulauskas SL, Finkelstein R: Depressive disorders in childhood, I: A longitudinal prospective study of characteristics and recovery. *Archives of General Psychiatry* 1984; 41:229–234.

Kovacs M, Gatsonis C, Paulauskas SL, Richards C: Depressive disorders in childhood, IV: A longitudinal study of comorbidity and risk for anxiety disorders. *Archives of General Psychiatry* 1989; 46:776–782.

Kraepelin E: *Manic–Depressive Insanity and Paranoia.* Edinburgh, Livingston, 1921.

Poznanski EO, Mokros HB, Grossman J, Freeman LN: Diagnostic criteria in childhood depression. *American Journal of Psychiatry* 1985; 142:1168–1173.

Preskorn SH, Weller EB, Hughes CW, Welles RA, Bolte K: Depression in prepubertal children: Dexamethasone nonsuppression predicts differential response to imipramine vs. placebo. *Psychopharmacology Bulletin* 1987; 23:128–133.

Robbins DR, Alessi NE: Depression symptoms and suicidal behavior in adolescents. *American Journal of Psychiatry* 1985; 142:588–592.

Winokur G, Clayton PJ, Reich T: *Manic Depressive Illness.* St. Louis, Mosby, 1969.

Assessment

Beck AT, Ward CH, Mendelson M, Mock J, Erbaugh J: An inventory for measuring depression. *Archives of General Psychiatry* 1961; 4:561–571.

Carlson GA, Kashani JH, Thomas MF, Vaidya A, Daniel AE: Comparison of two structured interviews on a psychiatrically hospitalized population of children. *Journal of the American Academy of Child and Adolescent Psychiatry* 1987; 5:645–648.

Chambers WJ, Puig-Antich J, Hirsch M: The assessment of affective disorders in children and adolescents by semistructured interviews. *Archives of General Psychiatry* 1985; 46:696–702.

Emslie GJ, Weinberg WA, Rush AJ, Adams RM, Rintelmann JW: Depressive symptoms by self report in adolescence. *Journal of Child Neurology* 1989; 3:114–121.

Endicott J, Sptizer RL: A diagnostic interview: The Schedule for Affective Disorders and Schizophrenia. *Archives of General Psychiatry* 1978; 35:837–844.

Feighner JP, Robins E, Guze SB, Woodruff RA, Winokur G, Munoz R: Diagnostic criteria for use in psychiatric research. *Archives of General Psychiatry* 1972; 26:57–63.

Gutterman EM, O'Brien JD, Young JG: Structured diagnostic interview for children and adolescents: Current status and future directions. *Journal of the American Academy of Child and Adolescent Psychiatry* 1987; 5:621–630.

Hamilton M: A rating scale for depression. *Journal of Neurology and Neurosurgery* 1960; 23:56–62.

Herjanic B, Campbell W: Differentiating psychiatrically disturbed children on the basis of a structured interview. *Journal of Abnormal Child Psychology* 1977; 5:127–134.

Herjanic B, Herjanic M, Brown F, Wheatt T: Are children reliable reports? *Journal of Abnormal Child Psychology* 1975; 3:441–448.

Herjanic B, Reich W: Development of a structured psychiatric interview for children: Agreement between child and parent on individual symptoms. *Journal of Abnormal Child Psychology* 1982; 10:307–324.

Kazdin AE, Petti TA: Self-report and interview measures of childhood and adolescent depression. *Journal of Child Psychology and Psychiatry* 1982; 23:437–457.

Petti TA: Depression in hospitalized child psychiatry patients: Approaches to measuring depression. *Journal of the American Academy of Child Psychiatry* 1978; 17:49–59.

Petti TA: The Bellevue Index of Depression (BID). *Psychopharmacology Bulletin* 1985; 21:959–968.

Poznanski EO, Cook SC, Carroll BJ: A depression rating scale for children. *Pediatrics* 1979; 64:442–450.

Poznanski EO, Freeman LN, Mokros HB: Children's Depression Rating Scale—Revised (September 1984). *Psychopharmacology Bulletin* 1985; 21:979–989.

Poznanski EO, Grossman JA, Buchsbaum Y, Banegas M, Freeman G, Gibbons R: Preliminary studies of the reliability and validity of the Children's Depression Rating Scale. *Journal of the American Academy of Child Psychiatry* 1986; 23:191–197.

Puig-Antich J, Chambers W: *The Schedule for Affective Disorders and Schizophrenia for School Age Children (KIDDIE-SADS).* New York, New York State Psychiatric Institute, 1978.

Puig-Antich J, Perel JM, Lubatkin W, Chambers WJ, Tabrizi MA, King J, Goetz R, Davies M, Stiller RL: Imipramine in prepubertal major depressive disorders. *Archives of General Psychiatry* 1987; 44:81–87.

Rush AJ, Giles DE, Schlesser MA, Fulton CL, Weissenberger J, Burns C: The Inventory of Depressive Symptoms (IDS): Preliminary findings. *Psychiatry Research* 1986; 18:65–87.

Spitzer RL, Endicott J, Robins E: *Research Diagnostic Criteria (RDC) for a Selected Group of Functional Disorders,* third edition. New York, Biometrics Research, New York State Psychiatric Institute, 1978.

Welner Z, Reich W, Herjanic B, Jung KG, Amado H: Reliability, validity and parent–child agreement studies of the Diagnostic Interview for Children and Adolescents (DICA). *Journal of the American Academy of Child and Adolescent Psychiatry* 1987; 5:649–653.

Family History

Akiskal HA, Down J, Jordan P, Watson S, Daugherty D, Pruitt DB: Affective disorders in referred children and younger siblings of manic-depressives. *Archives of General Psychiatry* 1985; 42:996–1003.

Delong GR, Dwyer JT: Correlation of family history with specific autistic subgroups: Asperger's syndrome and bipolar affective disease. *Journal of Autism and Developmental Disorders* 1988; 18:593–600.

Puig-Antich J, Goetz D, Davies M, Kaplan T, Davies S, Ostrow L, Asnis L, Twomey J, Iyengar S, Ryan ND: A controlled family history study of prepubertal major depressive disorder. *Archives of General Psychiatry* 1989; 46:406–418.

Biological Correlates

Carroll BJ: The dexamethasone suppression test for melancholia. *British Journal of Psychiatry* 1982; 140:292–304.

Coryell W, Schlesser MA: Suicide and the dexamethasone suppression test in unipolar depression. *American Journal of Psychiatry* 1981; 138:1120–1121.

Doherty MB, Madansky D, Kraft J, Carter-Ake LL, Rosenthal PA, Coughlin BF: Cortisol dynamics and test performance of the dexamethasone suppression test in 97 psychiatrically hospitalized children aged 3–16 years. *Journal of the American Academy of Child Psychiatry* 1986; 25:400–408.

Emslie GJ, Roffwarg HP, Rush AJ, Weinberg WA, Parkin-Feigenbaum L: Sleep EEG findings in depressed children and adolescents. *American Journal of Psychiatry* 1987a; 144:668–670.

Emslie GJ, Rush AJ, Weinberg WA, Rintelmann JW, Roffwarg HP: Children with major depression show reduced rapid eye movement latencies. *Archives of General Psychiatry* 1990; 47:119–124.

Emslie GJ, Weinberg WA, Rush AJ, Weissenburger J, Parkin-Feigenbaum L: Depression and dexamethasone suppression testing in children and adolescents. *Journal of Child Neurology* 1987b; 2:31–37.

Extein I, Rosenberg G, Pottash A, Gold M: The dexamethasone suppression test in depressed adolescents. *American Journal of Psychiatry* 1982; 139:1617–1619.

Giles DE, Biggs MM, Rush AJ, Roffwarg HP: Risk factors in families of unipolar depression, I. Psychiatric illness and reduced REM latency. *Journal of Affective Disorders* 1988; 14:51–59.

Giles DE, Roffwarg HP, Rush AJ: REM latency concordance in depressed family members. *Biological Psychiatry* 1987; 22:907–910.

Goldberg IK: Dexamethasone suppression tests in depression and response to treatment. *Lancet* 1980; 2:92.

Greden JF, Albala AA, Haskett RF, James NM, Goodman L, Steiner M, Carroll BJ: Normalization of dexamethasone suppression test: A laboratory index of recovery from endogenous depression. *Biological Psychiatry* 1980; 15:449–458.

Kupfer DJ, Foster FG: Interval between onset of sleep and rapid eye movement sleep as an indicator of depression. *Lancet* 1972; ii:684–686.

Lahmeyer HW, Poznanki EO, Bellur SN: Sleep in depressed adolescents. *American Journal of Psychiatry* 1983; 140:1150–1153.

McLeod WR: Poor response to antidepressants and dexamethasone non-suppression, in *Depressive Illness: Some Research Studies*. Edited by Davies BM, Carroll BJ, Mowbray RM. Springfield, IL, Charles C Thomas, 1972.

Poznanski EO, Carroll VJ, Banegas ME, Cook SC, Grossman JA: The dexamethasone suppression test in prepubertal depressed children. *American Journal of Psychiatry* 1982; 139:321–324.

Rush AJ, Giles DE, Roffwarg HP, Parker RC: Sleep EEG and dexamethasone suppression test findings in outpatients with unipolar and major depressive disorders. *Biological Psychiatry* 1982; 17:327–341.

Sackeim HA, Prohovnik I, Moeller JR, Brown RP, Apter S, Prudic J, Devanand DP, Mukherjee S: Regional cerebral blood flow in mood disorders, I. Comparison of major depressive and normal controls at rest. *Archives of General Psychiatry* 1990; 47:60–70.

Neuropsychology and Learning Disabilities

Brumback RA: Wechsler performance IQ deficit in depression in children. *Perceptual and Motor Skills* 1985; 61:331–335.

Brumback RA, Staton RD, Wilson H: Neuropsychological study of children during and after remission of endogenous depressive episodes. *Perceptual and Motor Skills* 1980; 50:1163–1167.

Denckla MB: The neuropsychology of social–emotional learning disabilities. *Archives of Neurology* 1983; 40:461–462.

Freeman RL, Galaburda AM, Cabal RD, Geschwind N: The neurology of depression: Cognitive and behavioral deficits with focal findings in depression and resolution after electroconvulsive therapy. *Archives of Neurology* 1985; 42:289–291.

Glosser G, Koppell S: Emotional-behavioral patterns in children with learning disabilities: Lateralized hemispheric differences. *Journal of Learning Disabilities* 1987; 20:365–368.

Heilman KM, Bowers D, Valenstein E: Emotional disorders associated with neurological diseases, in *Neuropsychology*. Edited by Heilman KM, Valenstein E. New York, Oxford University Press, 1985.

Livingston R: Depressive illness and learning difficulties: Research needs and practical implications. *Journal of Learning Disabilities* 1985; 18:518–520.

Reitan RM, Davison LA: *Clinical Neuropsychology: Current Status and Applications*. Washington DC, VH Winston, 1974.

Ross ED, Rush AJ: Diagnosis and neuroanatomical correlates of depression in brain-damaged patients. *Archives of General Psychiatry* 1981; 38:1344–1354.

Rourke BP, Young GC, Leenaars AA: A childhood learning disability that predisposes those afflicted to adolescent and adult depression and suicide risk. *Journal of Learning Disabilities* 1989; 22:169–175.

Rourke BP, Young GC, Strange JD, Russell DL: Adult outcomes of central processing deficiencies in childhood, in *Neuropsychological Assessment in Neuropsychiatric Disorders: Clinical Methods and Empirical Findings.* Edited by Grant I, Adams KM. New York, Oxford University Press, 1986.

Sollee ND, Kindlon DJ: Lateralized brain injury and behavior problems in children. *Journal of Abnormal Child Psychology* 1987; 15:479–490.

Tramontana MG, Hooper SR: Neuropsychology of child psychopathology, in *Handbook of Clinical Child Neuropsychology.* Edited by Reynolds CR, Fletcher-Janzen E. New York, Plenum Press, 1989.

Voeller K: Right-hemisphere deficit syndrome in children. *American Journal of Psychiatry* 1986; 143:1004–1009.

Weinberg WA, McLean A: A diagnostic approach to developmental specific learning disorders. *Journal of Child Neurology* 1986; 1:158–172.

Weinberg WA, Rehmet A: Childhood affective disorder and school problems, in *Affective Disorders in Childhood and Adolescence: An Update.* Edited by Cantwell DP, Carlson GA. Jamaica, NY, Spectrum, 1983.

Weinberg WA, Rutman J, Sullivan L, Penick EC, Dietz SG: Depression in children referred to an educational diagnostic center: Diagnosis and treatment. *Journal of Pediatrics* 1973; 83:1065–1072.

Weintraub S, Mesulam MM: Developmental learning disabilities of the right hemisphere: emotional, interpersonal, and cognitive components. *Archives of Neurology* 1983; 40:463–468.

PART II

Special Issues with Adolescent Patients

CHAPTER FOUR

Developmental Considerations

T. C. R. WILKES

INTRODUCTION

Psychotherapy with adolescents demands an awareness of the biological, psychological, and social development that occurs during puberty. This developmental period is usually a culturally bound transition from childhood to adulthood. Psychotherapy, directly or indirectly, will address developmental issues such as dependency, obedience to discipline, sexuality, separation from the family, and the development of a new "self" and "work" identity, including new associations with peer groups in the community. The ontogeny of the psyche also features increased control of the talionic impulse, the proclivity for demanding revenge for real or perceived insults, and results in an increasing tolerance of frustration and envy. The therapist working with adolescents must be prepared to recognize and negotiate these developmental vicissitudes.

The phenomenon of adolescent depression is complex, because in addition to the individual, the family will be undergoing a transformation influenced by the natural sequence of events in the life cycle. Depression, therefore, occurs superimposed on a shifting matrix of biopsychosocial developmental issues (see Rutter and Hersov, 1985): If the family or the therapist is rigid, ignores the developmental thrust, and insists on their own paradigms as the only ones that can be followed, there will be conflict, a poor fit, a cacophony versus a symphony. In some vulnerable individuals, this conflict manifests as a worsening of depression. Many adolescents proceed along their developmental paths without experiencing major depression or dysthymia, even under severe hardship. The biological, intrapsychic, and interpersonal resources of these youngsters outweigh the demands they are facing and no decompensation occurs. Many families will yield their social, economic, religious, and individual paradigms slowly and carefully, eventually allowing the adolescent to develop his own paradigm for life. However, some of these adolescents will still become depressed if their biological, intrapsychic, or interpersonal resources are overwhelmed. Therapists should remember that there is still much uncertainty about the cause of depression and other psychiatric disorders. Etiological theories may come and go, but phenomena remain. The cognitive therapy strategies of attending to the phenomenal field, seeking empirical validation, testing hypotheses, and pursuing logical analysis seem to be the most flexible, least harmful, and most likely to promote normal development.

Adolescents often present with troublesome behaviors. It is the therapist's job to assess these behaviors within the matrix of shifting biopsychosocial developmental issues. Are the behaviors a product of the adolescent's struggle for age-appropriate autonomy or are they the result of the adolescent's unique way of seeing the world? The adolescent's perspective may be unique because information processing and cognitive integration are influenced by factors such as the presence or absence of learning difficulties, placid or excitable temperaments, and stable or anxious attachments (Bowlby, 1984; Rutter and Hersov, 1985). Alternatively, the troublesome behaviors may be the manifestation of depression. For example, failing school grades or school withdrawal and increasing irritability, together with drug abuse and emerging promiscuity, are common manifestations of depression in adolescents.

The family context is crucially important when trying to assess the meaning of the troublesome behavior of an adolescent. What may be acceptable behavior by a family member at one point in time may no longer be appropriate later in the life cycle because the logical order has changed from the domain of childhood to that of adolescence or young adulthood. A parent asking a 3-year-old to go to bed should expect and will normally receive a different response than when instructing a 16-year-old to do the same thing. This discontinuous transformation from one developmental context to the next is important when assessing behaviors in families that exhibit a wide range of ages and developmental stages. Under these circumstances, latency-aged children may be treated as adolescents and adolescents may be treated as latency-aged children more by default and omission than by choice. When this occurs, the result is a poor fit between the developmental needs of an adolescent and the parenting style of the family.

COGNITIVE DEVELOPMENT AND LEARNING PROBLEMS

The adolescent's cognitive development will determine his ability to learn and to adapt to the environment. Piaget studied cognitive development or, more precisely, "genetic epistemology" (how knowledge is acquired) for many years. The resulting body of research has provided a basis for understanding discontinuous cognitive developmental stages in children and adolescents. Although many developmental specialists have challenged some of Piaget's findings (e.g., Donaldson, 1978; Case, 1988), his concepts and theories remain the most influential for the cognitive therapist working with adolescents. These include the concepts of schema, assimilation, accommodation, equilibrium, stages of sensorimotor development, preoperational period, concrete operations, and formal operations. These concepts will be discussed briefly because it is important in therapy to differentiate between cognitive development (inclusive of "ego defense mechanisms" and/or "cognitive distortions") and cognitive deficits.

Schemas

Piaget used the term "schema" to mean the structure or organization of actions as they are transferred or generalized by repetition in similar or analogous circumstances. So, schemas are cognitive or mental structures by which individuals intellectually adapt to and organize the environment.

Schemas are analogous to the paradigms, concepts, and categories or "cards in an index file" put forward by more contemporary developmental theorists. Each card represents a schema. At birth, a child has few schemas, such as grasping and other motor reflexes. But as the child develops, his schemas broaden and become more differentiated. They become less sensory and more numerous, and the network they form becomes increasingly complex and reflexive. Finally, these schemas become dissociated from their specific contexts. The good news for cognitive therapists is that many of these schemas are capable of undergoing change through the process of assimilation and accommodation.

Assimilation and Accommodation

The biological foundation of Piaget's developmental theory is clearly evident in his notions of assimilation and accommodation. These properties, called the "functional invariants," operate with the inherited neurological structure to influence cognitive development. Assimilation is the integration of external elements and stimuli into preexisting schemas, a process analogous to putting more air into a balloon. In this way, schemas grow but do not change. We assimilate new information constantly, often distorting facts to fit into our preexisting schemas. Cognitive therapy with adults is highly effective at challenging assimilation and the accompanying distortions.

Accommodation, on the other hand, occurs when the new stimulus is not fully integrated into existing schemas. Since the stimulus is not within the range of the child's, adolescent's, or adult's experience, the schemas are either changed to accommodate it or new schemas are created. This process accounts for development, a qualitative change analogous to a collection of balloons rather than just one large balloon. Cognitive therapists working with children and adolescents traditionally focus more on accommodation, the acquisition of new cognitive skills, than on assimilation, the correction of cognitive distortions.

Equilibrium

The processes of assimilation and accommodation are necessary for cognitive growth and development. But balance is required. Too much accommodation means that everything is categorized as different, making similarities difficult to identify. Too much assimilation means that everything is the same, making discrimination, choices, and appropriate judgments more difficult.

The presence of disequilibrium is called "cognitive conflict" and requires the child to seek balance. The individual ultimately assimilates all stimuli, with or without accommodation, to achieve balance, harmony, or accord. Usually a child's or adolescent's view of life will be internally consistent, even if not in harmony with an adult's view. For example, suppose an 8-year-old child breaks his mother's favorite mirror, and, sometime later, the mother falls ill and is admitted to the hospital. Because of the child's limited cognitive development, he will often perceive his "badness" as the cause for her hospitalization. He will not experience cognitive conflict because the course of events is consistent with his world view. He may, of course, experience guilt.

Periods of Intellectual Development

Now we review the developmental stages. However, the reader is cautioned to remember that these are only guidelines and theories, not facts carved in stone. Although other models of development exist, Piagetian theory meshes well with the concepts of cognitive-behavioral therapy.

During the sensorimotor period, which lasts from approximately birth to 18 months, schemas depend completely on perception and bodily movement. The important development during this period is the schema of object permanence, or the knowledge that objects in the external world have an existence independent of the child's action on them or interaction with them.

The period of preoperational thought, traditionally thought of as between 18 months and 7 years, is marked by the appearance of semiotic function, the ability to represent something by means of a signifier that is differentiated and serves only a representative purpose. This period marks the onset of language, mental images, and symbolic gestures. Children show deferred imitation in their play through the process of identification or modeling, a process that is still useful in therapy with adolescents. The child does not understand rules but often plays games as if, by himself, everyone can win. Piaget discusses this stage in more depth in his dissertation on children playing marbles. During this period, children are nonsocial but use symbolic play to help them adjust to their world and their feelings. Even adolescents use this mechanism during times of stress. At the end of the preoperational period, children become preoccupied with rules and winning.

The preoperational stage of cognitive development is highly limited because perceptual evaluation dominates the cognitive processes—"seeing is believing." During this period, children struggle with their egocentric view of life and have problems following transformations and centration; they often cannot see the forest for the trees. They may also have difficulty with irreversibility of thought, and conservation problems are beyond children at this stage. Thinking is often slow, plodding, and illogical. The preoperational period has been referred to as a period of "magical thinking," a time of nightmares and monsters, in which everything tends to be assimilated and thoughts are like facts, causing great anxiety and fear.

The onset of concrete thinking skills traditionally covers the age range of 7 to 11 years. This period is often heralded by the development of conservation; the child can discover what is consistent in the course of any given change or transformation. So, when faced with a discrepancy between perception and thought, the child can make logical, as opposed to perceptual, decisions. In addition, the youngster also begins to master reversibility, seriations, and the cognitive continuum. As the child learns to classify, he can recognize the difference between a class and its member; he can perceive both the superordinate and the subordinate class simultaneously. These logical operations evolve, as do all cognitive structures, out of prior structures as a function of assimilation and accommodation.

At the concrete operational stage, the child is logical, social, communicative, and much less egocentric. Although this level of cognitive development is clearly superior to the preoperational period, it is definitely inferior to the formal thinking skills of adolescents. The concrete operational child can solve concrete problems. However, hypothetical problems, problems that are entirely verbal, or problems requiring more complex or abstract operations are still beyond his developmental range.

Formal thinking develops around the age of 11 to 15 years and is characterized by the development of hypothetical deductive reasoning. The skills of working with propositions rather than concrete events and of isolating variables and examining various combinations of variables are achieved during this period. From this stage on, reasoning undergoes no more major qualitative changes, only quantitative ones. Thus, adolescents with formal thinking skills have the potential to reason as well as adults. However, not every adolescent develops formal thinking skills. Indeed, studies by many researchers have shown that no more than half of the North American population will develop all the skills of formal operations (Elkind, 1962; Kohlberg and Mayer, 1972; Kuhn et al., 1977). Because a large proportion of the adult and adolescent population will be limited to concrete operational reasoning, it is important for cognitive therapists to recognize the limits of the different developmental stages. This often means therapy needs to be focused on real-life events in the here and now.

The Interface between Cognitive Therapy and Adolescent Development

Adults and adolescents can appear to be the same superficially. Both can solve concrete problems, but only those with formal thinking skills can cope with the more complicated hypothetical reasoning required for abstract problems. How does this knowledge help the cognitive therapist who is treating an adolescent with depression? Knowledge of the cognitive development of adolescents facilitates communication between therapist and patient. Consider a 13-year-old who is cognitively delayed, operating with just a few concrete thinking skills. The therapist can successfully personify difficulties and fears in a concrete way and subject them to logical analysis, without insulting the youngster's intelligence.

"Splitting" is a term used by many child and adolescent mental health workers because it is so readily observed in this field where adolescents argue or attribute blame in a dichotomous fashion. It is either "yours" or "mine." Many adolescents experience mood swings with incredible urgency for immediate resolution. In therapy, the link between their catastrophizing thoughts and devastated feelings becomes obvious, and the presence of the black-and-white cognitive distortion is identified readily in this situation. By gently challenging the dichotomous mindset, which is often fueled by adolescents' "should" statements about how their world should be, adolescents can move away from the cognitively constricted position, no longer thinking in terms of "always" or "never" and seeing things as "maybe later" or "more or less" likely. Indeed, they can transcend the binary motif of labeling things as "pass" or "fail" to "more or less" helpful experiences. It is no longer a question of "either–or"; it can be "both" and a "win–win" situation created by altering the mindset. This process challenges the splitting that occurs so excessively with adolescents who have delayed cognitive development and works on the cognitive capacity of accommodation rather than assimilation, referred to in the earlier part of this section.

Another example of improved communication is the awareness that, for adolescents with delayed cognitive development who are stuck with preoperational and concrete reasoning, thoughts and fears are very real. Such beliefs will respond well to behavioral homework tasks. However, such adolescents may still have considerable difficulty identifying the difference between fact and fantasy or possibility and probability. The Socratic dialogue in cognitive therapy is invaluable in helping the patient see the difference. This technique is also useful in identifying the comparative difference between objects, subjects, and events. The ability to appreciate differences in general, and not just in specific instances, is important in both cognitive therapy and family therapy. Remember Gregory Bateson's (1972) fundamental principle that information is a difference and a difference is a relationship or change in a relationship. Both cognitive and family therapy use the appreciation of a difference to bring forth new perspectives and behaviors to respond to old problems.

Community schools follow a curriculum that assumes the development of these cognitive skills. Adolescents who fail to acquire them at the same time as some of their age peers often have academic difficulties and they naturally go through a period of uncertainty, anxiety, and even dysphoria. They may become inattentive, oppositional, or depressed whenever they are faced with school classes demanding more formal thinking skills than they are capable of mobilizing. Recognition of the adolescent's cognitive developmental level is the first step in planning an appropriate intervention strategy involving the school, the community, and the parents.

Finally, and perhaps most importantly, awareness of the complexity of cognitive development, particularly the Piagetian emphasis on "constructivist structuralism," reminds the therapist that the adolescent and his environment are constantly shaping each other in a dynamic interaction. Thus, the cognitive therapist avoids making the mistake of crediting all of the explanatory power to one part of this "drama." By avoiding blaming the family or the adolescent for the problem, the therapist suggests that a "multiple threshold theory" may be more helpful in understanding the adolescent depression than is a unifactorial model.

The presence of school difficulties or a history of developmental difficulties such as poor socialization at kindergarten or elementary school should alert the therapist to the presence of subtle learning difficulties. These may include problems with comprehension of the spoken word, sequencing, or prosody. Obviously, such problems can have profound effects on the psychotherapeutic relationship and the expectations of therapy. Therefore, it is often helpful early on to complete a developmental inventory to establish the adolescent's baseline skills.

The Weinberg lexical paradigm (Weinberg and McLean, 1986) and the binaural comprehension test (Green, 1991) are useful screening procedures to aid this part of the assessment. The former is a 10-minute office evaluation of the patient's lexical, reading, spelling, arithmetic, printing, and writing skills. Easily combined with a mental-state examination, it will identify the adolescent with dyslexia, receptive and expressive dysphasia, and any associated difficulty with sequencing and prosody. This knowledge, in itself, can be very helpful to the adolescent, who may be unable to operationalize his school difficulty into specifics such as dyslexia or a sequencing problem with auditory instructions. Instead he may use global statements such as "I'm just a dummy at math and anything that requires brains." Seeing the situation as stable, global, and as an internally attributed phenomenon is a strong predisposing factor for depression.

The depressed adolescent with learning difficulties, school problems, and mild attention-deficit hyperactivity disorder is a common referral to many adolescent clinics. Therapy must take into account the adolescent's information-processing limitations if intervention is to assist the adolescent in the developmental tasks of securing a new identity and coming to terms with intimacy. The forgetful adolescent who looks uninterested in therapy, constantly saying "What?" to authority figures may indeed have great resistance because of unresolved oedipal issues. However, the adolescent may also have major sequencing problems with a mild receptive dysphasia and hypoprosody. Intervention would need to include sharing of this information with the school counselor and devising an action-oriented, visually enriched, therapeutic milieu. Emphases in treatment will be placed on the associated cognitive deficits and impaired problem-solving skills. This attention would include training the adolescent in certain social skills, such as how to be appropriately assertive without being passively aggressive, how to start and finish conversations with peers and elders, how to recognize affect, and how to keep on track by maintaining a focus on the number one priority or goal. Hopefully, it becomes obvious how the screening for learning difficulties and the unique way of cognitive processing help to enrich the therapeutic milieu, facilitating the adolescent's success in the struggle for age-appropriate autonomy.

The binaural comprehension test is a research tool used to investigate corpus callosum transfer problems by giving the patient a series of stories through the left, right, and both ears alternatively, then assessing for recall. Some adolescents show clear comprehension difficulties when both ears are used, suggesting difficulty with processing. They may benefit from using an car plug. However, the point is that the neurodevelopmental state of the adolescent will profoundly influence therapy since it relies on the ability to communicate orally. The adolescent's cognitive development and cognitive skills will profoundly influence the way the family reacts and accommodates to the normal developmental crises of life. Many of the difficulties encountered by families and their adolescents may be the product of cognitive deficits and not cognitive distortions. This possibility must be taken into account by the therapist when preparing the formulation.

SUMMARY

Cognitive therapy with depressed adolescents, unlike cognitive therapy with their adult counterparts, must be keenly sensitive to developmental issues. The presentation of a depressed adolescent on a shifting bed of biopsychosocial issues is the essence of the difference between the two populations. When assessing a depressed adolescent, the therapist must try to identify the relative contributions of the major depression, the adolescent phase itself, and the adolescent's personality and temperament to the total clinical picture. Personality and temperament include degree of novelty-seeking behavior, attachment behavior, and learning style with the associated cognitive deficits. But the most important of these three factors is the developmental thrust of adolescence, which is separation–individuation. This process manifests as a struggle for a new identity, during which adolescents come to terms with their new strengths, sexual potential, and creative talents. The change is in their lessened dependence on their family of origin and their separation from childhood views and attitudes. The challenge is one of integration into the large community and society as a socialized but independent and creative individual.

When the adolescent's major depression is resolved, the therapist will still be left with the vicissitudes of the separation–individuation phase and how they are inflected through the adolescent's temperament and personality. This developmental phase, in itself, may present sufficient problems for the family and the adolescent to consult a mental health therapist. Thus, termination with the depressed adolescent may be more difficult because of a shifting therapeutic focus, which is in contrast to therapy with adults, most of whom have already resolved the issue of dependency and established a stable identity.

SELECTED READINGS

Bateson G: *Steps to an Ecology of Mind.* San Francisco, Chandler,1972.
Bowlby J: *The Making and Breaking of Affectional Bonds.* London, Tavistock, 1984.
Case R: The whole child: Toward an integrated view of young children's cognitive, social and emotional development, in *Psychological Bases for Early Education.* Edited by Pellegrini A. New York, Wiley, 1988.
Donaldson M: *Children's Mind.* Glasgow, Fontana Press, 1978.
Elkind D: Quantity conceptions in college students. *Journal of Psychology* 1962; 57:459–465.
Green P: *Monaural and Binaural Speech Comprehension.* Paper presented to the Canadian Psychiatric Association, June 1991.
Kohlberg L, Mayer R: Development as the aim of education. *Harvard Education Review* 1972; 42:449–496.
Kuhn D, Langer N, Kohlberg L, Hann N: The development of formal operations in logical and moral judgment. *Genetic Psychology Monograph* 1977; 95:115.
Piaget J: *The Origin of Intelligence in the Child.* London, Penguin Books, 1977a.

Piaget J: *The Moral Judgement of the Child.* London, Penguin Books, 1977b.

Rutter M, Hersov L (eds): *Child and Adolescent Psychiatry.* London, Blackwell, 1985.

Weinberg WA, McLean A: A diagnostic approach; to developmental specific learning disorders. *Journal of Child Neurology* 1986; 1:158–172.

CHAPTER FIVE

The Therapeutic Relationship with Adolescents

ELLEN FRANK

A. JOHN RUSH

THE THERAPEUTIC ALLIANCE

The therapeutic alliance refers to the working relationship between therapist and patient that facilitates the application of therapeutic techniques and constructive changes in behavioral, emotional, and cognitive patterns. This alliance is based on the nonneurotic, rational rapport that the patient has with the therapist and includes identification with the sympathetic, empathic, understanding part of the therapist. Various psychodynamic thinkers such as Melanie Klein and Otto Kernberg have identified a number of defenses against trust and the formation of this alliance. These defenses include denial, derogation, triumph, and reading negatives into what the therapist does. Denial refers to the patient's recognition of a fact while maintaining that the fact has "no meaning." Derogation refers to the patient's tendency to belittle the therapist and/or the therapy process. Triumph refers to the patient's belief that he does not need or want the therapist. The tendency of depressed patients to view neutral statements by the therapist or interactions with the therapist as attacks or accusations is referred to as reading negatives into the situation (Rush, 1980).

Every one of these defenses comes into play in therapy with depressed adolescents. Indeed, with the typical adolescent, almost all of them may be operating at once. Frequently, the adolescent denies that he has a disorder or even a problem. Rather, the problem is with his parents, his teachers, his siblings, perhaps his peers, but certainly not himself. Even the adolescent who denies that he has a problem will often feel the need to derogate the therapist and the therapy process. Statements such as "This is dumb," "You're dumb," and "This can't possibly help me," are frequently made, even by the adolescent who denies that there is any need for help (a classic example of how denial works). Along with the derogation of therapy and the therapy process, the adolescent will frequently believe that he does not need or want the therapist, indeed, does not need any help from anyone. Even those adolescents who are using all of these defenses to try to maintain as much distance as possible from the therapist and the therapy process may, nonetheless, engage in reading negatives into what the therapist says or does, with even positive statements being misinterpreted as negatives. For example, if the therapist compliments an adolescent girl on her appearance on a particular day, she frequently rereads that compliment to mean "I look only half as terrible as I did last week," not "I really look nice today." Selective attention and selective hearing are notable features of adolescent behavior in general. Not surprisingly, the depressed adolescent frequently selects the most negative statements or the most negative interpretation of statements to attend to.

Short-term therapies in general, and perhaps particularly with adolescents, demand careful and skillful management of the therapeutic alliance because these therapies create a demand for therapeutic change that is far more pressured than open-ended or nondirective approaches. That is, both the predefined time limit (usually between 10 and 20 weeks) and the therapist's role as a guide and prescriber of techniques create a focus on immediate issues and on change to be accomplished in short order.

We recommend a semidefined time limit with cognitive therapy for adolescents (see Chapters 7–9) to allow the therapist to modulate the intensity of the treatment based on the needs of the individual patient and family. Therapy with adolescents frequently creates an additional demand inasmuch as an alliance must be formed with the parents as well as with the adolescent. Negotiating this process can often be difficult, particularly when there is conflict between the parents and the child. Many adolescents and their parents may become uncomfortable with the pressure for rapid behavioral change and may respond by dropping out of treatment or failing to adhere to the therapist's directives or suggestions. Finally, in work with adolescents, one has the problem, rarely encountered with adult outpatients, that the adolescent may have been *brought* to treatment rather than have come of his own free will.

In those adolescents who are reluctant to come to therapy, reframing the problems in the manner described in Chapter 7 on the initial phase of treatment can often help to turn an adolescent who sees no need for treatment into one who can at least grudgingly acknowledge that the experiment is worth the risk. Indeed, framing the initial sessions as an experiment (and what could be more consistent with the cognitive approach?) frequently captures the attention and imagination of somewhat resistant adolescents.

Although a time-limited, more concrete, directive approach may actually increase optimism and adherence in adult patients and facilitate more rapid change than nondirective time-limited approaches, two factors may mitigate against this advantage with adolescents: First, adolescents have no particular expectations about what "therapy" consists of or how long it should last. Second, to an adolescent, 5 months often seems like an eternity. Thus, whereas a small number of adolescents will quickly form meaningful, stable therapeutic alliances in cognitive therapy, a substantial number will balk at this step. In these resistant cases, the therapist is required to focus on the development of the alliance itself, employing a range of techniques to nurture, shape, and establish a therapeutic relationship. Only after this critical step is accomplished can the therapist employ those techniques aimed at guiding the patient toward cognitive changes. For particularly resistant adolescents, the time limit itself may need to be modified or renegotiated as therapy proceeds.

The first section of this chapter provides guidelines for identifying those patients who will have difficulty forming a therapeutic alliance. Next, patient and therapist variables that may obstruct the formation of such alliances are discussed, including particular symptom patterns that may require modification of the usual cognitive approaches. Case examples are used to illustrate some of these points in greater detail.

The ideas and guidelines contained in this chapter have been developed largely from clinical experience. Few research data are currently available to test these notions. Although these concepts may apply to short-term therapies other than the cognitive approach, data are lacking to support the generalizability of these observations to other forms of short-term treatment. It is hoped that the notions contained in this chapter will provide some guidelines for the practitioner as well as hypotheses that can be empirically tested by psychotherapy researchers.

Most practitioners of short-term therapies with adults provide specific guidelines for patient selection, among which is the ability to rapidly form a therapeutic alliance. Psychodynamic (Zaiden, 1982) as well as cognitive (Beck et al., 1979), interpersonal (Rounsaville and Chevron,

1982), and behavioral (Lewinsohn et al., 1982) approaches all specify, to some extent, the inclusion or exclusion criteria for patients to be treated.

In work with adolescents, however, many of these guidelines for patient selection cannot be applied, since the contract is as much with the parents as with the patient, and the assumption in working with adolescents is that there will often be barriers to the formation of a therapeutic alliance. Nonetheless, it is essential that the therapist planning to engage in cognitive therapy with an adolescent make an assessment of how rapidly a particular patient will be able to form a therapeutic alliance. The therapist must also try to determine how rapidly he can expect to form an alliance with the family system and any other individuals, such as teachers, who may be critical to the success of the treatment plan. Family members and others may use the same defenses as the adolescent patient.

How might the clinician quickly assess a particular adolescent's capacity to form a therapeutic alliance? For purposes of discussion, evidence that bears on this question can be divided into that obtained from the clinical interview (including an assessment of the adolescent's developmental level) and that derived from the patient's history.

Depending on the adolescent patient's developmental level, cognitive therapy can vary markedly from an experience that is virtually indistinguishable from that with adults to something that verges on cognitive play therapy. Indeed, we would argue that many mature adolescents, especially girls who acknowledge their need for treatment, can often be approached in a manner that is identical to the approach the therapist would take with an adult woman patient. Treating these young women like age peers frequently draws on the most mature parts of their developing personalities. This concept leads to another important point: There is, especially in this age group, relatively little relationship between maturity and intelligence. Work with a fully emancipated, developmentally advanced adolescent of only borderline intelligence can proceed in a way that is no different from the way in which one would proceed to do cognitive therapy with an adult of borderline intelligence. Much of the focus of therapy is on mastery and pleasure sheets and concrete homework tasks. Any attempts at true cognitive interventions must take place within the therapy session, since the triple-column technique is well beyond the capacity of such individuals. On the other hand, bright but immature adolescents may prove to be much more of a challenge in terms of becoming engaged in the therapeutic process. Yet, once engaged, these patients may be able to participate fully in the most sophisticated cognitive techniques, although *issues* around which their cognitions are centered are much more childlike or "adolescent."

> Mary Beth was a slender, energetic 15-year-old who was referred for treatment after she had been raped by a girlfriend's older brother. The referral came from a crisis center that she had called on her own following the assault. At the time of the assault, Mary Beth had been doing "C" work in a program for educable mentally retarded children. Although of limited intelligence, she was quite mature and competent from a number of perspectives. She was well versed in the use of the public transportation system and willing to travel alone to the hospital, which was many miles from her home. She held down a 20-hour-a-week after-school and weekend job, which she had had for over a year when she entered treatment. When Mary Beth first presented, she had the full range of depressive symptoms, including depressed mood, a significant sleep disturbance, a weight loss of more than 5 pounds from her already thin baseline, and an almost complete loss of interest or pleasure in her usual activities. Over the strong objections of her parents (the reasons for which were never made clear to the therapist), she persisted in coming for 14 sessions of treatment. The triple-column technique was well beyond her cognitive or intellectual capacity. She was clearly unable to grasp the concept of thinking about thinking; however, when the concept of mastery and pleasure experiences was explained in simple language, she was able to grasp it and was able to read and write well enough to complete weekly activity schedules and to plan mastery and pleasure activities. The frequency of these experiences was targeted for increase with each week of therapy. By week 14, her depression had completely resolved.

When the therapy involves the use of homework assignments, the therapist will often begin by suggesting a relatively simple homework task. The patient's response to this task is often a useful clue to whether meaningful collaboration will shortly ensue.

In adult cognitive therapy, the first task asked of the patient is to read a five-page pamphlet, *Coping with Depression* (Beck and Greenberg, 1976), following the initial descriptive and medical diagnostic interviews. The first therapy session begins with a review of this task. Patients' responses to it vary from a meaningful "Yes, I can see how my negative thinking can make my situation worse," to a hostile "I don't think this approach has anything to do with me. Furthermore, I lost the pamphlet." Other responses might include "I read the pamphlet, and I got more depressed," or "I was too depressed to do it." Almost any homework assignment can evoke a similar range of responses in adolescents. The first response calls for a further probing of just what the patient learned from the assignment: Was it as helpful as initially stated, or is the patient simply acting in a compliant manner? The second, hostile comment suggests that the patient was somehow personally affronted at being asked to carry out the assignment and that he is angry at someone (probably the therapist). Here, a gentle exploration of the anger and cognitions associated with it is indicated. If the patient responds by escalating the denigration of the therapist or therapy, the therapist might have encountered a defense against trust and forming an alliance. If so, then forming a trusting relationship might become the central task of the first sessions of therapy. In this case, the fears, fantasies, and cognitions about the therapist and therapy must become the initial targets for treatment.

The adolescent who feels more depressed while doing the homework assignment but appears willing to participate in the therapy is perhaps expressing a fear of symptom exacerbation. We have found that many adolescents, particularly the older group, retain the fantasy that, if they succeed in "peeling away the layers of the onion," they will encounter something too horrible to confront and are, thus, quite fearful of the therapy process. The patient who seems to fear getting worse needs to be questioned further about the cognitions that occurred as he attempted to complete the homework assignment. Did the task seem too confusing, leading to the notion that "I can't even do this simple task; therefore, I'll never get better," or had the patient realized that negative thinking had been present for many years and had interfered with school and family to a much greater degree than initially thought? If so, it is likely that this is a patient who tries to perform the task and is able to express directly the pain and frustration that ensue. A therapeutic alliance is likely to develop with this adolescent.

The adolescent who was too depressed to complete the task is thinking globally and perhaps too pessimistically to initiate new behaviors. This patient may respond to the therapist's further exploration of this cognition and attempts to specify the details of how the depression stopped the patient. On the other hand, the adolescent may be attempting to establish a passive role, thereby placing all of the responsibility on the therapist to magically cure the problem without the patient's participation. Is this behavior an attempt to avoid establishing a therapeutic alliance so that, if therapy fails, the adolescent can blame the therapist or therapy, while avoiding further injury to his already negative view of himself? Again, further discussion about the details of this apparent noncompliance will determine whether it can easily be dispelled or whether it is the tip of an iceberg that points toward difficulties in forming a collaborative relationship with the therapist.

This brings us to the second interview-based observation, which portends the degree of ease or difficulty in forming a therapeutic alliance—that is, how easy it is to discuss in detail the reasons for noncompliance and convert the patient into a more willing collaborator. Can the patient report the negative expectations and fears associated with compliance? Does the adolescent take personally and respond negatively to such a discussion, or is he able to view the dialogue with some objectivity, to hear it as the therapist's attempt to help him review, observe, and respond to his initial negative cognitions? Patients who are severely ill do not easily establish the alliance and are more likely to respond negatively to such probing discussions. That is, such patients have more difficulty objectively evaluating the therapist–patient dialogue. The patient who is more likely to negatively personalize such discussions is even less able to form an alliance. Negative personalization can be countered by asking the patient to play the role of the therapist in rephrasing his or her own negativism.

Finally, since short-term therapies adhere to a time limit, the willingness of the patient to participate in agenda-setting and in the allocation of available time is often another clue to whether a therapeutic alliance can easily be formed. If the patient insists repeatedly over several interviews that there is not enough time for all of his problems, or if he repeatedly strays from the agenda and is offended at being drawn back to it by the therapist—perhaps commenting, "You don't care about me. You're preoccupied with time"—then the formation of the alliance should take precedence over methods aimed more directly at the ultimate objectives of therapy (e.g., cognitive change, interpersonal problem-solving, and so forth).

Time allocation can be particularly problematic with adolescents, who frequently have vague and distorted notions of time (e.g., 5 months may seem like an eternity). If the therapeutic hour does go quickly, and the adolescent has more that he would like to do or say, it is frequently difficult for the patient to understand why the therapy hour needs to end. This problem may be representative of a more general difficulty with limits characteristic of many adolescents. One approach to this problem is to ask the patient to write out what else needed to be said in the interval between the sessions; however, it is then imperative that the therapist begin the next session by reviewing this material.

In addition to interview behaviors, adolescents' histories often provide clues to their potential difficulty or ease in forming an alliance. Does the patient have relatively constant parenting figure(s)? Does he have a "best friend" with whom mutual intimate exchange has occurred for several years? All of these data give clues to the patient's capacity to form longer-lasting relationships and indirectly have implications for the formation of a therapeutic alliance. In the case of the patient who reports many broken relationships, taking a history of those relationships often provides a pattern of perceptions that lead to disruptions for that individual case. Such a history may also provide clues as to how this particular relationship, the therapeutic alliance, can be maintained.

A second relevant historical variable is whether the patient behaves impulsively. Does the patient, when confronted with interpersonal difficulties, leave the relationship? Does he make efforts to solve such difficulties; or are the feelings of rejection, anger, loneliness, and the like immediately converted into impulsive behaviors?

Sometimes the indicators of borderline, antisocial, or schizotypal features are obvious, even in these younger individuals. Adolescents who suffer from severe personality disorder are likely to have a difficult time forming a therapeutic relationship. In such cases, a revision of the time limit for therapy may be needed to allow sufficient time for the formation of an alliance before the particular depressive or Axis II symptoms are addressed. Alternatively, the therapist may decide to make the behavioral symptoms of the Axis II disorder the main objective of treatment, while treating the Axis I disorder with medication.

DIFFICULTIES IN FORMING THE THERAPEUTIC ALLIANCE

Three major groups of factors contribute to the formation of the therapeutic alliance: those attributable to the patient, those attributable to the therapist, and those attributable to the disorder. Because such contributors are manifold, we briefly illustrate each of these three groups by example rather than attempt an encyclopedic enumeration. For the practitioner of cognitive therapy with adolescents, it is important to keep in mind that any one of these factors (the patient, the therapist, or the disorder) can, at any particular moment, present obstacles. When such obstacles are encountered, they must be identified and dealt with differentially.

Patient Factors

Let us first turn to patient factors. One important variable is the patient's cognitive set. It is well known that depressed adolescent patients see themselves, their immediate futures, and those with whom they interact (including the therapist) in negative ways. One patient, who was particularly sensitive to the therapist's behavior, appeared upset when the therapist arrived 10 minutes late to the session. When queried, the patient reported thinking, "He isn't interested in me. I must be the worst patient he has." For the next session the therapist purposely arrived and began early. This time the patient reported her thinking as, "I must be sicker than all the other patients; that's why he's spending extra time." At the following session, the therapist was punctual to the moment. This time she reportedly thought, "He's just running a factory here. He's not taking a personal interest in me." Although these negative interpretations may be exacerbated by the presence of major depression, many patients will have a longstanding tendency to scrutinize closely and erroneously disparage any new relationship. In such instances, greater focus on these tendencies is required before and during the assignment of directive homework tasks. For such a patient, homework is likely to be viewed as a harsh demand without purpose and is likely to contribute to disruption of the alliance.

This brings us to a second patient variable—the response to homework assignments or directives in the interview. To ameliorate the potentially disruptive effects of such tasks, it is imperative that these tasks follow logically from the therapist–patient dialogue and that the rationale for such requests be clearly stated at the outset. Furthermore, the adolescent's participation in the creation of such tasks is essential, not only to improve the likelihood of adherence but also to ensure that the alliance is either strengthened or at least not weakened when such a request is made. Finally, once the adolescent attempts such tasks, the therapist should ask the patient, not simply about what he did or did not do, but about his feelings, thoughts, and attitudes about the undertaking. This review should be conducted at the beginning of each session in order to decipher the adolescent's feelings about the previous session and at the end of each session to review the transactions between patient and therapist in that particular session. Adolescents should especially be encouraged to share feelings of frustration, annoyance, hopelessness, and other negative emotions about the therapist and therapy. In this way, the therapist can gauge whether his behavior is viewed as or is actually contributing to a weakening of the alliance.

A third patient variable consists of the style by which the patient organizes and processes information. This style may or may not be associated with a particular personality disorder. Whereas some disorders are notorious for suggesting severe problems in interpersonal relationships (e.g., borderline, schizotypal), other personality styles (hysterical or obsessive–compulsive) can interfere with communication in a short-term approach and secondarily disrupt the alliance. For example, the relatively rare adolescent with clear obsessive–compulsive features may fail to be cognizant of the therapist's affective tone or may try to comply in too great a detail, thereby sidetracking the dialogue into a web of thoughts that have little or no emotional relevance. Those more commonly seen adolescents with a more histrionic style tend to think in global terms and balk, at least initially, at what appear to be picky details of homework tasks. Those with such personality styles will be more consumed with wanting to please, entertain, or win the approval of the therapist. Again, a greater focus is needed on the relationship itself and on how the adolescent's style of processing information affects the alliance.

A final barrier to the formation of the therapeutic alliance in the adolescent patient is the belief that the therapist cannot possibly understand the world he inhabits. The world of adolescents seems like "foreign territory" to many adults, and the adolescent patient may erroneously assume that the therapist is no different from any other adult.

Conveying to the adolescent that the therapist has some understanding of what that world is like (by drawing on the therapist's own experience as an adolescent—although many things have changed since then, many others have not—or by making reference to knowledge obtained in work with other adolescents) can help to break down the barriers between the therapist and the adolescent patient. On the other hand, if the therapist *assumes* that he understands the adolescent's world when he does not, this presumption will only support the patient's belief that no one understands what his life is like. Therefore, it is exceptionally important with adolescent patients that the therapist stop, inquire, and then inquire again when he does not understand what is being said, the nature of the conflict the adolescent is experiencing, or the importance of a particular achievement or function. Such inquiries have two positive alliance-building effects: (1) the process of inquiry, if handled tactfully, shows the patient that the therapist is interested; and (2) the inquiry puts the adolescent in the role of "expert," thereby diminishing the power struggle between the generations. In this respect, working with adolescents is no different from working with any patient who inhabits a world that is slightly different from the therapist's own. Thus, the therapist who works with individuals from an unfamiliar ethnic enclave, a foreign country, or a religious community must do a good deal of inquiry in order to understand the nature of the patient's life. Adolescents are no different in this respect.

A final problem in the adolescent patient, which is certainly not unique to adolescents but simply more prevalent in this age group, is difficulty in accepting the fact that they have a disorder. Getting the adolescent to accept the disorder leads to the adolescent's accepting the treatment and ultimately to maintaining the treatment gains. In talking with the adolescent about the disorder, the therapist must consider at least two important issues. The first is the timing of discussion about the disorder. Obviously, this discussion has to take place reasonably early in the treatment process if meaningful therapeutic work is to be done; however, sometimes just establishing the relationship must precede even talking about the disorder. The second issue in discussing the disorder with adolescents is helping them to see the difference between the full syndrome of depression, with its range of neurovegetative and cognitive symptoms, versus dysfunctional thinking that persists even after the major portion of the syndrome is resolved. The therapist must make it clear that continued work on dysfunctional thinking is an important part of the therapeutic process because it is this persistent dysfunctional thinking that may leave the adolescent vulnerable to recurrent episodes. As part of this discussion, it is important that the therapist acknowledge what he does *not* know about the disorder, its causes, and the vagaries of its treatment. Since the adult who does not "know it all" is likely to be a rare phenomenon in the adolescent's life, this simple acknowledgment may assist appreciably in the formation of the therapeutic alliance.

Therapist Factors

The therapist can contribute in numerous ways to the disruption or weakening of the alliance. The short-term directive therapist must constantly judge whether he is too active and directive (e.g., talking over the patient while failing to listen). This strategy is particularly tempting with the silent adolescent. Like the television interviewer, the adolescent therapist must learn to shape questions so that a yes or no answer is not possible, although, even when this strategy is employed, an adolescent who is determined to remain silent can frequently find two-word answers to even the most complex questions. On the other hand, the therapist may be too passive, hesitating to initiate action for fear that he has not fully understood the problem or patient. Perhaps the most useful guideline for reducing the probability of either error is to ask the patient his view when conceptualizing a problem or designing a task—to ask the patient whether the conceptualization seems realistic or whether the task appears feasible and reasonable.

In general, the degree of therapist activity/direction should be titrated against the patient's need for such direction. Early on in these therapies, a greater degree of directiveness is typical. Later, however, the patient will have acquired more understanding and familiarity with the techniques and approaches. Therefore, more patient and fewer therapist initiatives are to be expected during the latter phases of therapy. Indeed, when cognitive therapy is being practiced in its ideal form, whether the patient is an adolescent or an adult, the interchange typically sounds like a highly animated debate, with both participants contributing roughly equally to the interchange.

Many short-term directive therapies espouse particular techniques (e.g., thought stopping, cognitive reattribution, maintenance of schedules). The way these techniques are applied has implications for the alliance. Techniques may be misapplied in an impersonal, mechanical fashion, leaving the patient feeling uncared for. Alternatively, some therapists will prematurely switch from one technique to the next when the first appears ineffective. This strategy leads the patient to feel confused and frustrated, and confidence in the therapist may drop. On the other hand, dogged persistence with one technique that is clearly not helping can lead to similar feelings. Careful attention to these dangers, as well as continual dialogue with the patient about the therapist's reasons for persistence with or change of technique (and the patient's feelings about these events), is required.

Factors Derived from the Disorder

Let us turn to factors derived from the disorder itself that can impair the alliance. The contribution of personality difficulties that impair the formation of the alliance has already been mentioned. Where reality testing is impaired (e.g., with hallucinations or delusions) or where the patient is markedly suspicious, the therapist's directives may be confusing or misunderstood. In one study, Hole et al. (1979) attempted to modify schizophrenic delusions with direct cognitive techniques. These techniques exacerbated the delusions in some patients and led to marked hostility toward and suspiciousness of the therapist.

Where memory, concentration, or abstraction abilities are impaired, written instructions, telephone reminders, and a greater focus on specific, concrete, simple tasks and concepts are required. Within the session, a dialogue to summarize each step is often needed. Sometimes the therapist and patient need to create a written summary of the session. Depending on the developmental level of the adolescent and the nature of his particular relationships with parents or teachers, it is sometimes appropriate to ask another person to assist the patient in carrying out certain tasks. The therapist must constantly guard against jeopardizing the adolescent patient's sense of independence and desire for independent accomplishment; however, if these are not issues for the particular patient, the use of appropriate help for the seriously impaired, depressed adolescent may represent the bridge to the first concrete accomplishment and release from depressive symptoms.

Finally, not all disorders respond to short-term directive or even long-term nondirective approaches. Some depressions, perhaps those with endogenous or melancholic symptom features, may not respond at all or may respond only in part. The adolescent who has been sexually abused, either recently or earlier in childhood (see Chapter 11), is particularly likely to require additional treatment. The therapist must keep this fact in mind. When failure is encountered, the therapist should consider a revision in the treatment plan and even a new diagnostic evaluation.

SELECTED READINGS

Beck AT, Greenberg R: *Coping with Depression.* Philadelphia, Center for Cognitive Therapy, 1976.

Beck AT, Rush AJ, Shaw BF, Emery G: *Cognitive Therapy of Depression.* New York, Guilford Press, 1979.

Hole R, Rush AJ, Beck AT: Cognitive change methods with delusional patients. *Psychiatry* 1979; 42:312–319.

Lewinsohn PM, Sullivan JM, Grosscup SJ: Behavioral therapy: Clinical applications, in *Short-Term Psychotherapies for Depression.* Edited by Rush AJ. New York, Guilford Press, 1982.

Rounsaville BJ, Chevron E: Interpersonal psychotherapy: Clinical applications, in *Short-Term Psychotherapies for Depression.* Edited by Rush AJ. New York, Guilford Press, 1982.

Rush AJ: Psychotherapy of the affective psychoses. *American Journal of Psychoanalysis* 1980; 40:99–123.

Zaiden J: Psychodynamic therapy: Clinical applications, in *Short-Term Psychotherapies for Depression.* Edited by Rush AJ. New York, Guilford Press, 1982.

CHAPTER SIX

Family Involvement in the Adolescent's Cognitive Therapy

T. C. R. WILKES

GAYLE BELSHER

INTRODUCTION

A teenager does not exist in isolation but is actively engaged in several different social domains, including the family, the peer group, the school, and the community. Of these, the family is the primal group through which the adolescent is socialized into the currently accepted values and behaviors of society. Each family has its own unique story, mythology, or script that differentiates it from other families and sets certain expectations regarding the behavior of its members. Families are frequently unaware of this set of rules, paradigms, or schemas; they are like the silent assumptions of the individual. Although families are often too busy experiencing life to stop and think about the idiosyncratic sets of rules by which they function, it is this implicit governing paradigm that allows families to focus on problems, often solving them quickly and successfully. Without such a structure, the family would be in crisis and a new paradigm would eventually develop to replace the old one. But existing paradigms can cause families to ignore alternative solutions to problems in the name of efficiency or tradition. Furthermore, thinking about and articulating an existing nonfunctional paradigm in order to create a new more functional one may require more energy than a family is willing to expend. Because the family's paradigms may be the single most important contributing factor to a teenager's view of himself, the world, and the future, this chapter focuses on the family and its involvement in the treatment of adolescent depression.

GENERAL GUIDELINES FOR FAMILY INVOLVEMENT

Many people assume that cognitive therapy is synonymous with individual therapy. However, because the family provides an important context in which to view the adolescent patient, cognitive therapy with a depressed teenager should nearly always include family members. Decisions about which people to include and how often they should be involved will depend on factors specific to each case. Two of the most important considerations are the functioning and structure of the depressed adolescent's family unit. The role of family members, as well as the implications of family function and structure for cognitive therapy, are discussed below.

The Role of Family Members in Therapy

It is important to involve family members in the adolescent's initial assessment and to consult with them regarding treatment because families are an important source of emotional support and can help to confirm or refute the adolescent's perspective on his current difficulties. The family can also be an invaluable asset in operationalizing the adolescent's temperament or personality, which may be the focus of discussion at various times during therapy. Parents are overt or covert participants in therapy throughout the treatment process because they represent the source of many dysfunctional beliefs the adolescent may be harboring and can aid implementation of solutions to problems. Parents may even become "cotherapists" later in therapy when logical analysis is applied to the adolescent's dysfunctional beliefs and/or when homework activities are defined.

It is vitally important to include family members when the diagnosis of depression has an associated comorbidity such as attention-deficit hyperactivity disorder, schizoid personality disorder, or pervasive developmental disorder. In these cases, parents need education about the comorbid diagnoses as well as the depression to assist in setting appropriate expectations for the adolescent. When significant comorbidity exists, the scheduling of family sessions may occur on a much more regular basis than would be the case for a depressed adolescent without the additional psychiatric diagnoses. For adolescents with attention deficits, the therapist often relies on parents as "surrogate frontal lobes," and parents become an essential aid to solving problems and maintaining objectivity.

With respect to the adolescent's family, the cognitive therapist usually must decide "when," not "if," their involvement in therapy is appropriate. The frequency with which family members are included in the adolescent's therapy is not intended to reflect any etiological bias toward "individual" or "family" explanations for the depression. Rather, family involvement represents a pragmatic approach to therapy, allowing the therapist to maintain an accurate view of the adolescent within the relevant environmental context. The cognitive therapist transcends the issue of choosing between family and individual interventions by adopting the position that depression is a phenomenon with biopsychosocial contributors, all of which will be considered carefully and addressed where helpful.

Family Function in Relation to Therapy

Knowledge of family function is essential in conceptualizing the treatment plan for any teenager (Epstein and Bishop, 1981; Minuchin, 1974). It is important for the therapist to remember that families represent living systems with their own characteristic properties. One property that applies to the family is homeostasis, the tendency to maintain a steady state through negative or positive feedback. Extreme reciprocity among the family's component parts may make it almost impossible for family members to effect change in their system or to place themselves outside the family system. A second important characteristic is that the family represents a superordinate level of abstraction, different from one individual's or even the sum of all individuals' difficulties and strengths (Tomm, 1984). As such, the family has power to exert influence that is much greater than the sum of its individual members' effects. Similar to the difference in power between one soldier and a platoon, the family group can achieve objectives that one member could not. Agents of change exist in a hierarchy of logical types: the individual, the family, the community, the country, the continent, the world. To address one as if it were the other usually results in confusion and chaos.

The fact that a family is a homeostatic system of a higher order of magnitude than any individual has clear implications for treatment of the depressed adolescent. Consider, for example, a depressed adolescent who has an active perfectionistic schema. Because this schema is often generated and supported by the family's belief system, family members will tend to undermine the therapist's work with the adolescent unless they are invited to participate in a cost–benefit analysis of their existing schemas. Only by involving family members in the adolescent's therapy may they adjust their expectations, perceptions, and values from those consistent with a "product-oriented" thinking style to those characteristic of a more "process-oriented" thinking style (Burns, 1980). Such a shift in family values would accommodate the belief that "you should try your best and pursue excellence," while it introduces greater perspective with the caveat that "the pursuit of excellence is as important as the product."

In addition to producing cognitive change, family involvement in therapy often facilitates behavioral change in the depressed adolescent. When faced with a seemingly impossible task, which demands more resources than the individual adolescent has available, he may succeed only by using the composite resources and help of the entire family. For example, many adolescents are stimulus-dependent, unable to focus on tasks independently. Family members can facilitate more time on task and faster completion of tasks by applying their greater resources in this domain.

Family Structure in Relation to Therapy

Family structure refers not only to the cohabiting members of one family unit but also to the families of origin of the adolescent's parents (Minuchin and Fishman, 1981). Grandparents are often active participants in families, particularly in those that include small children. Grandparents may contribute greatly to the smooth running of a family by helping its members to meet their basic needs including shelter, food, and income. They may also be involved in affective struggles as couples separate from their respective families of origin and establish new sets of rules or paradigms for regulating such issues as intimacy, violence, sex, religion, or family economics. The paradigms with which grandparents operated often become counterpoints for the new beliefs held by the next generation of families. Thus, although grandparents and an adolescent's immediate family may live in separate residences, the influence of grandparents' beliefs, expectations, and values on the younger family tends to be extensive. Often, grandparents' standards become the "gold standards" by which new generations of families measure their own performance. The cognitive therapist must remain cognizant of family structure and the potential influence of the previous generation, inviting significant grandparents to treatment sessions, if necessary, during times of major paradigm shift in the adolescent's immediate family.

Indeed, in spite of being powerful family members who influence the establishment of a belief system, sometimes grandparents are more likely than the adolescent's own parents to see that a change in family beliefs is necessary. As such, grandparents can be good allies for the therapist, assisting parents with logical analysis of anachronistic values. In addition, grandparents can be good parental allies, helping to control the behavior of depressed adolescents who have the comorbid diagnosis of attention-deficit hyperactivity disorder.

Because grandparents often have the power to exert significant influence, they can also potentially hinder rather than help implementation of treatment recommendations. For example, some grandparents may demonstrate considerable resistance to the use of medication in conjunction with psychotherapy, as might be recommended for a depressed hyperactive adolescent. If grandparents are actively involved in the adolescent's family, the therapist must include them in discussions about treatment planning lest they, either alone or in alliance with a subgroup of the family or the adolescent himself, mount a significant campaign of resistance to therapeutic intervention.

Later in the family's life cycle, grandparents or other relatives who have become ill or otherwise dependent may be living in the same house as the adolescent and his parents. With three generations cohabiting, any conflict between the rules or expectations of the two older generations may become more obvious, for example, the grandparent offending the parents by upholding a rigid and conservative stance regarding an adolescent's privileges. It is essential that the cognitive therapist note family structure because it influences the family rules and expectations that guide the adolescent's behavior. Family structure may also help to define limitations of the adolescent's role in shaping the family paradigm.

An increasingly common phenomenon in North America and the United Kingdom is the single-parent family. Some adolescents perceive this type of family structure as an opportunity to gain a sense of mastery and as a factor to facilitate their independence. Others view it as a threat or a sign of deprivation and restricted opportunity. They may perceive the necessity of becoming involved in the day-to-day chores of the household as unfair and unjust, thinking, "Kids should have parents to do these sorts of things for them." The adolescent's viewpoint depends on the set of beliefs or rules he has adopted. On the other side of the generation gap, the adult in a single-parent family will often struggle just to maintain the family unit, using coercion, negotiation, or sacrifice depending on which strategy best achieves the family's instrumental tasks.

When working with single-parent families, the therapist often finds the missing parent is absent in body only. This parent's expectations, intentions, and interests often are keenly experienced by the adolescent as well as the remaining parent. In cases where the adolescent's depression appears to be associated with the behavior of the absent parent, it is important, and sometimes vital, to test this assumption by including the absent parent in therapy, after seeking permission from the custodial parent. Sometimes it may become necessary to meet with only the separated parents in order to develop a joint parenting plan for containing the adolescent's depression. In some cases, the absent parent may be recruited by the adolescent as a coconspirator against the custodial parent who is trying to enforce some rules. This kind of triangulation needs to be avoided by clearly identifying responsibility for and ownership of the problem. In yet other cases, the absent parent may desire inappropriate involvement in therapy in an attempt to reinstate the marital relationship, again a situation to be avoided. Finally, there are situations in which the absent parent is living away from the family because of an alcohol problem or history of inappropriate sexual behavior. In such cases, the absent parent should be included in therapy only if there are clearly defined advantages for the overall treatment plan.

The Interrelationship of Family Structure and Function

Family structure and function are often related and must be considered jointly when one chooses therapeutic interventions (Haley, 1971). Consider, for example, a family of four that consists of two parents and two adolescents living in the same residence. The goal of the family is, of course, to ensure adequate environmental support for appropriate growth and development of all its members. A therapist might assume that the goal of economic maintenance of the family would be achieved by the parental subsystem. However, the male adolescent may be working and providing not only valuable economic support to the family but also vital nurturing and emotional support for an alcoholic father. Similarly, the female adolescent may be providing most of the nurturing and emotional support in a reverse parenting arrangement with her depressed mother. To avoid disruptive interventions that are based on the therapist's own ethical judgment on how a family should function, the therapist must assess carefully the role of different family members in day-to-day functioning in areas as diverse as economic and emotional support.

Before making any therapeutic interventions, the cognitive therapist should remind himself that the depressed adolescent is subject to influence both as an individual and as a member of the family group (Bandura, 1978). The therapist should consider the potential impact of a particular intervention on both the individual and the family because interventions that threaten family function or structure may cause the family to activate homeostatic mechanisms that will serve to maintain the status quo. As an illustration, consider a 17-year-old boy who was the eldest of three children. He presented with depression 4 months after a motorcycle accident. During therapy, the adolescent revealed that the "accident" was not accidental; it was his solution to a "no win" situation. He had a particular gift for academics, but his family was having difficulty making the family business succeed, so he was expected to graduate from school and then join his parents in their business endeavor. He had hoped that after the accident somebody would realize his dilemma and understand that he would rather die than choose between his family and a career of his own. Therapy had to proceed carefully, exploring the family structure and function. In particular, the therapist focused on the parents' expectations of their eldest son concerning the family business. A cost–benefit analysis of their beliefs helped them to consider alternatives in a nonthreatening way. This discussion necessitated the inclusion of all family members, including the patient's two younger siblings, as they might have been expected to take on his role if he chose a career other than the family business.

Flexibility in the family's definition of roles and generational boundaries is essential to ensure appropriate growth and development of children from infancy through adolescence to eventual adult maturity. Developmental issues vary between early and late adolescence. In particular, late adolescence involves highly personalized decisions regarding issues such as age-appropriate independence, responsibility, separation from parents, and selection of a career or sexual partners. Families often experience considerable conflict over the timing and appropriateness of these choices. Such conflict may heighten parents' awareness that their children no longer "need" them in the same ways as when they were younger and that the parental role is changed forever. For some parents, this realization is associated with the development of depression and the "empty nest" phenomenon when the youngest child of a family leaves or is preparing to leave home. Alternatively, for blended families or foster parents, the independence and separation of the adolescent from the family may be viewed as an opportunity for the new family to consolidate without the added complication of a child from a former relationship. Here, adolescents may perceive the parents as "letting go" too easily, leaving them before they have time to leave their parents. Such themes demonstrate the importance of realizing that the adolescent is part of a family system and that one part of the family cannot fully be understood in isolation from the other parts. Indeed, the structure and idiosyncratic functioning of each family make critical contributions to the behavioral, cognitive, and emotional repertoire of family members and to the movement of the each individual along the paths of life.

COMMON THERAPEUTIC PROBLEMS WITH FAMILIES

Therapists treating depressed adolescents face two common classes of problems: hidden agendas and social control. Hidden agendas refer to the parents' or the adolescent's unspoken reasons for seeking therapy, including the presence of serious parental psychopathology, marital dysfunction, or child-custody disputes. Problems concerning social control arise when the parents or the adolescent is involved in a conflictual relationship with the child-welfare service or the police regarding such issues as drug use or promiscuity, for example.

The Adolescent's Hidden Agendas

In some cases, the depressed adolescent may agree to seek help for his depression primarily because he wants to draw professional attention to serious parental psychopathology or family problems. This situation may present as an urgent request by the family itself or by the general practitioner for assistance in treating the depressed or acting-out teenager. However, arranging an appointment with the adolescent's family may become a major task, ostensibly because one or another parent is always out of town or busy with work or with some other commitment. Parents may even engage in behaviors such as dropping the adolescent off for treatment sessions while they go shopping. This logistic difficulty suggests that the family does not wish to be involved or inconvenienced by the adolescent's therapy, and it presents a major problem for the therapist who needs to confirm that the adolescent is indeed depressed. It also introduces a significant obstacle in trying to identify the meaning of the adolescent's depression for the family and how its members might be able to help the adolescent. Such families can be very effective at forcing the therapist to keep a narrow view of the problem and continue treating the adolescent in isolation. If therapy proceeds without family involvement, there may be some initial improvement before a plateau is reached and the therapist feels "stuck." Eventually the therapist may feel completely isolated or even despairing. This scenario often reflects the adolescent's dilemma, the core issue of which will have been experienced by the therapist who wants to effect change but cannot in the absence of parental willingness to participate in achieving the goal.

Management of cases that present with hidden agendas requires great energy and determination on the part of the therapist. In order to mobilize the family, it is often useful to employ questions such as "Will you help me treat your son's depression?" or "Is it possible that your son is protecting you by being depressed?" or "Is this family so busy that the only way your son can get your attention is to be sick or attempt suicide?" Asking questions like these will usually capture enough of the parents' attention to achieve at least one family session during which the therapist often learns that the adolescent's depression is only part of the psychopathology in a very troubled family. The adolescent may be unable to openly verbalize concerns about family problems but silently hopes that the family will be invited to participate in treatment and that the professionals will ask "the right questions" or do "the right thing" to make life better. By using Socratic dialogue to operationalize the problem of depression and explore what makes it better or worse, the therapist helps to uncover terrible dilemmas that the adolescent may be facing. Sometimes sexual or physical abuse is disclosed. Questions such as the following may be useful in revealing the adolescent's hidden agenda: "What goals or priorities is this family working on at this moment?" "Where does this family want to be in 5 years, and who will be doing things differently then?" "Does anyone else know what it is like to be as depressed as your son?" "Does anyone have a theory about the cause of his depression?" "Are you expecting your son to cope the same way you coped . . . by ignoring things?" Questions may uncover hidden feelings of guilt or depression in family members other than the adolescent.

If the therapist becomes aware of an adolescent's hidden agenda to gain help for his parents or family, he must avoid being seduced into treating only the parents, forgetting about the adolescent's depression. Occasionally, it is appropriate to treat the parents, but more often it is best to explore parental problems in the context of a family session and later refer the parents to another treatment agency. The therapist must remember that the adolescent did present with depression, and careful monitoring of his continued well-being is essential. Whenever parental or family problems are revealed, therapists should ask themselves,

"What relevance does this issue have for the adolescent's depression?" By focusing on the adolescent's depression, the therapist gains license to address personal issues within the family or the marital dyad with less likelihood of antagonizing defensive parents.

The following case example demonstrates how treatment of an adolescent's depression can unmask one type of hidden agenda, which is to acquire treatment for one or both parents. Stacey was a 15-year-old girl, the oldest of three siblings living with two parents. During the initial assessment, it was revealed that her mother was an alcoholic and her father was being treated for cancer. Stacey's parents appeared to be engaging in considerable denial regarding their own problems and felt ashamed that their daughter was depressed. They seemed to wish that Stacey could deny her own frustrations and disappointments, much as they were doing. Stacey, however, was deeply concerned about her father's increasing social isolation and her mother's increasing alcohol intake. It was apparent that Stacey's desire to fix her parents, whom she had effectively "lost," and her sense of hopelessness in accomplishing this task were major factors contributing to her depression. When the problems of her parents were identified during therapy, Stacey made a rapid recovery, returning to her former emotional health within a month. In spite of her recovery, the family continued to see the therapist for several months and focused on finding solutions for the many parental problems that were affecting the family. This strategy helped Stacey to clarify the limits of her parents' and her own responsibilities, thus further alleviating her sense of helplessness.

A second type of hidden agenda for some adolescents is the desire to gain a coconspirator who will help to defend their wishes or points of view against those of a domineering parent. For example, Leslie was a 17-year-old girl in a family of four. Her father was a professional man with severe obsessive–compulsive personality traits and many perfectionistic expectations for all of the family members. His perfectionism caused considerable marital conflict, and the constant tension at home was terrible. Leslie and her younger brother had increasingly withdrawn to their bedrooms to avoid witnessing the conflict between their parents. Leslie's father was angered because she did not pursue his perfectionistic style, which was manifest in his consuming concern for productivity and success in the acquisition of material possessions. Her father's overbearing view jeopardized expression of her own beliefs so seriously that she presented a mask to her parents, denying her own thoughts and feelings at home. However, when Leslie encountered the support of her school counselor, she revealed severe depression and suicidal ideation. The school counselor brought Leslie's depression to the attention of her parents, who were ashamed and angered that their child would be depressed. They claimed to provide everything she could want. A family meeting was eventually scheduled after much persistence by the therapist. It was clear that Leslie's parents were emotionally divorced from each other, although legally still married. They revealed that a marital separation was imminent, but they had planned to wait until Leslie had graduated from high school. Leslie's father's demands for perfectionism were identified as a major factor in both the marital conflict and in Leslie's depression. His obsession with materialistic gain was identified as a significant obstacle to spending time with his children or wife. By seeking help from her school counselor and the therapist, Leslie had acquired a surrogate voice with which to challenge her father's rigid belief system and domineering personality.

A third type of hidden agenda for some depressed adolescents is the desire for help with problems that have arisen in relation to their secret lifestyle. Invariably the "secret" involves sex and/or drugs. The sexual problems may range from deviant masturbation behaviors to frank prostitution. Alternatively, there may be fears of contracting AIDS as a result of homosexual behaviors or sexual experiences with known intravenous drug users. If the adolescent has been involved in prostitution, there may be a history of sexual abuse, sexual assault, or extreme coercion from a dominant delinquent peer group. Depressed adolescents with such histories often have significant comorbidity such as posttraumatic stress disorder. They may also have families that endure a chronic chaotic lifestyle with blurring of boundaries and inappropriate regulation of intimacy.

Adolescents with secrets often do not reveal them unless therapists ask the right questions and demonstrate that they will assist the formation of a working alliance, even though the adolescent initially may be angry and distancing. One effective strategy to employ during the initial session is to invite the adolescent to "paint a picture" with words, actions, or drawings that illustrates the kind of life he is leading. In addition, the adolescent's personal journal, poems, or other writings can be rich sources of clues to hidden lifestyles. When family members are present, the therapist must design the session so that part of the time at the beginning or end will be reserved for the adolescent alone, to allow appropriate disclosure. The importance of time with the individual patient is paramount when dealing with adolescents who have the comorbid diagnoses of attention-deficit hyperactivity disorder, pervasive developmental disorder, schizoid personality disorder, posttraumatic stress disorder, or conduct disorder.

A fourth type of hidden agenda for some adolescents is their unspoken intent to acquire the therapist as an ally in order to coerce their parents into meeting various demands. Adolescents may claim that their depressive symptoms or suicide attempts should convince parents to lift all restrictions or relieve them of all responsibilities. In these cases, the involvement of family members is essential. Even if some parental compromise is granted, the therapist should stress that, just because the adolescent is depressed, it is not reasonable to excuse all responsibilities or accountability for his behavior. In short, parents are advised not to be held hostage or terrorized.

The Parents' Hidden Agendas

When treating depressed adolescents from single-parent families, the therapist may encounter a variety of parental hidden agendas. One of the most difficult is the nonverbalized intent of a single parent to gain professional support for some aspect of a child-custody or maintenance dispute. For example, the hidden agenda may relate to the amount of time or money that the absent spouse contributes to the parenting of the depressed adolescent. Clues to hidden agendas of this nature are statements such as "John's depression seems to be worse ever since his father left," or "If only his father could provide more financial support and pay the school fees." In such cases, the therapist must exercise great caution to avoid triangulating the adolescent in the parents' disagreements. The therapist can avoid this problem by clarifying the arrangements and responsibilities for parenting, paying particular attention to which parent provides the placement on weekends and holidays. If the parental agreement is unclear, an appointment scheduled with only the adolescent's parents may be indicated, particularly if the lack of clarity is perceived by the depressed adolescent as a sign of rejection or lack of personal worth. Whenever parents are invited to sessions and whatever the issues are, it is essential that the relevance of the discussion to the adolescent's depression be clear for all parties.

When issues concerning the absent parent arise in therapy with singleparent families, the therapist must realize that each spousal party will have his or her own reactions to the loss and the major life transitions that follow a marital separation (Bowlby, 1984; Guidano and Liotti, 1983). Thus, a second hidden agenda of single parents may be their attempt to gain treatment for their own adjustment disorders under the guise of seeking treatment for the adolescent's depression.

A third hidden agenda common with single-parent families is the desire to conscript the therapist to fill the "gap" left by the absent parent. If this motivation is suspected, the therapist must clarify parental expectations tactfully and redirect the parent to more appropriate resources such as Uncles at Large, Aunts at Large, Big Brother, or a variety of agencies that provide community youth workers.

Sometimes parents involved in highly conflictual relationships with acting-out adolescents seek therapy for their teenager's depression with a hidden agenda concerning implementation of a desired resolution to the behavior problems. In some cases, parents may have decided that they cannot continue to live in the same home as their adolescent and seek treatment for the adolescent's depression as the first step in gaining access to an inpatient treatment program or a custody placement through child welfare. Again, the therapist must remain sensitive to these potential issues, clarifying unspoken motivations so that frank discussions can ensue.

Finally, it should be remembered that parents, as well as the adolescent, have pride that occasionally inhibits their ability to admit their marital or personal problems. The parents' hidden agenda in seeking treatment for the depressed adolescent may be to get involved in family therapy themselves as an indirect way of addressing their own difficulties.

Problems of Social Control

Depressed adolescents may present with antisocial behaviors such as promiscuity, stealing, drug abuse, or vandalism. When such behaviors are sufficiently numerous and frequent, the diagnosis of conduct disorder, in addition to depression, is warranted. When therapists discover a history of behavior problems in adolescents who have had multiple foster-home placements, the adolescent's depression may be associated with self-injurious behaviors and represent part of a disturbed personality warranting the additional diagnosis of borderline personality disorder. The antisocial behaviors of adolescents may cause considerable perturbation in their families and the community, so much so that the therapist may be urged to contain troublesome adolescents with outpatient or inpatient psychotherapy. Parents may even attempt to use threats of seeing a therapist as a means to control their adolescent's behavior with statements such as "If you stay out late again, you will have to see the psychiatrist." For some families, the diagnosis of depression is viewed as a fortunate circumstance because it can then be labeled the cause of the adolescent's behavior problems, which parents mistakenly assume will vanish when the depression is treated. However, this is a dangerous position for any professional to take because no therapist can be responsible for an adolescent's behavior. Much to the disappointment of many parents, they are ultimately the ones legally accountable to the community if the adolescent's irresponsible behavior continues, even if it is in the context of a psychotic illness.

Although an adolescent in trouble with the law may indeed be depressed or worried, the therapist should realize that the adolescent's emotional distress may stem primarily from concern about the consequences of his antisocial behaviors. Some adolescents are astute enough to recognize the possibility of psychotherapy as a "soft option" and readily endorse the symptoms necessary for a diagnosis of depression in order to defer legal action. When a "con" of this sort is suspected, the therapist should test this hypothesis by inquiring about the symptoms of depression and about previous episodes of depression, not only with the adolescent but also with family members, school counselors, and significant others. Even if a bona fide episode of depression is diagnosed, mental health workers need not be paternalistic and should not substitute treatment for punishment. The two can coexist nicely, communicating to the adolescent some important lessons about accountability and mutual respect. Therapists may find it particularly challenging to instill a sense of respect for others in cases in which the depressed adolescent has a comorbid diagnosis of conduct disorder because these patients sometimes view compassion and understanding as a sign of weakness and fear. Careful exploration of the adolescent's belief system and persistence in addressing maladaptive cognitions will be required in such cases.

Some parents may seek therapy for their adolescent in an attempt to bypass the juvenile court system or the child-welfare system. Parents may wish to protect their adolescent who has serious behavioral problems, as if the teenager were an innocent 6-year-old, not the young adult he actually is. In such cases, it is important for the therapist to explore with the parents the consequences of continuing to accommodate their adolescent in this way. For example, the therapist might ask, "What will you do in 5 years' time if your adolescent has failed to learn the lessons of accountability and self-responsibility?" In other words, the therapist should pursue a cost–benefit analysis of the family's current parenting style, focusing on the future as well as the present point in time.

If parents are unable to provide effective parenting to contain their adolescent's behavior, then residential placement outside the home may be appropriate, and the therapist should share this recommendation with the adolescent and his family. The requirement for placement occurs most frequently in chaotic, lower-socioeconomic-class families who have been involved with multiple agencies often because they have been "shopping around" for the expert who will agree with them. In these complicated families, the therapist must liaise actively with other agencies, establish appropriate and realistic expectations about therapy, and emphasize that, although the adolescent is depressed, people should still expect him to know the difference between right and wrong and hold him accountable for his actions. The therapist also must be aware that some adolescents may deliberately behave in such a way as to coerce authority figures to move them from one residence to another when they become bored with their current placement or do not want to assume responsibility for their behavior, an expectation levied after they are integrated into their new home. Some adolescents perceive the assumption of such responsibility as a loss of their specialness.

When treating adolescents who have been removed from the parental home, the therapist needs to clarify the goals of therapy with the adolescent, the family, and the different agencies involved. It is important to operationalize the meaning of "appropriate behavior" to help the family and the larger social service system perceive positive signs of the adolescent's growth so that they do not focus exclusively on the negative aspects of the adolescent's behavior. Contracting for therapy must be specific, for example, four or six sessions followed by a review to see if therapy is addressing the established goals. When contracting, it is important to anticipate missed sessions and the consequences of such. For example, it may be agreed that the adolescent can "fire" the therapist but must do so in person and in such a way that all other interested parties are informed of the decision.

With chaotic dysfunctional families, family involvement in the adolescent's therapy may be contraindicated. Sometimes separation of the adolescent from the family helps to minimize the adolescent's dependence on unreliable and/or damaging caretakers. This is particularly the case when adolescents are being physically or sexually abused in their family of origin. In other situations, parents may be frankly uninterested in pursuing anything other than a superficial contact with the therapist, adamantly stating their belief that the adolescent needs to be "fixed" but denying that the adolescent's problems are related in any way to themselves or to the family.

Application of Cognitive Therapy Techniques with Families

When dealing with problems of hidden agendas or social control, it is useful for the therapist to remember that the cognitive techniques used with individuals are also applicable with families and professional agencies. In particular, the development of an agenda, definition of problems, and identification of priorities are highly constructive strategies. Communication of the cognitive therapy model is central. Graded-task assignments may have dramatic results in some families. Wilkes and Rush (1988) discuss the application of the mastery and pleasure technique with enmeshed families to enhance an individual's sense of self-efficacy. The technique of pro–con analysis can assist adolescents who are removed from their homes to adopt realistic views about their new residential placements. The use of a cognitive continuum can help to challenge dichotomous thinking about a "good old home" versus a "new bad home," for example. During specific times of crisis with a depressed adolescent, eliciting the thoughts, emotions, and behaviors of family members or child care workers can help to decatastrophize a situation. Alternative perceptions of a crisis situation can be pursued through logical analysis, reframing, and the use of metaphors. Examples of these and other techniques are presented in Part III.

It should now be apparent that cognitive therapy need not be restricted to individuals but can be practiced with couples, with a family, or within an institution. Although the therapist may wish to hold private sessions with the adolescent when secrets are being discussed, it is essential to remember that the adolescent lives in a larger community and that the therapist's responsibility is to assist successful integration of the adolescent into the various systems that are superordinate to him. Efforts toward this integration are enhanced by using Socratic dialogue in respectful exploration of the adolescent's and others' beliefs.

SELECTED READINGS

Bandura A: The self system in reciprocal determinism. *American Psychologist* 1978; 33:344–358.
Bolwlby J: *The Making and Breaking of Affectional Bonds.* London, Tavistock, 1984.
Burns DD: *Feeling Good.* New York, William Morrow, 1980.
Epstein NB, Bishop DS: Problem-centered systems therapy of the family, in *Handbook of Family Therapy.* Edited by Gurman AS, Kniskern DP. New York, Brunner/Mazel, 1981.
Guidano VF, Liotti G: *Cognitive Processes and Emotional Disorders.* New York, Guilford Press, 1983.
Haley J: Approaches to family therapy, in *Changing Families.* Edited by Haley J. New York, Grune & Stratton, 1971.
Minuchin S: *Families and Family Therapy.* Cambridge, MA, Harvard University Press, 1974.

Minuchin S, Fishman C: *Family Therapy Techniques.* Cambridge, MA, Harvard University Press, 1981.

Tomm K: One perspective on the Milan systemic approach. *Journal of Marital and Family Therapy* 1984; 10:253–271.

Wilkes TCR, Rush AJ: Adaptations of cognitive therapy for depressed adolescents. *Journal of the American Academy of Child and Adolescent Psychiatry* 1988; 27:381–386.

PART III

Macrostages and Microtechniques in Therapy

CHAPTER SEVEN

The Initial Phase of Cognitive Therapy: From Assessment to Setting Goals

T. C. R. WILKES

GAYLE BELSHER

INTRODUCTION

The initial phase of therapy is crucial because it lays the foundation for several aspects of the work to follow. The number of sessions devoted to the initial phase may vary from patient to patient but, with all adolescents, it should include diagnosis and assessment of the problem, development of a cognitive case formulation, contracting, socialization into the cognitive model, and the establishment of goals and priorities. Each of these issues is discussed in the following subsections.

DIAGNOSIS AND ASSESSMENT

The diagnosis of depression is central to the process of developing a shared "world view" among the adolescent, the family, and the therapist (see Kendell, 1975). Although criterion variance continues to be an issue in adolescent psychiatry and the diagnosis of major depressive disorder in adolescents is less reliable than in adults, adolescent depression does have considerable construct validity. Furthermore, a depressive syndrome that has considerable content validity can be described to the family if assessment of the adolescent includes use of multiple diagnostic criteria such as those included in the Research Diagnostic Criteria (Spitzer et al., 1978), the *Diagnostic and Statistical Manual of Mental Disorders*, fourth edition (American Psychiatric Association, 1994), or the Weinberg criteria (Weinberg et al., 1973; Petti, 1978). If the parents have a history of depression, the predictive validity of the adolescent's diagnosis of depression may be enhanced, and such a history immediately helps to reframe the disobedient, rebellious behavior of some adolescents into a nonjudgmental phenomenon, "the depressive syndrome." Reference to a family history of depression also helps to demystify the diagnosis of depression and set the stage for parental involvement in therapy with the adolescent.

When discussing the diagnosis of depression, it is important to separate the adolescent from the disorder by asking a question such as "How long have you been fighting against the depression?" In this way, the diagnosis is not used as a dehumanizing and restrictive label but, rather, as a liberating experience because the name of a treatable illness is provided to the family. The adolescent is discussed as a victim of the depression, which can be "beat" with appropriate treatment. Questions used at this time can be empowering, for example, "Did you know that 90% of people who are treated for depression get better? What will be the first sign that you are getting back to your old self again?" This approach primes the adolescent to look for signs of improvement rather than signs of depression.

Once the crucial distinction between the "adolescent with depression" and the "depressed adolescent" is made, therapeutic work can begin immediately with the introduction of certain cognitive therapy constructs, such as how the depression affects the adolescent and the family. The therapist will want to ask, "What adjustments has the family made to accommodate the depression?" or "What steps have the family and the adolescent taken to beat the depression in the past?" and "When did the depression take over?" Such a Socratic dialogue emphasizes that the disorder is not a character flaw and that it can be treated successfully. This approach demonstrates the difference between primitive thinking and mature thinking, as illustrated in Beck et al. (1979).

Asking questions that imply that the disorder can be overcome is an intervention founded on the learned helplessness model of depression (Abramson et al., 1978). This model posits that, when individuals lack a perception of control over their lives, they may show signs of depression. In particular, Abramson and colleagues proposed that internal, stable, and global attributions for negative events contribute to one's perception of "helplessness" and depression. It is common for therapists to see this attributional style in depressed adolescents, who often perceive negative events as the result of some "permanent defect" in themselves that will "ruin their whole life." Such depressogenic attributions also reinforce the negative cognitive triad of the self, the world, and the future. Socratic dialogue is useful during the assessment phase of therapy in order to raise the possibility that the adolescent's views may not be the only ones possible. Instead, a "bad event" such as the diagnosis of depression can be perceived as a problem external to the adolescent that is likely to change in the near future.

COGNITIVE FORMULATION

The cognitive formulation is based on information derived from the initial assessment. It focuses on the adolescent's key automatic thoughts and "ideas about his own ideas," or the underlying assumptions and attitudes that appear central to the depressive syndrome. In essence, the formulation is a written explanation of the problem, highlighting cognitive factors that are hypothesized to play a role in the development and/or maintenance of the adolescent's depression. The formulation will, therefore, suggest priorities for treatment and guide the timing of interventions that may be vital to the success of therapy. For any individual patient, there is no single formulation; rather, the hypothesis changes constantly based on new information about recent developments in the adolescent's life.

Although the development of a cognitive formulation is an essential step in therapy, it is sometimes omitted by therapists, leading to subsequent therapeutic confusion. The formulation helps to clarify the therapeutic process by serving as a constant reminder that cognitive therapy is theory-driven and that new information must be related to theoretical constructs in order to best direct subsequent therapeutic interventions. Because of their age-appropriate dependency, adolescents are part of a complex social system to a greater extent than adults; and they are continually influenced by their interactions with the family, peers, and community, as well as by their own ideas. Change in one part of this system has subsequent effects on other parts of the system, which may hinder or promote cognitive, emotional, and behavioral adaptations. As such, the cognitive formulation should reflect the influence of the social system on the adolescent's views of himself, his world, and his future. It is vital that the therapist understand how the adolescent sees himself relating to his world, bearing in mind that his perception of this relationship will depend in part on his perceptions of himself and the world as somewhat separate entities. The following case vignette illustrates how a cognitive formulation might be developed from relevant information acquired during the assessment process.

Assessment Information: Fifteen-year-old Jessica presented with depression, a Children's Depression Inventory (CDI) rating of 47, and suicidal ideation. Some key cognitions that she verbalized were the beliefs that she was "no good," "unlovable," "ugly and fat," and "may as well die." Closer examination of her history revealed that she had been sexually abused at home and subsequently was separated from her family of origin. She had been relocated six times; her parents had separated, and her relationship with her mother had deteriorated to the point of frank rejection. Jessica stated that she anticipated future rejections from her peers and future homes. She reported that she perceived herself as unlovable and thought the world was rejecting and punishing her because of her role in the parental conflict.

Cognitive Formulation: Jessica's depression was apparently precipitated by her perceived rejection by her family of origin. Her belief that her family rejected her appeared to be based on another of her beliefs, that her sexual abuse caused her parents' marital difficulties and subsequent separation. As a result, Jessica felt guilty and worthless and had many self-deprecatory cognitions. Her five unsuccessful foster placements helped to confirm her belief that she was unwanted and doomed to experience a life of continued rejection. Her sense of isolation was perpetuated by her passivity, a symptom of the depression, and by her anger, a symptom of her repeated grief reactions. Jessica's isolation and anger, in turn, impaired her development of socialization skills. Her key assumptions seemed to be that she also was the cause of her family's breakup and that she was then and remains unlovable and unworthy. Her secondary assumption was that she could be happy if people loved her.

The formulation presented above is not the only one that could be written for Jessica. Although different therapists would develop slightly different formulations for a particular case, all of them should include a description of the way in which the adolescent perceives his life experiences and how these perceptions may contribute to an unrealistically negative view of himself, the world, and the future, or to a pervasive sense of helplessness.

The formulation of any case suggests multiple interventions at several levels, including the family, peer group, and/or individual. In Jessica's case, interventions at all of these levels were attempted. She was, of course, reluctant to join a therapeutic peer group and experienced a great deal of anticipatory anxiety associated with the belief that she would be "rejected" and considered "funny or odd." However, she did attend group therapy, where she was not rejected, and she even reported having a pleasant time. This positive experience served to illustrate the dysfunctional nature of her thoughts because her primary assumption about her "unlovability" had been examined through the process of collaborative empiricism.

Another example of a cognitive formulation is illustrated below.

Assessment Information: Fourteen-year-old John presented in a depressed state with self-destructive behavior. He had had a long history of being unsuccessful with his peer group at school. He also had a history of disruptive behavior in the home, and his parents often had to reprimand him. John's mother reported that he had always struggled with learning disabilities and poor physical coordination and that he had difficulty separating from her as a young child. His parents reported considerable anxiety because of their own problems, which they related to his father's proclivity for upholding perfectionistic standards. Some of John's key cognitions included "I hate school," "I'll never have friends," "I'm no good," and "Nothing works out."

Cognitive Formulation: John's beliefs about himself were probably central to his depression. He appeared to hold the conviction that his worth or "goodness" depended on good performance with his chores at home and on popularity with his peers at school. However, it was likely that John's learning disabilities and poor physical coordination in combination with his father's perfectionism resulted in repeated negative experiences of "failure" at home. Apparently, school has also been an experience in "failure" for John. His bids for popularity have lead him to attract attention by being silly or doing outrageous things, behaviors that seemed to have alienated people rather than have won their friendship. Currently, John's attitude about himself appeared to mirror that of the community and family toward him.

Based on the formulation above, one of the initial interventions that could be made would be to change John's environment by changing his school. This action would remove one precipitating factor, the persecution John experiences from his peer group. The family's perfectionism predisposed John to depression by setting inappropriately high expectations, which he had no way of meeting because of his learning difficulties. As such, the father's perfectionism could be confronted by reframing his dichotomous "competent versus incompetent" view of people as "happy versus depressed." A strategy that would not be recommended would be to challenge John's negative self-statements without the family's involvement. This is because John is a dependent person in a larger contextual environment that continually provides negative feedback, so challenge in such a way would be unlikely to effect any major change outside of the clinic office.

It is important to realize that the initial formulation is not intended to be the "absolute truth." It is merely a provisional reflection of some of the key factors that are operating in the patient's cognitive domain. However, by writing a formulation, the cognitive therapist is better able to determine the point at which interventions will be most likely to achieve change or relief from the depression. The therapist must always remain aware of the dynamic interplay between a patient's knowledge of the self and his knowledge about others. This so-called "looking glass effect" was put simply by Popper and Eccles (1977), who stated, "Just as we learn to see ourselves in the mirror, so the child becomes conscious of himself by seeing his reflection in the mirror of other people's consciousness of himself."

Development of a cognitive formulation provides an eloquent way of exploring the diagnosis of depression. The negative cognitive triad can be used to illustrate how an individual's negative view of himself, his world, and the future tends to result in the avoidance of social contact, the consideration of suicide, and the general feeling of inadequacy, for example. In short, the four D's of depression—desertion, deprivation, defeat, and a sense of being defective (Beck, 1976)—are acknowledged and then identified within the framework of the adolescent's cognitive domain. Similarly, the cognitive errors seen in depression can help to explain the depressed adolescent's acute sensitivity to parental comments, which are especially likely to be perceived as criticism. A formulation can also help to explain the relationship between maladaptive cognitions and behaviors. For example, as high school graduation nears, final exams and the impending separation from friends or favorite locations may lead to cognitions such as "I'm dumb," or "I'm stupid," or "I'll never have another friend again," or "I never have a good time." These cognitions, in turn, might result in negative behaviors such as running away, passivity, and irritability.

The cognitive formulation often includes mention of dysfunctional family beliefs and assumptions. However, where discussion with the family is concerned, it is often helpful to use Socratic dialogue to operationalize dysfunctional "rules" that may predispose to depression, rather than to discuss dysfunctional "beliefs" or "assumptions" per se. Examples of perfectionism, intense ambition, and competitiveness are often quite evident in the families of depressed adolescents. With family members, it is also important to emphasize that depression is a complex phenomenon that has biological as well as psychological contributors. No single influence predominates; instead, all are considered important and reciprocally connected in a complex ecological system.

CONTRACTING

Contracting can occur only when the family, the adolescent patient, and the therapist have achieved at least a partially shared "world view" of the problem. Indeed, failure to reach this consensus will often undermine therapy as competing agendas surface later. For example, the parents' or therapist's ideas about the underlying cause of the depression may be competing with different ideas held by the adolescent or other family members. Such a lack of consensus can result in therapeutic sabotage, either by the parents or by the adolescent himself. To avoid this possibility, the therapist sometimes will need to spend considerable time exploring multiple perceptions of the problem. In addition, the therapist must be able to answer the question "How do the adolescent's and the family's perceptions differ from the therapist's own perception of the problem?" This is a key consideration because resolution of contradiction in the "story" or "explanation" of the depression can lead to immense cognitive, behavioral, and emotional change in a very short time.

As a consensus definition of the depression is developed, the therapist begins to relate the adolescent's problem to an agreement for therapy. The contract for therapy must, of course, address the problem by specifying expectations about the number of sessions, the role of the family in helping the therapist, and the importance of regular review sessions. This information would usually be communicated to the family within the first session.

Intervals between sessions may vary tremendously, depending on the severity of the depression and the degree of family support. For example, severely depressed adolescents requiring hospitalization, or those with limited family support and moderate depression, can often make excellent progress with one session every 1–2 weeks. As the symptoms become less intense and the homework tasks more complicated (thus requiring more time to complete), intervals between sessions may be as long as 4–6 weeks, depending, of course, on the degree of family support.

SOCIALIZATION

Socialization involves communicating the diagnosis of depression and the cognitive therapy model to the adolescent and his family. As such, socialization into therapy really begins during the assessment phase; by the time contracting is completed, a collaborative relationship should be well established.

Socialization requires consideration of the adolescent's cognitive and behavioral assets as well as his liabilities. An adolescent's level of cognitive development determines how he processes information. For a patient who has developed formal thinking skills, the traditional way of explaining the cognitive model of emotional disorders will pose no difficulty. However, many adolescents will still be operating with concrete or preoperational thinking skills and will find it difficult to "think about their thinking." In clinical practice, it is evident that many adolescents are not thinking much about anything; they appear to be impulsive and, in fact, may be relatively deficient of the cognitive errors found in their adult patient counterparts. This lack of formal thinking and deficit in cognitive skill often result in an adolescent's difficulty identifying the consequences of his actions and considering how other people may feel.

For impulsive, "nonthinking" adolescents, the therapist's exploration of mood shifts and automatic thoughts is often not appreciated, meaningful, or even helpful. Instead, the adolescent without formal thinking skills may respond better to the operationalizing of a belief or assumption. In practice, "operationalizing a belief" translates to (1) identifying the rules or assumptions operating in the family or individual patient and (2) exploring the effect of these rules or assumptions on the adolescent and other family members. For example, an adolescent may have been identified as a "klutz" or a "rebel" in the family. Using Socratic dialogue, the therapist and patient would explore the observable or "measurable" effect of these constructs. The process of defining the meaning of a particular construct in observable terms facilitates challenge of cognitive distortions. Considering the "klutz" or "rebel" mentioned above, would the family ever see the "good" side of the adolescent—the "conformer" or the "perfectionist"? Or would family members insist on seeing only evidence to support the negative constructs? This tactical approach illustrates the cognitive model by example and may be more appropriate for an adolescent who lacks formal thinking skills than the more abstract approach used with adult patients. As cognitive distortions are made apparent through a Socratic questioning process, the adolescent's family members become more aware of their own assumptions and expectations, and how they are reciprocated.

June was a 16-year-old adolescent living in a large blended family of five children. She presented with depression, school failure, and verbal conflict with her father. She was accused of being lazy, irresponsible, and moody. Through careful questioning by the therapist, however, the family was encouraged to describe aspects of their daughter's behavior that contradicted their negative views. For example, the family reported that June often helped her mother with the younger children and that she also helped with the shopping. In fact, she was so good at finding bargains at the supermarket that she often saved the family money. When June's father praised her or spent more time with her, she became withdrawn, upset, or confused. In response to the therapist's questions about her behavior with her father, June revealed her concern that her father did not like the other children as much as he liked her. She felt that she was depriving them of time with their father. To correct the situation as she saw it, June tried to be nice to her sisters and brothers by helping her mother do things for them. But she was so helpful that she became intrusive, and her behavior often resulted in arguments or the withdrawal of family members. As the interview unfolded, it became apparent that everyone had different perceptions of June's depression. Through Socratic dialogue, the problem of June's depression and the initial focus on her lazy, irresponsible behavior changed to a focus on how the family could regulate the father's involvement with the other children and help June rediscover the "good side" of herself.

Another method of socialization into the cognitive therapy model uses metaphors and stories. For example, the power of thought and belief is illustrated implicitly in a children's story, *The Emperor's New Clothes*. Another story, *The Ugly Duckling*, illustrates how personal thoughts and beliefs may painfully misrepresent reality and color future expectations. It also illustrates an important point in problem resolution, the role of second-order change superseding first-order change, or "reframing." One of the main differences between novice and experienced cognitive therapists is the ability to use the power of the metaphor and reframing. Because adolescents, more than adults, will have difficulty with abstract concepts such as "thoughts" and "beliefs," it is fortunate that they often find communication in metaphor to be easy and fun. Teachers have long capitalized on the pedagogical aspect of stories, and therapists, likewise, must welcome the opportunity to use stories if the adolescent presents them. Similarly, adolescents and children will frequently act out their emotional dilemmas through play, allowing the therapist to infer how their cognitive domain is constructed. By observing how an adolescent interacts with his family and how the family responds, the therapist can collaboratively examine the assumptions underlying the family's behavior and then encourage the family to experience new, helpful, and more realistic cognitions.

The therapist must listen carefully for opportunities to introduce discussion that will help socialize the adolescent or family members into the cognitive therapy model. The therapy excerpts presented below demonstrate the socialization process with adolescents of various ages and cognitive developmental levels.

Example 1

The following example concerns a 16-year-old female adolescent who presented for outpatient therapy approximately a month after being discharged from an inpatient adolescent psychiatry program. The discussion occurred toward the end of the first session with her. Note that the therapist used the patient's vague reference to her own thinking as the stimulus for "socialization" dialogue.

   T: Can you say what you think you might like to accomplish with me?
   P: Haven't really thought about it. I don't know.
   T: You haven't gotten that far yet?
   P: No. And I sort of think this month gave me enough time to push everything aside again.
   T: Do you think you're feeling better now than you were a month ago?
   P: A bit.
   T: Well maybe we can work on strengthening the things you've learned to do to make yourself feel better. Does that sound like something you might want to pursue here?
   P: Well, just the way I can deal with my. . . . (*silence*)
   T: The sadness? Or with what?
   P: Just with my . . . with whatever's going on with me inside. When I take a different mind and action . . . just so I know what to do if I was in a situation.
   T: What kind of situation?
   P: Learning how to deal with my thoughts . . . and all that.
   T: Your thoughts hurt you quite a bit?
   P: A bit.
   T: Thoughts make you sad?
   P: Uh huh.

T: Angry?

P: Uh huh.

T: Well, I'd like to work with you on dealing with your thoughts if that's one of the goals that you have. Because I agree that thoughts have lots to do with the way you feel. I think a major part of depression and learning to cope with depression is learning to control the kinds of thoughts that we have. Certain kinds of thoughts can really feed depression, it's like keeping the fire stoked up, you know. Does that make any sense to you?

P: Uh huh.

T: Do you have any experiences where you know that you've kind of been making yourself sadder by thinking something?

P: Uh huh.

T: You've done that?

P: I've done that, yeah.

T: OK. That's good if you already have that realization because lots of people don't know that about themselves. They have no idea that their thoughts can affect how they feel. But if you already know that, then it's going to make our work easier, and we can start to focus a bit on your feelings and how they might be connected to your thoughts.

P: OK.

Example 2

The following example concerns a 15-year-old male adolescent who had been asked to keep records of his anger and sadness for the week following his initial assessment. Note how the therapist uses the patient's homework to introduce the important role of thoughts in contributing to emotional distress, thereby promoting socialization into the cognitive therapy model.

T: David, we talked about you keeping track of anger and sadness. Did you use the calendar that I gave you?

P: Uh huh.

T: Is that what you brought there?

P: Uh huh. That's about it. (*Points hesitantly to pages brought.*)

T: Good. Could I have a look at it?

P: You won't be able to read anything. (*Hands pages to therapist.*)

T: Sure I can. You did lots of work! Wow! Terrific! (*looking at records*) So, angry on some days, more often angry than sad. Did you do this every night?

P: (*Shakes head "yes."*)

T: So each night you wrote it down? This is just great. By doing this, did you start to be aware of your feelings more?

P: Not really. Whenever I got mad I would write it down. But I wouldn't pay much attention to it.

T: But at least you did pay attention enough to write it down when you felt that way. Good for you. I'd like to spend some time by understanding each day, and what you wrote down. The reason I wanted you to keep track is so that I can talk with you about what was going on and see if together we can understand what was running through your head at the time. You know, like the first thought that occurred to you.

P: Like my ideas about it?

T: Right, because sometimes that first thought, that automatic thought, like I said before, is one that's going to make you feel down. So it's not a helpful thought to you. I suppose you don't know you're doing it.

P: No. I just get mad or sad.

T: Right, that's how it seems. If you knew what ideas were making you that way, you'd stop, I'm sure. It's just that you don't even know you're doing it. And we all have some of those ideas. When you're feeling down and depressed you could be using quite a few of those negative thoughts that are automatic. So my job is to help you to discover them, and we can do that by talking about these things that you wrote down.

Example 3

With very young adolescents, metaphors or stories are often useful aids to the process of socialization. The following example concerns a 13-year-old female adolescent who did not understand the therapist's first attempt to explain the cognitive model. As such, the therapist employs a hypothetical situation that the patient understands quickly.

T: Maybe I've not been clear about what I'm trying to do with you. Sometimes we think that things happen to make us mad. Right? And what I want you to consider is the thought that you had that might be making you mad. OK? So depending on what you're thinking, the same thing could happen and make you feel very differently at different times.

P: Uh huh.

T: Can you give me an example of that?

P: Um. . . . (*silence*)

T: OK, let me see if I can help with an example. Say somebody knocks on the door and it's a stranger, right? And you open the door. You could have one of many different thoughts. What if you look at him and you say, "Uh oh, this guy looks like the picture of the murderer I saw in the newspaper and who's on the news"? What kind of feeling would you have then?

P: I'd be scared.

T: Good. What if your thought was, "I think I see the mail truck down at the corner"? What kind of feeling would you have?

P: The mail person, oh, that person. I'd feel safe.

T: So you wouldn't particularly feel scared. What if your thought was, "Maybe this is the package I've been waiting for." What would you feel?

P: Probably excited.

T: Yeah. Yeah. So you see it's not the guy ringing the doorbell who makes you feel scared or excited. Right? Tell me what kind of thoughts you would have if you opened the door and something made you feel sad.

P: Um. . . . If some person had a dead cat or something, and asked me if it was my cat or something like that.

T: OK. Good. So somebody may have lost their cat or something like that. Or maybe you thought that somebody was going to tell you your cat was gone. Good. So you see sometimes what we think affects how we feel. So let's try again with that situation with your homework. You made a mistake. What kind of thought about that mistake might make you really angry at yourself?

Example 4

Family members are socialized into the cognitive therapy model in much the same way as are individual adolescents, by focusing on the important relationship between emotion and cognition. The following example concerns a 14-year-old, Lynn, who lives with her father and her older sister. Her father's commonlaw spouse of 8 years (Shelly) moved out of the home about 4 months earlier. During the assessment interview, the therapist learned that the onset of Lynn's depression occurred shortly after her "stepmother's" departure. Lynn's father is primarily concerned about her withdrawal and increasing refusal to interact with himself and her sister. The following discussion occurred during the first family session following the initial assessment.

T: Do you have any ideas why you spend so much time alone in your room?

P: I don't like getting close to anyone.

T: What's hard about getting close to anybody?

P: It's just that everyone I got close to before, they would always leave. So I keep them away now. (*Begins to cry.*)

T: You say everyone. Do you mean your dad's girlfriend, Shelly?

P: (*Shakes her head "yes" through the tears.*)

[Here, the therapist continues to discuss the patient's relationship with Shelly for several minutes.]

T: (*to dad*) The reason I'm talking to Lynn about Shelly in some detail is that, whenever we have losses and we're hurt, then we don't want to repeat that experience. Does that makes sense?

Dad: Sure, of course. I know Lynn was very close to Shelly and misses her a lot.

T: And if the way we interpret a situation is to think, "When I get close I get hurt," then the obvious solution is not to get close to anybody. But that can cause problems in families. For example, Lynn wants to be in her room and alone all the time. Sometimes Lynn is going to feel like pushing you away. You want to be close, but she's going to want to push you away. And those family problems that come up, can come from the belief "If I get close, I'm going to get hurt."

D: I can see how that could happen.

T: Does that make sense to you, Sandy [older sister]?

Sister: Yeah. If I thought that way, I'd stay in my room too.

T: Right, you probably would. Well one way that therapy tries to help is to ask, "How true is that belief?" And we'll take a real live example, like Lynn and Shelly. We'll talk about Lynn's belief that "If I get close, I'm going to be hurt."

P: I guess I could try to see her [Shelly].

T: OK, I guess you could try that. What if you and Shelly can't immediately agree on a good time that you want to see each other? What would you think of that?

P: I'd probably think that she was trying to avoid me.

T: That would be your first automatic thought, right? "She's trying to avoid me." And after you had a chance to think about it, might there be some other explanations?

P: Maybe she had other plans.

T: "She had other plans." OK, that's one explanation. That's a possibility, isn't it?

D: Maybe she had a work commitment.

T: That's possible. (*to Lynn*) What might be some other explanations?

P: (*silence—no response*)

T: (*to Lynn*) Suppose you and Shelly disagreed on a specific date to see each other. (*to dad*) Lynn's first inclination is to interpret it as Shelly doesn't want to see her. So Lynn interprets that disagreement as rejection.

D: I can see that.

T: But what I tried to point out and what's very important, especially in depression, is to know that those first interpretations can be what contributes to depression a lot of the time. So we need to look for other interpretations. Lynn came up with one that was a little bit more acceptable when she thought Shelly might have had other plans.

D: Uh huh.

T: Another possible explanation was she had a work commitment that day.

D: Or any other commitment.

T: OK. Your dad came up with another interpretation. For example, Shelly might have another commitment with her friends or family. It doesn't mean she doesn't want to see you. It just isn't convenient at that particular time. That could that be another explanation, right?

P: I guess so.

T: Lynn, the reason I'm talking with you about this is because a lot of times I talk to people who feel bad, and they might think people don't want to see them and they feel hurt. Maybe they feel rejected. Sometimes those feelings come from wrong ideas that they have. And if they start to test the ideas out, they find which ones are right and which ones need changing. So that's one of the ways we might help you work with your depression to see if we can help you adjust those first thoughts that go through your mind because sometimes those might be the ones that are making you feel so bad.

Clearly, one important aspect of socialization into therapy concerns the timing of interventions. The aphorism "One can lead a horse to water but can't make it drink" is very true for adolescents. Sometimes adolescents will have their own agendas to communicate before they will be receptive to the cognitive therapy model. When this is the case, the therapist must be prepared to wait and must avoid forcing techniques on an unwilling patient. Frequently, several sessions or even weeks are required for the therapeutic relationship to develop, especially in the case of adolescents who have experienced multiple placements in foster homes. These adolescents often have learned to be cautious of the "trust me" and "it's in your best interest" attitude held by adults.

SETTING GOALS AND PRIORITIES

Psychotherapy without goals or priorities is like a ship without a navigator, at the mercy of the prevailing elements. One of the distinguishing features of cognitive therapy is its emphasis on agendas, goals, and the ability to prioritize. Making the diagnosis of depression is useless in psychotherapy unless the diagnosis is operationalized. The therapist accomplishes operationalization of the depression by determining the answer to questions such as the following: How is the depression affecting the adolescent's life? What is the adolescent missing because of the depression? How long does he expect it to go on? What would he do if not depressed? Do his ambition and the continual frustration of goals have any bearing on how he feels now? If the adolescent were less ambitious, would his depression be less severe and frequent? Questions that explore the effect of depression on the adolescent's life lead the therapist to establish short-term and long-term goals in a collaborative manner with the adolescent. Objectives need to be explicit and are often written down in detail.

The importance of identifying a number-one priority can be illustrated with the example of a high school student who is trying to compete in track and field events, participate in army cadets, socialize with his friends in the mall, and go hiking in the mountains at the same time. It is impossible to pursue all of these activities simultaneously; the patient must prioritize in order to avoid frustration, despair, and fatigue. Most depressed patients obtain a great deal of subjective relief when they have a clear plan and a priority list. Often their resources have been overwhelmed by their own internal demands as well as the external demands of life, so prioritization of goals helps to provide a sense of control.

The difficulties involved in helping the adolescent identify a number-one priority can be addressed by using a circular pie chart, as is often used with adults. The center of the circle is the adolescent, and the points on the circumference represent the various difficulties with which the patient is struggling.

Joan, a 16-year-old separated from her parents, presented with depression and sleeping problems and was unsure of what to do in her complex life. She complained of feeling so depressed that she could not get to sleep at night or concentrate on her school work. She did not know what to do with her boyfriend and wondered, "Should I run away with him?" She wondered whether she should leave her foster mother and return to her real mother. Joan felt as though she were in a bind and complained that she even dreamed of arguing with her mother and her boyfriend and being left by both of them. In addition, she was frightened about her impending court appearance the next month. She felt so irritable and tearful she did not know what to do first. When anyone tried to help her, she usually fought with the person. A circle (Figure 7.1) was constructed during the session. Through a series of questions, the therapist led Joan to consider the impact of the depression on the other areas of her life in the diagram. In particular, discussion focused on some of the thoughts Joan had that seemed to decrease her motivation, increase her indecision, and threaten her self-efficacy. By the end of the session, Joan was able to decide to work on "beating her depression"

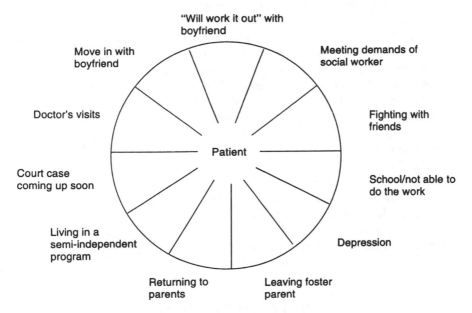

FIGURE 7.1. Circle of impact of Joan's depression.

since it appeared to be affecting all the other aspects of her life. A number-one priority had been established, and a contract for 10 sessions was made with her without any fights.

SUMMARY

The initial phase of cognitive therapy with adolescents includes diagnosis, assessment, formulation, contracting, and socialization into the cognitive therapy model (see Bedrosian, 1981; Kendall and Hollon, 1981; Trautman and Rotherman-Borus, 1988; Wilkes and Rush, 1988). Having taken these steps, the therapist, adolescent, and family can focus on setting goals and priorities for therapy. One of the many unique features of cognitive therapy is the emphasis on developing operational definitions of large problems so that they can be reduced to smaller, more manageable ones. This process complements the emerging cognitive skills of adolescents and enhances their capacity to challenge dichotomous thinking with an awareness of less extreme alternatives. Prioritization and setting goals also help to regulate the adolescent's affect, reducing impulsivity and the sense of urgency.

When the initial phase of cognitive therapy is completed effectively, therapy itself is largely completed because adolescents and their families have already begun to transform their thinking styles. In addition to an awareness of problems, solutions are sought and found. Rather than a dark veil of despair, there is a sense of hope. With some adolescents, the initial phase of therapy is especially difficult because they have been "forced" into treatment by their parents and have difficulty forming a therapeutic alliance. In such cases, the therapist must be patient and must be prepared for initial rejection by the adolescent and his "testing" of the therapist's commitment to therapy. More time is needed to overcome such reluctance with adolescents than with their adult counterparts, and the therapeutic alliance may be extremely fragile during the process. Although the therapist must be patient and flexible during this period, he must persist calmly with the Socratic dialogue, focusing on key cognitions and silent assumptions, generating alternative perceptions, and making homework assignments.

SELECTED READINGS

Abramson LY, Seligman MGP, Teasdale JD: Learned helplessness in humans. Critique and reformulation. *Journal of Abnormal Psychology* 1978; 87:49–74.

American Psychiatric Association: *Diagnostic and Statistical Manual of Mental Disorders,* fourth edition. Washington, DC, American Psychiatric Association, 1994.

Beck AT: *Cognitive Therapy and the Emotional Disorders.* New York, International Universities Press, 1976.

Beck AT, Rush AJ, Shaw BF, Emery G: *Cognitive Therapy of Depression.* New York, Guilford Press, 1979.

Bedrosian RC: The application of cognitive therapy techniques with adolescents, in *New Directions in Cognitive Therapy: A Casebook.* Edited by Emery G, Hollon SD, Bedrosian RC. New York, Guilford Press, 1981.

Guidano VF, Liotti G: *Cognitive Processes and Emotional Disorders.* New York, Guilford Press, 1983.

Hudgeons RW: *Psychiatric Disorders in Adolescents.* Baltimore, Williams & Wilkins, 1974.

Jarrett RB, Rush AJ: Psychotherapeutic approaches to depression, in *Psychiatry,* Vol. 1. Edited by Cavenar JO. Philadelphia, Lippincott, and New York, Basic Books, 1985.

Kendall PC, Hollon SD (eds): *Assessment Strategies for Cognitive-Behavioral Interventions.* New York, Academic Press, 1981.

Kendell RE: *The Role of Diagnosis in Psychiatry.* Oxford, Blackwell, 1975.

Petti TA: Depression in hospitalized child psychiatry patients, approaches to measuring depression. *Journal of the American Academy of Child Psychiatry* 1978; 17:49–59.

Popper KR, Eccles JC: *The Self and Its Brain.* New York, Springer International, 1977.

Rush AJ, Shaw BF, Khatami M: Cognitive theapy of depression, utilizing the couples system. *Cognitive Therapy Research* 1980; 4:103–113.

Seligman MEP: *Helplessness: On Depression, Development and Death.* San Francisco, Freeman, 1975.

Spitzer RL, Endicott J, Robins E: Research Diagnostic Criteria: Rationale and reliability. *Archives of General Psychiatry* 1978; 36:773–782.

Trautman PD, Rotherman-Borus MJ: Cognitive behavioral therapy with children and adolescents, in *American Psychiatric Association Annual Review,* Vol. 7. Edited by Frances AJ, Hales RE. Washington, DC, American Psychiatric Press, 1988.

Viederman M: The psycho-dynamic life narrative: A psychotherapeutic intervention useful in crisis situations. *Psychiatry* 1983; 3:236–246.

Watzlawick P, Weakland JH, Fisch R: *Change.* New York, Norton, 1974.

Weinberg WA, Rutman J, Sullivan L, Penick EC, Dietz SG: Depression in children referred to an educational diagnostic center: Diagnosis and treatment. *Journal of Pediatrics* 1973; 83:1065–1073.

Wilkes TCR, Rush AJ: Adaptations of cognitive therapy for depressed adolescents. *Journal of the American Academy of Child and Adolescent Psychiatry* 1988; 27:381–386.

CHAPTER EIGHT

The Middle Phase of Cognitive Therapy: Intervention Techniques for Five Steps in the Therapeutic Process

GAYLE BELSHER

T. C. R. WILKES

INTRODUCTION

The middle phase of cognitive therapy begins after the diagnosis of depression has been communicated to the family and a thorough assessment of problems related to the depression has been completed. By the time the middle phase of therapy begins, the therapist will have met individually with the adolescent as well as with the entire family, and a cognitive formulation for the case will have been prepared. All family members will have been introduced to the theoretical model underlying cognitive therapy and will understand that discussion will focus on the examination of thoughts and beliefs likely to exacerbate the adolescent's depression. In addition to communicating the theoretical model, therapists will have already established a "contract" regarding the number and frequency of therapy sessions, the family's participation in therapy, and such issues as payment for therapy, when applicable.

During the middle phase of therapy, as with the initial and final phases, the "key principles" that were discussed in Chapter 2 continue to apply. These principles will not be reiterated here, although they are evident in the examples throughout the chapter. Rather, the purpose of the current chapter is to review more specific techniques that have been found useful for eliciting, evaluating, and changing maladaptive depressogenic cognitions. Because the participation of an adolescent's family in some therapy sessions is nearly always recommended, we have attempted to include examples that demonstrate the application of each technique not only in individual sessions but also in family sessions.

Because all interventions will not be equally applicable or effective with all depressed adolescents, the techniques presented in this chapter should not be applied in a rote, mechanical fashion. It is essential that the therapist remain sensitive to the cognitive development of the adolescent, the particular life circumstances of the adolescent, and the potential role of the adolescent's family, as well as any comorbid diagnoses. Furthermore, it is crucial that the therapist use various techniques in a purposeful, goal-directed manner. To assist in conceptualizing the therapy process and determining which techniques are most applicable at what stages in "working through" the depression, the discussion that follows has been organized into five sequential steps that generally occur during the middle phase of cognitive therapy.

The first step in the sequence involves increasing adolescents' awareness of their own emotional variability. Having accomplished this goal, the therapist proceeds to the second step, which focuses on helping adolescents discover the automatic thoughts that occur in response to their most distressing life experiences. The third step often overlaps with the previous one and involves the identification of beliefs or "schemas" that are hypothesized to engender automatic thoughts. Once automatic thoughts and/or beliefs have been identified, the fourth step focuses on evaluation of these cognitions in order to determine the degree to which they are realistic and adaptive. Depressed patients will typically reveal unrealistic and maladaptive thoughts or beliefs, which then become the focus of the fifth step, cognitive change.

Although the primary objective of the current chapter is to provide examples of therapeutic techniques useful at each of the five steps in the process described above, a sixth step will sometimes be required in conducting therapy. In this optional step, the focus becomes problem-solving. One indication for problem-solving is when the evaluation of thoughts or beliefs fails to reveal unrealistic or maladaptive cognitions. Instead, discussion of a particular circumstance elicits thought processes and emotional responses that appear to be quite reasonable, given the event or situation described. In such cases, interventions directed at various members of the patient's social system are often required. In other words, the target of intervention shifts from the adolescent's cognitions to his environment. A second indication for problem-solving is when skill deficits rather than cognitive distortions appear to be contributing to the depression. When this is the case, therapists may need to address the deficit through instructional means or by referring the adolescent to additional forms of therapy such as social-skills training. When therapists do engage in problem-solving, it is particularly important that the principles of collaborative empiricism and Socratic dialogue be observed so that the therapy remains consistent with the cognitive model in which the patient is the "expert" and the therapist is a helpful assistant in the process of change. When there is evidence of both realistic problems and maladaptive cognitions, the therapist may combine the goal of problem-solving with that of cognitive change.

To demonstrate the types of issues that arise and some of the techniques that can be applied to problem-solving, a few brief examples are included at the end of this chapter. However, our discussion of problem-solving should be regarded as less comprehensive than that of the previous five steps, which represent the "essence" of cognitive therapy. Likewise, this chapter does not address the remediation of skill deficits in any substantial way, and readers are referred to alternate sources of information dedicated more specifically to this topic.

Therapists working with depressed adolescents and their families will quickly discover that the steps in cognitive therapy are seldom pursued in the exact progression in which they are presented in this chapter. Rather, the sequence of five steps should be viewed as a template from which deviations will be appropriate and necessary. For example, with younger adolescents, the elicitation of automatic thoughts is often more difficult than the identification of maladaptive beliefs; consequently, the therapist may spend relatively little or no time on the former. However, some adolescents are quick to identify automatic thoughts and propose alternatives that would be less emotionally distressing to them. In such cases, the amount of time spent evaluating the thought may be minimal because the patient sees it as "obviously" distorted as soon as it is detected and immediately begins to explore changing the maladaptive cognition. In general, younger adolescents will require more time with the first step, increasing awareness of emotional variability, before progressing to later steps in the cognitive therapy process. Within one session, it is important that the therapist move flexibly "forward and backward" through the sequence of steps as necessary. This flexibility requires a clear conceptualization of the overall process of cognitive therapy and an ongoing assessment of the adolescent's progress with respect to steps in this process. Also, thorough familiarity with the techniques appropriate to each step in the therapy process will allow the therapist to combine or modify techniques in the most advantageous manner for the adolescent in question.

STEP I: INCREASING AWARENESS OF
EMOTIONAL VARIABILITY

Early in the therapy process, it is important for adolescents to learn that there is some variability in the degree to which they feel "depressed." Although some adolescents will claim initially that they are "always depressed" about "everything," careful exploration of daily events in their lives typically reveals some situations that trigger more intense feelings of depression than others. Identification of these precipitating situations is important for two reasons: First, it demonstrates to the adolescent that life is not equally depressing at all times, a cognitive intervention that, in and of itself, helps to challenge the binary motif. Second, the identification of precipitating situations allows the therapist to begin focusing the adolescent's attention on the thoughts that accompany the times of greatest emotional distress.

In addition to understanding that there is variability in depression, another important aspect of early therapy is helping the adolescent identify and label other emotional states. Some adolescents who have been diagnosed as depressed do not directly acknowledge feeling "depressed." Instead, their primary concern may be extreme feelings of anger or anxiety, for example. The identification of different emotional states and the situations that precipitate them is important because the content of maladaptive cognitions typically varies with the emotion felt. Therapists will be able to guide their patients in identifying maladaptive cognitions much more effectively if they have an accurate description of the emotional states that the adolescent experiences.

Usually, older adolescents will have less difficulty than younger ones in labeling their emotions or seeing a relationship between precipitating situations and degrees of emotion experienced. However, therapists must be constantly aware of potential discrepancies between chronological age and cognitive development. Some 16-year-old patients will demonstrate cognitive abilities much like adult patients; others will demonstrate reasoning capabilities much more like a typical 11-year-old child. One of the challenges of cognitive therapy with adolescents relates to this issue of working with the patient at a speed and level that are appropriate to his developmental stage. The necessity of matching therapy to the cognitive development of the patient cannot be overemphasized because the adolescent's awareness of emotional variability is the foundation for subsequent steps in therapy, and it is crucial that the therapist assess the patient's ability to detect such emotional variability and relate it to his life experience.

Therapists will usually find it helpful to chart the relationship between situations and emotions for the patient and/or themselves. Initially, a two-column chart might be developed with the patient during the course of a session. Later, it is useful if the adolescent keeps his own records during the time between therapy sessions. An example is presented in Table 8.1. Some adolescents will be unable to relate life situations to degrees of emotional distress without considerable help from the therapist. The techniques discussed below can assist the therapist to collect the information needed to complete a two-column chart, if one were developed.

Mood Chart

A mood chart involves a more global assessment of variability in emotion than the two-column record presented in Table 8.1. When an adolescent has difficulty remembering or explaining what specific situations have resulted in heightened levels of emotional distress, the therapist may have to begin with a review of "generally good" versus "generally bad" days in the previous week. Most adolescents will have some idea about the events that contributed to the "best" as compared to the "worst" day over some reasonably short retrospective period of time. Alternatively, it is often possible to focus the adolescent's attention on one particular emotion, asking him to assign a rating for that emotional state to each day in the week between sessions. Of course, it is more helpful if the adolescent is able to record, even briefly, the significant

TABLE 8.1. Situation Feeling Chart

Situation	Feeling (emotion) (0 = lowest, 10 = highest)
I received a poor mark on an arithmetic test.	Depressed—7
Three of the friends I invited to a sleeping party didn't come.	Sad—8
Dad wouldn't let me go skiing with him on the weekend.	Mad—8
Mom made me do my homework so I missed my favorite program on TV.	Mad—8
My sister wouldn't let me use her sweater.	Sad—3
I didn't get the part I wanted in the school play.	Sad—5
We had to come home from vacation two days earlier than I was planning.	Sad—4

event(s) that contributed to his emotional rating for each day. A variation of this technique is to request three emotional ratings per day: one for the morning, another for the afternoon, and a third for the evening. We have found it useful to give the adolescent a "calendar" format with space for the ratings and space for a brief note about daily events or circumstances. The calendar can be used to record ratings for more than one emotional state; but, with younger adolescents, focus on one emotion at a time is sometimes necessary.

Example

A young boy has been asked to keep a record of his global index of anger for each day in a week. His homework involves nothing more than a rating between "0" and "10" for each day. When presented with the patient's daily ratings, the therapist explores the events that have contributed to the fluctuations in anger over the preceding week. The mood chart completed by the boy is shown in Figure 8.1.

Cognitive Continuum

Therapists employ a cognitive continuum any time reference is made to a quantitative assessment of an abstract concept such as "distress" or "change." Patients can be asked to consider their feelings on a scale of "0" to "10" or to use a proportion rating, for example. Alternatively, a visual representation of a continuum can be used with adolescents whose thinking skills are more concrete. A continuum is also implied any time the therapist uses descriptive words that challenge the idea of a binary classification, for example, "better and worse," rather than "good and bad." Demonstrations of change are easier if the change is evaluated along a continuum because even a small amount of improvement can still be regarded as movement in the right direction.

Example

The young adolescent boy whose mood chart was shown in Figure 8.1 has a diagnosis of attention-deficit hyperactivity disorder in addition to depression. A central aspect of his depression is anger at himself for his impulsive behaviors and extreme mood swings, particularly his short temper. The patient's homework from the previous week was to keep a

In the space at the top of each square, rate the amount of
___ANGER____ (emotion) with numbers 0 to 10. In the remaining
space, write what you were doing, where you were, or who you were
with to remind you what was going on at the time.

Remember that: 0 = lowest   10 = highest

	Mon	Tue	Wed	Thurs	Fri	Sat	Sun
am		0	0	0	3 / M	5	0
noon		0	0	4	3	5	0
pm	3	0	0	0	0	5	8

FIGURE 8.1. Mood chart.

"mood chart" in which he would record global ratings of anger each day
of the week. In the following excerpt, the therapist reviews the patient's
homework, emphasizing the idea of a cognitive continuum of anger. By
using the continuum, the therapist is able to help the patient construct
an agenda for the session.

    T: Good work (*looking at homework*). It looks like you had quite a
few different feelings around here. (*pointing*)

P: Yeah. Here (*pointing*) I'm mad at my brother because he went in my room and he used my desk and everything. He didn't ask me.

T: OK. (*looking at the week's record*) Then you had a couple of days that nothing really happened to upset you? Here (*pointing*) you were mad because?

P: I was mad at my grandpa because I'll be talking to him and he'll be walking away. And he'll be talking to me and he'll walk into the other room. I just can't hear all of it when he does that.

T: OK. And then what happened on this day here? That looks like you were a little upset; you gave that day a 3 [on a 10-point scale].

P: Yeah.

T: A little upset about what?

P: I think a little upset. I put an "M" there because I was mad. I would have to wait an extra day to get a gerbil, and I was sort of mad at that.

T: OK. You had to wait an extra day to get your gerbil?

P: Uh huh.

T: And how about Saturday? What happened? You gave that day a 5.

P: I was OK on that day . . . nothing really happened.

T: Oh, so should this one really be a 0?

P: Yeah.

T: And then that's another day (*pointing to record of emotional ratings*) when you were quite mad. You said 8 out of 10.

P: I was real mad at dad. About my school and stuff. Because I've been asking him for help, and he thought I could do it. I could do some of it, but other things I couldn't. I was getting real mad and frustrated.

T: Let's see. We have to decide which one of these we should start talking about. Which one do you think was the most troublesome to you?

P: The one with dad.

Emotional Thermometer

A thermometer is a concrete symbol of graded measurement that will be familiar to adolescents. For developmentally younger patients, the introduction of an "emotional thermometer" may be easier to grasp than a cognitive continuum without the symbolic metaphor. As with the cognitive continuum, the therapist's goal is to challenge the binary motif, showing that degrees of feeling an emotion covary with the nature of the precipitating situation.

Example 1

In the first example, the idea of an emotional thermometer is introduced with a very young girl. To keep the illustration as simple as possible, the therapist does not associate number ratings with the degree of emotion felt, but rather, refers to emotional intensity as "high," "medium," and "low" on the thermometer. In the following excerpt, the therapist attempts to demonstrate that (1) there are degrees of sadness, and (2) there is a relationship between degrees of sadness and different precipitating events. The patient in this case is a 13-year-old girl who lives with her mother, separated from her father.

T: Let's pretend that your feelings are on a thermometer. OK? And way down here (*pointing to a thermometer drawn on a page*) is "none" and way up here is "lots," like the most sad you've ever felt.

P: OK. I guess so.

T: Maybe it would help if we put some anchors on here. Can you think of what situation has made you about the saddest, one of the things that really, really made you very sad.

P: I guess maybe my dad. He always gets me sad.

T: What does he do?

P: He never calls me, and he should call me because I'm always the one that calls him. And when mom yells at me for stuff that I don't do.

T: OK, mom yelling at you, dad not calling you on the phone. Give me an example of something that would make you about halfway up there [on thermometer].

P: When Randy [brother] gets mad at me.

T: Now that doesn't make you as sad as when your mom gets mad at you?

P: No.

T: OK. Randy gets mad. How about something that would put you low down, almost at none [on sadness thermometer]?

P: When a friend tells me they're angry with me. I feel a little sad.

T: So you'd just be a little sad if a friend got angry. But less sad than if your brother got mad? And your mom and dad are at the top. Right?

P: Uh huh. Dad can make me the saddest.

T: Does the amount of sadness go up and down according to what the situation is?

P: Yes.

T: OK. So can you give me an example of that?

P: Like, if mom says something to me in front of my friends, or if my dad says he's not going to visit me or something like that.

T: That he's not going to visit you. OK. Now where would that be on the scale?

P: The very top.

T: What kind of things could your mom do to make you really sad, at the top?

P: Well, making comments about my friends.

T: And what could your brother do that would make you sad say at in the middle?

P: Tell me to leave him alone or to get out of his room.

T: Now if he tells you to get out of his room, how sad does that make you?

P: Pretty sad because I feel like he doesn't want me around. In the middle.

T: You know one of the things that sometimes happens for a lot of kids is that there's very little difference between being here (*pointing to low end of thermometer*) and being up there (*pointing to high end of thermometer*). They frequently spend a lot of time up at the top. And that gets very painful to be really sad all the time. Right?

P: Uh huh.

T: One way to keep the amount of sadness where it belongs is to try and think about how sad is this worth getting. "Is it something to be very *very* sad about or just a little bit sad?"

P: Yeah.

T: Because probably you can have different amounts of sad depending on the situation, or what you think about it.

Example 2

Number ratings are attached to the thermometer to convey the idea of graduations of emotion. Word labels are also attached to further convey the idea of a continuum. The young boy in this case is frequently angry at himself or others. The anger contributes to his depressogenic view of himself and his "world" of relationships.

T: You know, what I want to do with you is make something called a feeling thermometer. Now, being mad is the feeling that is one of the big problems for you, right? So let's pretend there's mercury in here (*drawing a thermometer on a page for patient*). And this is how mad you can get. Zero is not made at all. Ten is the very, very maddest that you have ever been. In between there's a 1, 2, 3, 4, 5, 6, 7, 8, 9. See if you can think of a situation that's made you feel just a little bit made, say just annoyed, say around maybe a 2. Tell me about something that might make you feel about a 2.

P: Um. . . . Like if I'm playing a sport and I'm trying hard or something like that.

T: OK. So say you're trying, what sport do you play?

P: Baseball.

T: Baseball. Miss a ball in game? And that kind of annoyed you a little bit but not enough so that you really get angry. OK, let's go a little bit higher than that. Say a 5. Still pretty far from being furious. But beginning to get angry.

P: Um. Probably if I fail a test or something like that.

T: OK. That makes you angry?

P: Uh huh.

T: Fail a test, that makes you angry. OK. Let's go a little higher than that.

P: My brother, he'll take my stuff, and he won't ask me to use it, and then he makes a mess of my room. He uses the stereo in my room, and then he won't pick up his mess. That makes me pretty mad.

T: OK. Where would you put that?

P: Um . . . about 7.

T: Seven. OK.

P: And then when I talk to him, he'll say, "Well I didn't think you'd mind." And then that makes me really mad.

T: Does that make you even madder?

P: Um . . . yeah. When he says, "Well I didn't think you'd mind."

T: "I didn't think you'd mind" will bring anger up to where? About an 8?

P: Yeah. The thing is he didn't ask me.

T: OK. And then let's get to 10 which is the very maddest you've ever been, furious.

P: Well if my mom tells me to do something, and then I start doing something else and get sidetracked. An hour or two goes by and she says, "Tony, have you done this 'cause I really need it to be done." I get mad at myself because she told me an hour ago and I didn't do it.

T: Would you put that all the way up here at 10, being furious?

P: Yeah. 'Cause I get real mad at myself when I forget stuff. Short patience. I get mad easily.

Emotional Pie

An emotional pie is a pictorial version of a mood chart. It requires that an adolescent evaluate himself with respect to two or more emotional states by indicating the proportion of a circle that would correspond to each emotion. An emotional pie could be used to describe the adolescent's global view of his emotions over a period of a week; or several emotional pies could be used, one for each day of self-observation. For younger adolescents, concrete images of space increasing or decreasing in size may be easier to relate to change in emotional states than the abstract concept of a numbered rating scheme, such as would be employed with a mood chart.

Example

A 13-year-old girl has difficulty describing her emotions and has consistently been unable to identify any notable events in her life when asked about the past week. She is apparently unaware of any relationship between current circumstances and various emotional reactions. Or perhaps she has some awareness of the relationship but feels unable to express it verbally. Because of the difficulty encountered when attempting to discuss the girl's feelings and the circumstances that precipitate them, the therapist asks her to describe herself with reference to a circle drawn on a page.

T: How have you been feeling the past week?

P: OK.

T: Did anything especially good or bad happen to make you feel happy or sad?

P: I don't know.

T: We talked last time about your mom not having a job, and how you were kind of noticing that she seems more grumpy than usual. Did she get a job this week?

P: No, not yet.

T: Do you have some upsetting feelings when you think about your mom and the fact that she doesn't have a job?

P: Yeah, sometimes.

T: What words would describe your feelings?

P: I don't know.

T: Do you know what the word "worry" means?

P: It means you're scared.

T: Right. Do you ever worry about your mom?

P: Uh huh.

T: Do you worry about your mom a lot?

P: No, just some of the time.

T: (*drawing a circle on the page and showing patient*) Could you show me with a piece of pie in the circle how big your worry about your mom is?

P: (*Takes pencil and draws a segment.*)

T: Now we've talked about you being depressed too, haven't we?

P: Yeah.

T: What would be some words that mean the same as "depressed"?

P: Sad and crying.

T: OK, good. If this amount of you is worried (*pointing to the "worry" segment of the emotional pie*), could you draw another piece to show me what part of you is sad right now?

P: (*drawing in another segment*) There.

T: Is the rest of you (*pointing to the emotional pie*) happy or just OK?

P: OK.

T: All right. Let's write a "W" in the piece for "worried," and an "S" in the piece for "sad," and "OK" in the rest (*writing letters in the segments of the emotional pie*). If your mom got a job this coming week, do you think this piece of you that is worried (*pointing*) would get smaller, or bigger, or stay the same?

P: Get smaller.

T: OK. Good. Can you think of anything that would make it get really big?

P: If my mom and dad fight a lot.

T: Do they do that sometimes?

P: They used to, but not now.

T: How come this piece of pie (*pointing to the "S"*) shows that you're sad?

P: I'm sad when I'm bored.

T: If you had lots of interesting things to do, would this piece of pie get smaller?

P: Yeah.

T: What else would make it get smaller?

The therapist continued to make reference to the drawing of an emotional pie throughout the session, exploring the sizes of the pieces and relating increased or decreased size to circumstances in the patient's life. For homework, the therapist drew seven circles on a page, labeling each one for a different day of the coming week and provided a legend for the patient to use in drawing and labeling segments of the emotional pies to indicate her feelings for each day. Shown in Figure 8.2 are two of the self-descriptive graphs that the patient returned the following week. They were used to further explore the girl's emotional variability, relating it to circumstances in her school and family life.

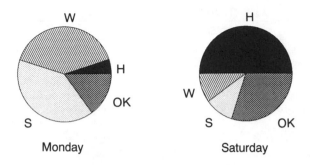

FIGURE 8.2. Emotional pie.

STEP II: DETECTION OF AUTOMATIC THOUGHTS

Once adolescents have gained an awareness of the association between events in their lives and their emotional reactions to these events, the therapist can begin to explore the cognitions that accompany emotional distress. Because the goal of cognitive therapy is to change maladaptive cognitions, the thoughts associated with depressed mood must first be detected and then evaluated to determine whether change needs to occur. The second step in the cognitive therapy process concerns the detection of automatic thoughts.

Thought Chart

A thought chart is a useful way of summarizing situations, emotions, and automatic thoughts. The therapist himself may wish to develop this chart based on conversations with the adolescent in session. Various techniques for eliciting automatic thoughts through dialogue are demonstrated below. Alternatively, some adolescents will be able and willing to develop such a thought chart themselves by recording events that occur throughout the week between therapy sessions. An example of such a chart produced by an adolescent patient is shown in Table 8.2.

Cognitive Replay

Cognitive therapists often ask patients to keep records of distressing situations, emotions, and automatic thoughts, which can then be exam-

TABLE 8.2. Thought Chart

Situation	Feeling (0–10)	Thoughts
Tues: missed bus on way to school so was late.	Mad—3	I'm always goofing up. Now my day is ruined.
Tues: fouled out during basketball practice so got sent to change room early.	Depressed—5	I'm so stupid. I lost the game for our team. Everyone is angry with me. I'll have a bad reputation in the whole city.
Wed: nothing.		
Thurs: fight with mom about going to a movie.	Angry—6	She never lets me do anything. She's mean.
Fri: OK.		
Sat: fight with best friend on phone.	Mad—5 Sad—8	Why did I say that? I'm always opening my big mouth. Now I've lost her. She hates me. I've ruined everything.
Sat: sister won't drive me over to a friend's house.	Angry—4	She never does anything for me. Nobody likes me.
Sun: homework takes all afternoon.	Depressed—7	If I weren't so dumb, this would take no time. What's wrong with me?
Mon: nothing.		

ined in session. However, adolescents tend to live very much "in the moment" and can become impatient with the somewhat tedious task of keeping records of things gone by. Some adolescent patients are reluctant to write down much of anything because they assume that it must be "right" or "the way the therapist wants it." Rather than risk failure or disappointing the therapist, they avoid the homework request altogether or make minimal attempts to complete it. Cognitive replay of past events is using dialogue in session to gain the necessary information about some particular distressing situation and the emotions associated with it so that the goal of identifying automatic thoughts or underlying beliefs can be pursued.

Example

A 17-year-old male high school student with a history of school difficulties has found it hard to identify his own thought processes without the help of the therapist. However, he is able to introspect about his thoughts if guided by the therapist in session. Furthermore, by the end of the excerpt, the therapist asks about the cumulative meaning of his thoughts, and he is able to state the belief that he is a "failure."

P: Sometimes I'm in a bad mood for no reason. Everything's OK, and there's nothing really wrong in my life at the moment. I didn't get a bad test mark or something. It's just an average day. I'll just be in a bad mood. I don't know why that is.

T: Is it an all day thing?

P: There will be a period that I'll be OK, because I'll be with my friends. But as soon as I think about going home, or homework or something, then I'm a hard person to get along with.

T: What do you think triggers it?

P: Well, school plays a major part in it. Major.

T: Thinking about homework, studying?

P: Assignments, tests.

T: What automatic thoughts are associated with those activities? When you think of the fact that tonight you've got to do some homework?

P: I plan it out in my head: "I'll go home and do my homework for an hour and then I'll have the rest of the night to do whatever I want." But then the homework is always left out and I'll say, "I don't feel like doing this; I'll just hang around for a while and then I'll do it after dinner." After dinner comes and I say, "I'll do it at 8 o'clock."

T: OK, there's a point where you get into a bad mood about it. Do your thoughts at that point begin in the early afternoon, midafternoon, after school?

P: Yeah, after school. After school for sure.

T: OK, what's going through your head at that time that puts you in a bad mood?

P: I usually say, "I'm not going to do this. I don't feel like doing this." That's what I think is my automatic thought.

T: "I don't feel like doing this."

P: After I might say to myself, "I don't even know where to begin."

T: "Don't know where to begin."

P: So I don't want to try.

T: When you decide you're not going to try or have thoughts like "I don't really feel like it and it's too hard and I don't know where to begin anyhow," what's the cumulative thought about? If you had to make a single statement about all of this stuff, what would it be that you're saying to yourself?

P: I feel like a failure.

T: You feel like a failure?

P: Yes.

Cognitive Forecasting

Cognitive forecasting refers to the technique of predicting emotions and thoughts or hypothetical future events. It is similar to the technique of cognitive replay except that the focus changes from past to future situations. Young adolescents, in particular, sometimes become impatient with discussing past occurrences. "Out of sight, out of mind" seems to be their unspoken motto, and attempts to engage them in detailed replay of a past event can be difficult. Perhaps a "reliving" of the emotionally provocative event is too painful for them initially, or perhaps they fear criticism of their emotional or behavioral response to the situation. When analysis of past events is difficult, the therapist may make more headway by switching focus to a future hypothetical situation. The imaginary situation can be created so as to include the relevant characters and issues as the real situation the patient is reluctant to discuss. Even young adolescents who have relatively little to say about some event in the past will often be quite willing to engage in discussion of the imaginary situation revealing what they would likely feel and think given a certain set of circumstances.

Example 1

A young boy's parents are separated. He lives with his mother but has been wanting to see his father, who often works out of town. The future circumstance is one likely to occur in his own life, and he quickly reveals the nature of his catastrophic thinking.

T: Let's talk first about your dad. Did you talk to him this week?

P: I tried but he wasn't home. I'll phone again next week when he's back from working out of town.

T: What do you think you might be feeling when you dial this time?

P: Probably nervous again, I would wonder if he's home this time.

T: What would be so bad if he's not home?

P: Then I'd start to get worried that something might have happened to him.

T: What would you be worried about?

P: Well, since he is in construction, I would think that something happened with the dump truck, or he broke his leg in a ditch or something.

Example 2

A young girl has frequent feelings of rejection by her peers at school. The hypothetical scenario quickly reveals her depressogenic thoughts about herself.

T: Well, if somebody said "No," she couldn't go shopping with you, what are the thoughts that would run through your mind?

P: I'd think that she didn't like me.

T: You'd think she didn't like you. That would be your conclusion?

P: Well maybe not that. But I'd take it she's thinking, "Get away from me. I don't want to be seen near you."

T: And after you thought, "She doesn't want to be seen with me," then what would be your next idea?

P: I would probably think that I'm no fun to be with. Or that I'm the last person who she would want to hang around with.

T: Anything else?

Offering Hypotheses

When offering hypotheses to an adolescent, the therapist essentially guesses at what the patient might be thinking in a particular situation. Sometimes patients will endorse an example offered by the therapist and can be encouraged to add other thoughts of their own. Often, patients will not acknowledge that any of the thoughts offered are their own but, instead, will correct the therapist's suggestions.

Example

A 16-year-old female adolescent is upset about the impending move of the family, which will necessitate a change in her school. She is initially unable to explain what is disturbing to her about this situation, but the discussion results in a statement of her belief that moving is a never-ending pattern over which she has little control.

T: How do you see starting a new school as one of the disadvantages of moving?

P: Well, I just started at this school this year. I'm just getting to know students in my school, and now I have to move again.

T: And you will have to meet new teachers and students in September. Is that difficult? Is that hard for you to do?

P: No, but I just get sick of moving all the time.

T: Some people get sick of moving because they don't like putting stuff in boxes. Is that it?

P: No, that doesn't bother me.

T: But I'm just trying to know the thing that makes you really sick about it. Is it the problem of choosing classes that's hard?

P: No.

T: No? Is it getting involved with new students? Or meeting them?

P: Uh huh, yes.

T: Partly that?

P: Yeah, because I'm wondering if I will go to this new school for one semester and then change schools again.

T: Why would you do that again?

P: Every semester it seems I change to a different school. So I think, "Here we go again, moving all the time."

Third-Person Perspective

When the therapist adopts a third-person perspective, someone (real or hypothetical) other than the therapist and patient is introduced as the focus of discussion. The goal is to have the adolescent identify the similarities or differences between himself and this third "other." In general, this technique is possible only with older adolescents who are developmentally able to put themselves in the position of another person. It is sometimes a useful way of eliciting dysfunctional automatic thoughts because imagining the thoughts of some other person may be less threatening than revealing one's own. Of course the therapist must eventually get the patient to relate the discussion of the third person to his own life.

Example

A 16-year-old male who is socially immature is just beginning to develop an interest in girls, but depressogenic cognitions about himself inhibit action toward his desired goal and reinforce his social isolation, in general. The therapist knows from previous discussion that one of the patient's favorite solitary activities is to write stories, so he uses the third-person perspective technique to elicit the patient's thoughts about his own unsatisfactory social situation.

T: One of the things I wanted to ask you about today is how you did on your two make-believe characters. Did you enjoy doing it?

P: Yeah (*referring to homework notes brought with him*). Well, the first one I called Brett Sinclair. He goes on a lot of dates, and he's in grade 11. He's 16 years old. He's very sure of himself and very confident, and when he's asking some girl for a date he feels excited and there may be some anticipation, and maybe he's just a little bit nervous. And some of the thoughts running through his head might be, "Whatever happens happens. This might be the most exciting night of my life," and maybe even "Don't' get your hopes up too high."

T: Uh huh. What about your other character?

P: The second one I called Frank Brown. He's shy and quiet, and he's kind of reserved. He's also 16 in grade 11. He barely has any self-esteem. He's not confident. He's not really sure of himself, and when he's asking for dates he might have doubts, and he assumes and anticipates what the girl might say. Or he might not even try because he thinks the girl will always say "No." I came up with a lot of thoughts like "Oh, she'll never like me, why should I try? Why should I think she likes me? She hates me. Why won't she go out with me? What's wrong with me? If nothing was wrong with me then she'd go out with me." And the last one, "Why can't I be someone like Brett? He acts so cool and how come I can't be like him?"

T: Wow. You did do a lot of thinking about those two imaginary people. When you were getting into the character of Frank Brown, did you draw on your own self to make him up?

P: Yeah, I kind of wrote him like myself.

T: What about Frank Brown is most like you?

P: Shy, quiet, reserved. The thoughts "She'll never like me. Why should I try?" Maybe even sometimes, "I'm so stupid to even think that she likes me." And "Why won't she go out with me? What's wrong with me?"

T: So are all of those thoughts ones that you've had of yourself?
P: Uh huh. That's what I think.

STEP III: IDENTIFICATION OF BELIEFS

Like their adult counterparts, adolescent patients are usually not aware that their beliefs influence their interpretations of events or situations in their lives. Automatic thoughts tend to be specific to particular life experiences. In contrast, beliefs are more general and will typically influence the interpretation of a wide variety of different situations. A set of beliefs concerning a particular topic can be thought of as the patient's "schema" regarding the topic. For example, a "perfectionistic schema" might consist of the following beliefs related to the topic of perfectionism: "An imperfect job is not worth doing"; or "Anything less than perfect is intolerable"; or "Perfection is the only way to demonstrate one's worth." This relatively small set of beliefs related to the topic of perfection could be expected to engender a much larger set of automatic thoughts in response to the specific life circumstances encountered. For example, an adolescent who was reprimanded by his parents for improper behavior during a dinner party might have the automatic thought "I'll never be a decent human being." After an argument with a girlfriend, he might think, "This just demonstrates that I'm a bad person." If a teacher's comments on a school assignment indicated ways to improve the work, he might think, "I'm stupid." A tactical error made during a baseball game might lead to the thought "I can't do anything right." Normal differences of opinion with others might be interpreted as "I'll never get along with people." A sequence of events leading to automatic thoughts such as these might eventually lead to the conclusion "It's hopeless. Why bother trying?" In effect, the automatic thoughts that could occur in response to specific situations are virtually limitless.

When the goal of therapy is to examine the potential role of maladaptive cognitions in contributing to emotional distress, the therapist should be aware of both the patient's automatic thoughts and the underlying beliefs that engender them. The stage of cognitive therapy that explores the adolescent's belief system need not necessarily occur after an extensive exploration of automatic thoughts. In actuality, the identification of thoughts and beliefs often occurs simultaneously, or the therapist moves back and forth, alternately focusing on one and then the other. When automatic thoughts are the focus in therapy, the therapist should be constantly forming hypotheses about the patient's beliefs that might apply across the various situations discussed. When beliefs are the focus in therapy, discussion will focus on the adolescent's general way of viewing things, and questions will often relate to the patient's reasons for reacting in certain ways or the meaning he attaches to certain events.

The identification of beliefs is particularly important when family members are involved in the depressed adolescent's therapy. Over a period of years, children have usually been socialized into a family belief system that may be resulting in the adolescent's depressogenic interpretations of family experiences. Alternatively, the conflicting belief systems of adolescents and their parents can lead to conflictual interactions, which are themselves interpreted in depressogenic ways. The techniques discussed below may be useful in attempting to identify beliefs, which can then be examined to determine their potential role in the adolescent's depression.

Down Arrow Technique

The down arrow technique (called "vertical arrow" by Burns, 1980) refers to a series of questions about the emotional significance of a particular past or anticipated event (or interpretation of it). In essence, the therapist repeatedly asks, "So what?" after each successive patient explanation. Of course, the words "So what?" would seldom be used. Instead, there are varied ways of asking the same question and guiding the focus toward what the therapist anticipates will be a key belief related to the depression. The therapist must show considerable sensitivity when using this technique so as not to frustrate the adolescent with the same question over and over, suggesting that he is not answering the question the first time or that the therapist is not listening. Skilled rewording usually overcomes this potential obstacle to the elicitation of underlying beliefs, which is the goal of this technique.

Example 1

The therapist uses a series of questions that begin with "Why" or words that mean the same. Note the sequence ". . . so horrible, . . . so awful, . . . so terrible, . . . so devastating" that is employed. The down arrow technique succeeds in eliciting a depressogenic belief held by the patient, which is essentially "If one person turns down an invitation from me I'll always be lonely and sad because I'm nothing."

T: Why would you hesitate to ask a girlfriend home from school?

P: Because I wouldn't be sure how she'd react. Or how she'd take it.

T: What do you think are the possible ways she would react?

P: Well, the worst thing she would say is "No way" and walk off.

T: OK, if she said "No" and walked away, what would be so horrible with that?

P: Well it's going to hurt a little because if she just says "No" and nothing else, and then walks off; it feels like a door slammed in your face.

T: So it would hurt a little bit. Yes, I think so. What would be so horrible about that amount of hurt?

P: I don't like to get hurt.

T: Well, I can understand that. But what is the reason that a "No" would be so awful?

P: Because it would mean that she didn't want to see me.

T: So, one person doesn't want to see you. Why's that so terrible?

P: Because no one else would want to be my friend either.

T: I'm not sure that's true. But let's just suppose no one wanted to be your friend. Why would that be so devastating?

P: It would mean I'll always be lonely and sad. I'm nothing.

Example 2

The therapist uses a series of questions that begin with the words "What does it mean that . . . ?" When the patient encounters difficulty with this series of questions, the therapist uses a variant, providing more specific guidance to the adolescent by asking, "What does it mean to you about yourself. . . ?" Eventually, the down arrow questioning succeeds in eliciting the patient's depressogenic belief that "I'm not special."

P: No one said anything until this year about thinking that I might be depressed, which shows that it isn't as personal as I would like it with the teachers or with anybody.

T: What did that mean to you because I'm not sure? Help me understand it. What did it mean to you that none of your teachers said anything about the possibility of you being depressed?

P: Well, now that I think about it, I've probably been depressed for a long time, for years, and no one said it. No one noticed until this year.

T: And what does that mean to you, that no one noticed?

P: No one's paid any attention.

T: What does that mean to you that no one's really paying attention.

P: I wish they were.

T: You wish they were. What does it mean to you that you think they weren't?

P: I don't like it, of course.

T: Why not?

P: It's just if no one is paying attention then you don't like it.

T: What does that say to you about yourself when you think nobody was paying attention to you?

P: I was just there. You know what I mean?

T: What do you mean?

P: I mean they always talk about being lost in thousands of kids and no one knows your name and they hardly know your face.

T: You said you felt nobody was paying attention to you, and I heard you say you didn't like it. What does that mean to you about yourself?

P: I wasn't special.

T: You weren't special, that's what it means?

P: Yeah.

Genogram Probe

The genogram probe refers to the process of focusing discussion on the beliefs of family members other than the adolescent patient. The belief system of a family can exert powerful influences either to support or to unwittingly sabotage the work being done by the adolescent in individual sessions with the therapist. Most often, family members will be unable to state their core beliefs, which, in turn, often give rise to depressogenic automatic thoughts that may exacerbate the adolescent's depression. The therapist will need to inquire about the views of parents and/or siblings in the household and will often find it useful to explore beyond the immediate family to include parents' families of origin. The goal of using a genogram probe is to compare the family beliefs to those of the depressed adolescent. Sometimes the family beliefs will appear to be inadvertently reinforcing the patient's maladaptive beliefs. In such a case, the therapist must work to alter both the adolescent's and the family's belief systems. Sometimes the family beliefs will differ from the depressogenic beliefs of the adolescent patient, and the therapist will find it useful to involve family members as "cotherapists" in assisting the process of change in the patient.

Example 1

This example demonstrates how an entire family of four can hold the same basic belief that "anger is bad" for various different reasons. The discussion not only reveals the beliefs held by the adolescent's family members, but also includes reference to both parents' families of origin. The patient is a 14-year-old female referred for therapy after she impulsively attempted carbon monoxide self-poisoning with the family car. After the session in which the family beliefs about anger were expressed, the therapist hypothesized that the patient, like her parents and brother, had come to believe that anger was a bad thing. As such, when she did feel angry or expressed displeasure with something, she was overcome with guilt for violating the family's implicit code. From her perspective, anger may be "taboo" and to feel or express it may mean risking parental rejection or self-recrimination.

Mom: I don't think any of us really deals with anger in the house at all. I'm afraid of it. When I was raised, there was a lot of anger in my house. My dad was very angry. He yelled and screamed at my mom.

T: What did the anger mean to you?

M: It was really scary. My dad would get very violent. I guess there was a fear that the whole family would fall apart or that he might hit somebody like my mom or us. And I felt responsible somehow because I was the eldest and I always took on a lot of responsibility. So I'm very afraid of anger. When Sandra [daughter] gets angry, I'm afraid. And I don't think that's very helpful for her when I feel that way.

T: What do you think your fear is when Sandra gets angry?

M: I just don't know what she'll do because her anger is channeled destructively a lot of times. That really scares me. With the car exhaust, she was really depressed, and when she gets angry then quite often she'll get depressed after.

T: I hear you saying that just as you felt responsible for keeping everything calm in your childhood home, you again feel responsible for keeping things calm and keeping Sandra placated in some way so she's not too depressed or too angry because that somehow falls onto you to look after these things.

M: I don't really know what to do. She won't talk to me usually when I'm trying to find out what's wrong.

T: It is interesting that one of the things Sandra said herself that she was aware of was the need to talk more about how she was feeling. (*to patient*) Is it OK if I tell them a little bit about you and Bob [boyfriend]?

P: (*Shakes her head "yes."*)

T: OK. For example, when Sandra and Bob would have some difficulty, one of his requests was that she be more open explaining when she gets angry and what she's angry about. She thought that if she could learn to be more expressive instead of just acting angry, it would help the relationship. Sounds like that's not only true with Bob but maybe the people Sandra lives with too.

Brother: [older brother is 18] I didn't used to talk about my problems either. I'd hold things inside of me. My mom would talk to me for hours trying to get things out of me. I've been doing a lot better with that because Adele [girlfriend] tells me when I'm mad at her I need to tell her I'm mad at her. I wouldn't talk to her at first, but now I do tell her right away when I'm mad at her and why.

T: So your girlfriend has had the same complaint about you as Bob has had about your sister. Is that right?

B: Yeah. I guess so.

M: It's the same with Dave [husband]. I didn't know he was angry at something last week, and he told me 2 days after why the wrath of Dave came down. But for 2 days he's angry at me, and so I think no wonder Sandra [daughter] reacts like this. Our house is full of people who do this, who have trouble with anger.

T: Well you [mom] did some explaining about your history with anger. I'm wondering a little bit about Dave [husband], about your history with anger.

Dad: Well I never realized it much, but I've had it pointed out to me my father was the same. That could be where it comes from.

T: Your father was a punitive or angry man?

D: Well he would hold things—kept it all to himself.

M: His [Dave's] mother was more punitive, but his father would escape. He would go to the garage or he'd escape some way, which is what I see Sandra actually doing when she gets angry and refuses to discuss things.

T: (*to patient*) What would be so bad about just really getting angry, instead of being mad in silence?

P: Because they [her parents] get mad at you when you do that.

T: You mean they get mad if you get angry?

P: No, I mean they get mad if I yell.

T: Well, if you're angry don't you have the right to express that?

P: They don't like it.

M: (*returning focus to husband*) I think how Dave expresses it is by criticizing others or putting people down. If something's wrong he blames somebody else. He can get angry, but I don't want to be blamed for what's going on.

T: (*to patient*) Is blaming how anger is expressed in your house?

P: Yeah.

T: Does your mom get angry?

P: Yeah. She usually tells you though when she's angry. She doesn't yell.

T: She says, "I'm mad because you did this . . ."?

P: Yeah.

T: And does that feel like blame to you?

P: No, mom doesn't blame me.

T: How is your dad different?

P: He makes it my fault.

T: (*to dad*) So what you hear them saying is you can get angry. Go ahead, it's fine. But you have to be careful how much you're pointing a finger at people when you're angry. I guess that's what they're saying.

M: Well I think Dave is really uncomfortable discussing his feelings though. So I think I'm afraid of his anger because when he gets angry I don't know what he's going to do. He often does the same thing as his sister. His sister's husband says he hates their house because it's so scary. He actually takes the children and they leave because he gets so scared of his wife's anger.

T: (*to mom*) Are you afraid when Dave gets angry?

M: Oh yeah.

T: Well, what do you think will happen?

M: I'm afraid of him . . .

T: That he'll punch you?

M: I'm not sure what. He breaks things or throws things or he gets physical when he's angry too. And when both of them [daughter and father] are angry, it's really scary because of all the tension. I'm afraid they are going to kill each other some day because they both want to be physical instead of thinking in a positive way to resolve the conflict.

T: Would it be OK for voices to get raised when people are angry?

M: Sure as long as they're not hitting each other. But not swearing and not feeling as if your life is in danger, that they're going to get hurt or I'm going to get hurt.

T: By getting loud? Animated?

M: That would be all right. I guess that would be anger that I could manage.

[Discussion continues to explore family beliefs on the expression of anger.]

Example 2

The adolescent's mother spontaneously describes her belief about her parental responsibilities in response to the therapist's inquiry about her heightened affect in the session. Through further discussion, the therapist learns that the patient and his mother appear to hold a common belief that the adolescent is irresponsible and largely incompetent. The fact that this belief appears to be common to the two of them probably reinforces the boy's dependency on his mother and exacerbates his depression because his sense of self-efficacy is repeatedly challenged. The excerpt concerns an 18-year-old adolescent who lives at home with his parents and has had problems keeping jobs and managing money. Just prior to the following excerpt, it had been revealed that the patient had "borrowed" some money from his mother to cover credit charges, but both are keeping this a secret from his father.

Mom: I think if I could go back and do some things over I'd try to be a lot more open. And I wouldn't let this pattern of secrecy get started. I take responsibility for that.

T: How do you think it would be different if you were more open in your family?

M: I think it wouldn't be as stressful. I think I realize that I always want to be little mother hen going around and making everything OK.

T: You look after people?

M: Yes, a lot. So I think if I could approach things different, maybe some things would've been different. But I think I take the caretaker role a lot. Really, I'm always making sure everybody's OK, everybody's happy. I guess I seem to think that I can take care of everybody.

T: On the other side of that though, it sounds like, when things are not going well, you feel it's your fault.

M: Yeah, I think I'm like that too. I blame myself a lot.

T: But if you're responsible for everything and you think you're at fault when things go wrong, I wonder if it makes it hard for Bruce [patient] to feel independent or to be on his own and do his own thing. I wonder if he feels overly dependent and that affects his depression?

M: Sometimes I don't honestly know what he'd do without me.

P: Sometimes I really do need a hand. After all, she is my mom. (*Mom begins to cry.*)

T: (*to mom*) How are you coping with the belief "I'm responsible for things not going well"?

M: I guess I don't have an answer for that (*crying more*).

T: How do you think it's affected you to have that belief?

M: I'm sure it's not healthy for me.

T: When you think that you need to make everybody happy, to make things go well, how do you feel?

M: It just goes back to my own family for me. I was always looking after things for people when I was at home.

T: The reason that I'm sort of pushing you to look at your beliefs is that they can generate negative feelings, like worry or guilt, which are dysfunctional. And if you see your belief about looking after people as dysfunctional or one that is irrational, then you might know where to start making changes that could be helpful to you and to Bruce, to his depression.

Example 3

The therapist elicits a father's beliefs about parental duty to protect adolescents. Unlike in the previous example, the adolescent's and her father's beliefs are different and, as such, lead to considerable conflict. In essence, father believes that his daughter is somewhat irresponsible and emotionally unstable, a view the patient does not share. Father's beliefs about his daughter affect not only her activities but also her developmentally appropriate wish to individuate. As her father repeatedly challenges her sense of independence and self-efficacy, her depression worsens. Note how events in the family's history have influenced father's beliefs. Father and daughter are the only two people living in the household.

T: (*to patient*) I've heard your dad say he's scared you'll actually commit suicide. (*to dad*) Is that what you're telling me?

Dad: No, I'm scared she's doing all these things so that she can accidentally kill herself. So she doesn't have to make a decision to go out and do it. In some way in the back of her mind. . .

T: You're scared that she might end up in situations where she would accidentally die and in some way secretly have a wish to die?

D: Yeah, sort of subconsciously. Because she doesn't want to make that decision. She gets all depressed and instead of sitting down and talking to somebody, she tries to kill herself. See, this is another thing that her mother was like. If she had a problem, she didn't want to admit it to anyone. Sometimes I sit there and think it's easier for Jennifer [daughter] to do this so no one can say, "You're a coward." Instead she has an accident to kill herself.

T: (*to dad*) I hear you saying that you see similarities between Jennifer's mother and Jennifer.

D: Uh huh. I do.

T: You saw your wife die in a car accident, and you're wondering if she had some unconscious wish of death. She had a depression in her adolescence too. Is that right?

D: Yes, she did. They have a lot of similarities.

T: (*to patient*) I hear your dad has some deep-seated concerns for your safety. Those are legitimate, I think. Your dad does care for you and is worried. (*to dad*) What I think is important for us though is that you may be trying to save Jennifer from a worry that is yours, not from a danger that's hers. I think it would be important to try and find some way to trust that Jennifer is not your late wife.

D: I'm not totally rigid with Jennifer. If she wants to go off and do her thing with her friends, I don't say, "No you can't do that." I respect her opinion. I respect her abilities. I think I rarely veto any decisions. I haven't since she was little because I always wanted her to be able to think things out. But it's my job to protect her.

T: Is it, at age 17?

D: Well, it starts when they're born. You learn to provide for them, to protect them. Like you don't let your kids play on the street because that's not right. So it progresses as they grow up.

Offering Hypotheses

When the therapist offers a hypothesis about a belief that may be held by the patient or family, essentially a suggestion is made for the adolescent and/or family members to consider. The suggestion may be accepted as stated or revised to more accurately reflect the actual family belief. Alternatively, individual family members may endorse their own specific variations of the belief suggested by the therapist.

Example

The therapist offers a hypothesis about parents' beliefs that may be influencing their overinvolvement with their adolescent son, the patient. The patient in question is an exceptionally talented 17-year-old, very mature for his age, who has been pursuing a "career" in figure skating since a young age. He has won several international competitions and is struggling to balance the demands of this pursuit while completing high school. His parents are very supportive of his skating but appear to be overly involved and anxious about their son's various life pursuits. Their anxiety, in turn, may be contributing to their son's feeling of inadequacy, which is central to his depression.

T: (*to dad*) Let me ask you, in general, does Brian take on big jobs that have the potential to bring disappointment or depression?

Dad: No, I don't think so. But I think it's reasonable at the same time that he may be a little bit like myself. I remember when I went to University I had difficulties getting organized to achieve a lot within a reasonable time. I was wasting lots of time. He doesn't want to be reminded he's 17, but I think it's still very young to reach the stage where you can really organize yourself to maximum efficiency.

T: And maybe being in high school that's to be expected. I would hope that there is some room for not being a perfect time manager in high school.

D: Sure. But he has a lot on his plate.

T: You see, the demands of perfection can be oppressive.

Mom: That's right. But I think what my husband means is that what Brian is up to is much more difficult than for most kids in high school. When the pressure gets too great, he can get into trouble like last summer.

T: I'm wondering if Brian has changed since last summer, if he is more willing to handle the math, more willing to set skating aside sometimes. Is it a demonstration of his ability to juggle things appropriately?

D: Oh, I think he's capable. I think it's just hard on him. I think unnecessarily difficult.

T: (*to patient*) I hear the concerns of your parents, who seem to be speaking about the demands on you and the pressure you may feel.

P: Uh huh.

T: (*to parents*) I hear your concern. I also see the need for somebody to experience, to be allowed the independence that goes with growing up and with being responsible. He needs to be allowed to make some mistakes. If he's not a perfect teenager, that would be normal. Actually to be a perfect teenager you'd make some mistakes.

P: That's the one thing I wanted to bring out of this conversation. Last week, I got mad at the attitude my parents have. Because I made some mistakes this summer, I got the feeling that they think I didn't learn anything and that I don't have the strength to refuse what I think is wrong, that I don't know what is wrong.

M: No, no, Brian.

P: Well, it feels like you don't trust me. You always think something bad is going to happen.

T: I'm wondering if one of the prevailing ways of thinking in your family is to assume the worst. Perhaps that has had an impact on Brian and his depression and your relationships with your son. Maybe some change in family thinking style needs to occur.

P: I would think probably "yes," but I can't see that happening.

T: Well, you may be right. It may not happen equally for everyone.

P: I've been trying to change the way I think and in that respect things are easier at home. I try not to predict the worst when I'm with my parents, but I don't want to be the only one that's changing.

T: I agree. That's why I have a strong interest in working with parents as well as kids because I wonder if there's an idea in your parents' heads that's driving their behavior. Is it possible that your parents think, "Adolescents don't know what they're doing," or "Independence is dangerous." Maybe there's something in their minds that is influencing them to interfere in your life in ways that you find frustrating.

[Discussion continues to explore these two potential parental beliefs.]

STEP IV: EVALUATION OF AUTOMATIC THOUGHTS AND BELIEFS

Once the adolescent's thoughts and/or beliefs have been identified, the next step in the cognitive therapy process is to evaluate these cognitions to determine whether or not they are maladaptive. The therapist should not assume that cognitions are maladaptive just because they are associated with emotional distress. Sometimes the thoughts associated with life events or the beliefs regarding some issue are perfectly reasonable in spite of the fact that emotional distress is associated with them. For example, thinking that one is being mistreated and responding with anger or depression would be a realistic response to the experience of abuse. In such cases, cognitions such as "This treatment is wrong," or "I am being mistreated," would be regarded as adaptive because they could lead to behavioral or environmental change. Under such circumstances, the therapist would be doing the adolescent a disservice to focus on changing thoughts or beliefs about the situation. Instead, intervention would most appropriately focus on solving the problem of abuse. Various techniques for evaluating cognitions are discussed below.

Identifying Cognitive Distortions

Cognitive distortions are habitual ways of interpreting information that alter reality so that an unnecessarily negative view of one's self, circumstances, or future is generated. Various taxonomies for describing distortions have been proposed, each offering slightly different labels and definitions (e.g., Beck et al., 1979; Burns, 1980). In our work with depressed adolescents, we have found the taxonomy described by Burns to be extremely useful. For application with an adolescent population, therapists may find it helpful to discuss "thinking errors" rather than "cognitive distortions" and to substitute the "adult" examples in Burns's work with ones containing more "adolescent" content, such as those demonstrated below. With older adolescents, an effective way of introducing the distortions is to relate one or more of them to the patient's description of his own life experiences and then to assign some reading to see if the adolescent can identify any additional maladaptive thinking patterns in the coming weeks. With younger adolescents, the therapist will usually need to take a more active role in identifying one or two central distortions during the course of a therapy session.

The identification of cognitive distortions is also a useful technique to employ with the parents of depressed adolescents. Families often have habitual ways of interpreting things, some of which may distort reality in a way that is harmful to the patient or the parents themselves. When therapists help parents evaluate their own automatic thoughts by identifying cognitive errors, it is important to point out the potential impact of the parents' thinking styles on the adolescent patient.

Ten cognitive distortions, written with examples typical of adolescent patients, are described below. The list has been adapted from Burns (1980), although the order of presentation has been changed to reflect what are often the most commonly identified distortions with adolescents (those earlier in the list). In addition, the names of several distortions have been altered to make them more comprehensible for a younger patient population.

1. Binocular Vision

Binocular Magnification. Normally when you look through binoculars, things look bigger than they are in reality. This thinking style is especially dangerous when you focus on difficulties or disappointments in your life because binocular vision can make negative things seem unbearable. Instead of being a disappointment, something can seem disastrous. A slight difficulty can seem like an impossible problem. In other words, you tend to see things as catastrophes. Some adolescents specialize in this thinking style after they have experienced bitter disappointments. When things get magnified in this way, you may become overly upset or give up trying when it is not necessary.

> Michael has some arithmetic homework to do before school the next day. Sometimes he has difficulty with school work, so even though he has the whole evening to get the three questions done, he begins thinking the task is far too enormous to accomplish in the short amount of time available. He concludes that completion of his homework is impossible. He has thoughts like "This is too much for me," and "It's a lost cause so why should I even try."

Clues to Michael's binocular vision are the following words: "enormous," "impossible," "too much," "lost cause."

Binocular Shrinking. If you look through binoculars another way, things can be made to look much smaller than they are in reality. This type of binocular vision causes the most problems when it is used to distort positive things about yourself or your life because you do not give yourself the credit you deserve or you disregard pleasant events as "nothing." Instead of feeling good about a special accomplishment, you might view it as nothing unusual. Or instead of thinking that someone worked hard to arrange something special for you, you might view their efforts as nothing out of the ordinary.

> Carla has recently changed schools and has met only one girl in her new location. This friend discovers Carla's birthday is coming soon. To help Carla meet some other kids, her friend organizes a surprise birthday party to which everyone comes. Carla does not think much about the event and dismisses it as "no big deal." Because she views the party this way, she makes no attempt to show her friend that it is appreciated and she continues treating everyone at her new school like strangers, in spite of their friendliness toward her.

Clues to Carla's binocular vision include the following:

- She does not think much about the party afterward.
- She views the event as "no big deal."
- She does not tell her friend that the party was appreciated.
- She makes no attempts to repay other people's friendliness with some of her own.

2. Black-and-White Thinking

This style of thinking is the tendency to see things in only two extreme ways. For example, experiences are great or terrible, life is good or bad, people are best friends or worst enemies. Words that are clues to this kind of thinking include opposites like "always–never" and "all–none." Black-and-white thinking typically is not realistic because things usually are not *totally* one way or another.

> John gets a poor mark on his science test. Although he has received some decent marks in the past, he sees the poor mark as evidence that he is "a complete failure in school." He has thoughts like "I'm totally useless at school work," and "I'm a disaster as a student."

Clues to John's black-and-white thinking are the words: "complete failure," "totally useless," "disaster."

3. Dark Glasses

Dark glasses block out brightness so that what you see is a "blackened" version of the real world. This thinking style occurs when you focus on the undesirable aspects of some situation or when you pay attention only to the most negative information and ignore what is more positive. By wearing dark glasses, what you think about yourself or your life tends to be the worst view instead of a balanced view that includes both the favorable and unfavorable parts of the whole.

> Matthew enjoys listening to the latest popular music and has a large collection of his own that includes most of the current bands. For a school dance, he volunteers to bring his collection of music and be the disc jockey. After the event, he hears that most students think his selections for the dance were good but that, in the second half of the evening, he was a little too slow changing from one song to the next. Some people feel that his slowness in getting the next selection playing resulted in a few kids losing their enthusiasm for dancing and sitting down or finding other things to do. Matthew concludes that the dance was a "flop" and decides that he will never again volunteer to be the DJ. Over and over in his mind he remembers things like "I was too slow," and "People got bored waiting for me to get the next song playing."

A clue to Matthew's use of dark glasses is the fact that he ignores the following comments about his night as DJ:

- "He has a huge collection of music."
- "He generously gave a lot of his time to the dance."
- "He made really good selections."
- "His timing for part of the dance was great."
- "Most of the kids didn't lose enthusiasm for dancing at any time during this evening."

4. Fortune Telling

Predicting the Future. One type of fortune telling occurs when you make predictions about what will happen in the future without enough evidence. This thinking style is a problem if you predict negative things about the future because it can lead you to start acting as if these negative things had already happened. Even though your prediction might be wrong, you start feeling bad and do something or give something up that is not necessary.

> Lisa really wants to get a part in the school play. A few days before the rehearsal to select actors, she starts to think that her chances of being picked are small because a lot of girls are going to try out. Eventually, she concludes that there is no point in going to the rehearsal because she would not be successful anyway. Instead, she plans something else for that day. Lisa has thoughts like "There are too many girls for me to get a part," and "I don't stand a chance."

Clues to Lisa's fortune telling were the following predictions she made without enough evidence:

- "There are too many other girls."
- "I won't get a part."
- "I don't stand a chance."

Mind Reading. This is a type of fortune telling in which you predict what other people are thinking without enough evidence to back up your conclusions. You can end up feeling very bad about yourself or other people by using this thinking style if you assume the worst about their opinion. The problem is that you might be wrong and suffer bad feelings or even lose a friend because you jumped to a conclusion without getting enough information.

> Aaron misses a chance to score in the last minute of a basketball playoff game. The spectators from his school groan because the bas-

ket would have won the trophy for their school. After the game, he starts avoiding his teammates and other school friends because he concludes that everyone blames him for blowing the whole year. He has thoughts like "The coach wishes he kept me on the bench," and "Our team captain has decided that he will never give me a chance again."

Clues to Aaron's mind reading are the following assumptions he made about other people's opinions without adequate evidence:

- "The coach wishes . . ."
- "The team captain has decided . . ."

5. Heart Talk

When you listen to your heart talk, you allow your feelings to decide what the reality of the situation is. For example, just because you feel like a nerd, you conclude that you are, in fact, a nerd. Sometimes, an occurrence will feel like a disaster, and so you decide that it actually is a disaster. But in reality, your feelings can often be misleading, so if a more realistic assessment of the situation were made, the facts would not support your conclusion that you are a nerd, or that a particular event is a disaster.

Brett is invited to spend the weekend with his friend's family visiting their ranch. He has a great time riding horses and thoroughly enjoys the trip out of the city. After several miles of driving back home at the end of the weekend, he remembers that he had left his jacket with his house key in the pocket hanging in the barn at the ranch. Although his friend's father does not seem to mind going back for it, Brett feels terribly embarrassed about what he thinks is a disaster and concludes that he is an irresponsible goof-up. He has thoughts like "I'm an idiot," and "Something's wrong with my head."

The clues to Brett's emotional reasoning are the following:

- Based on feeling embarrassed, he makes the following erroneous conclusions: (1) the trip is a disaster, (2) he is an irresponsible goof-up, (3) he is an idiot, and (4) something is wrong with his head.

- Brett ignores the reality of the situation that: (1) they have not traveled very far when he remembers his keys, (2) his friend's father does not mind going back.

6. Personalizing

This thinking style occurs when you take personal responsibility for things that are not your job or things that are not in your power to control. Even though part of the responsibility might be yours, you tend to forget that the other part belongs to someone else. Sometimes you might even take responsibility for things that are beyond anyone's power to control. When things do not work out the best way, you tend to blame yourself even for things that you could not possibly have controlled.

> Ellen invites several of her friends to a party at her home. The barbecue starts off well, with everyone having a good time. Then two of her guests get into an argument about one of the teachers at school and will not speak to each other for the rest of the party. Furthermore, an unexpected storm blows in so the backyard volleyball game gets interrupted, and all the food has to be moved into the house where her younger sister becomes a pest. Ellen decides she has let everyone down by having a bad party. She has thoughts like "It is my job to ensure everyone has a good time," and "Why can't I have a successful party?"

The clue to Ellen's personalizing is the way she blames herself for the following things beyond her control: the two friends arguing over a teacher, the two friends deciding not to speak to each other, the storm, the interrupted volleyball game, the move indoors, her younger sister being a nuisance.

7. Overgeneralizing

This style of thinking occurs when you use one example of something to draw conclusions about lots of other things, or all similar circumstances. Just because one experience is unpleasant, it does not mean that life in general is not going well. Even if you have had several disappointments, you will be overgeneralizing if you see life as one big letdown.

Rosanne dates a boy from her school a few times, but they have several arguments, and she eventually refuses to go out with him any more. She concludes that guys are hopeless. Her thoughts includes things like "One is as bad as the rest," and "Jason's just like all the others."

Clues to Rosanne's overgeneralization are the following pairs of words: "one" . . . "the rest" and "Jason" . . . "all the others"

8. Labeling

Just as a label on a box of cereal summarizes the contents of it, a label on a person summarizes what that person is like. The problem is that people are much more complicated than cereal boxes, so one label cannot possibly capture all aspects of the person. Labels cause the most problems for your emotional well-being when they are negative, because negative labels erroneously suggest that the entire person is "bad." Labeling yourself and labeling other people are both summaries that are not accurate.

Daniel has a part-time job stocking shelves at a supermarket. Most of the time, his boss is a nice guy. But one day when Daniel finishes putting a huge box of cans on a shelf, his boss insists that he stay late in order to move them to a different location in the store. Daniel concludes that his boss is a "jerk" with no feelings for anyone else. Daniel has thoughts like "The guy is just a complete dictator," and "What a pig." The more he rehearses these ideas, the angrier he becomes.

Clues to Daniel's labeling are the following single words that he used to describe his boss as a whole person: "jerk," "dictator," "pig."

9. Disqualifying the Positive

When you disqualify the positive, you turn something positive into something negative instead. This style of thinking is especially dangerous because two things happen: first, you miss out on the positive thing that occurred in your life and, second, you experience something negative that is a creation of your own mind.

Jessica has received some money for her birthday and spends it on some new clothes for herself. When she wears one of her new sweaters to school, a friend tells her she looks especially nice and that her sweater goes well with her other clothes. Instead of being pleased, Jessica concludes that most of the time she looks awful and decides that her friend probably just wants to borrow the sweater for her own use. She has thoughts like "I'm not attractive," and "No one likes me for who I am."

The clues to Jessica's disqualification of the positive include changing the following positives into negatives:

- "You look nice" changes into "I usually look awful."
- "You have a nice sweater" changes into "I'm not attractive."
- "Your sweater suits you" changes into "No one likes me."

10. Should-y/Must-y Thinking

With this thinking style, you beat yourself up or beat other people up with ideas about what should and must be done. Rather than thinking it would be better if you did something or it would be nice if someone else behaved a certain way, you insist that you or other people act in the way you think is best. By demanding in your own head that something be the way you want it, you set yourself up for being unrealistically angry at yourself or someone else. Sometimes by demanding that you behave a certain way, you set yourself up for being unrealistically guilty.

> Andrea knows that her mother is expecting several guests for Thanksgiving dinner and will have a lot of work to do for the meal. She realizes that her mother would probably appreciate her help to entertain the younger children for a few hours so that her mom can concentrate on the meal preparations. When a friend asks Andrea to go to a movie that day, she readily accepts the invitation and forgets all about the big Thanksgiving dinner. Later she concludes that she should have said "no" and should have helped her mother. She has thoughts like "Caring children must be thoughtful at busy family times," and "Good daughters must remember to offer their help." The more she tells herself what she should and must do, the worse she feels about the situation.

Clues to Andrea's should-y and must-y thinking are the following words: "should" have said no to her friend, "should" have helped her mother, caring children "must" be thoughtful . . . , good daughters "must" remember. . . .

Discussion of Adolescent Thinking Distortions

Most adolescents find identification of the distortion an extremely interesting and useful technique. Reading the "menu" of 10 distortions presented above is often an exercise that captures their attention quickly, as if the examples hold some secret about themselves. Even when the therapist names a single distortion to describe what appears to be a systematic style of thinking, adolescents typically understand and apply the idea to several situations in their lives, although younger patients may require the additional use of a concrete metaphor such as is presented in the first example below.

Example 1. In the first example, the patient is a 13-year-old developmentally delayed male. The therapist identifies for him the "dark glasses" distortion first by giving a definition and then by using a metaphor the boy is likely to understand.

T: One of the things that I noticed through this session is that there was a tendency for you to focus on the negative.
P: I always focus on the negative.
T: OK. What's the price you pay if you do that?
P: Thinking negatively.
T: And, what else?
P: Being negative.
T: And what effect does that have on your real life if you do that?
P: I don't know. I get really upset.
T: It makes you upset?
P: Yeah.
T: What does it do to your real-life relationships with family and school people?
P: It doesn't make me feel real good; I feel bad.
T: Right. Well one of the things I'm concerned about is that it sets up a self-fulfilling prophecy. If you think negatively about someone, usually you'll see it. If the mind's primed, you seem to confirm your view and so it kind of narrows you down. So you can always confirm negative views if you look hard enough. You know what I mean? So I am concerned that, if you have that style, it sets you up for problems. And so I want to help you focus on seeing positive things.

P: I can't, it's hard.

T: Sometimes it is. But I just want to emphasize that I see you being a real specialist by focusing on negatives, and I'm going to have to get rose-tinted spectacles and bring them in here. That way you can come here looking through rosy spectacles so you can see the good things as well as the bad, OK? So try and keep that as a balance.

Example 2. With adolescents who are more able to adopt a "metaposition" than the boy in the previous example, therapists often find it useful to have the patients themselves identify the distortion. In the following example, the therapist has written down some of the key statements made by the patient during the session and reads them aloud for him to evaluate later in the session. Although the distortion is black-and-white thinking, the therapist adjusts the label so it is appropriate for the patient in question. The pattern of "always–never" thinking is identified as problematic.

T: One more thing before we stop [at the end of the session]. Tell me if you see a pattern in this. OK? (*Reads some of the patient's statements during the session back to him.*) "We never have money. I never get anything. Nothing's ever gonna work."

P: It keeps going down. I mean the thoughts just slip. That's kind of sad but then there's no hope.

T: Right. You've got it. And what's the word in there that really makes it like there's no hope?

P: "Never."

T: So if you were just thinking to yourself, "This is bad," you would not be real happy. OK? But if you were thinking to yourself, "This is never going to change," what would that do to you?

P: It would make me feel worse because I'd think never.

T: Yeah. Now one thing that you should know is that we've talked about you having depression. Right?

P: Uh huh.

T: Depression is an illness that can really affect the way that you think. And the way that you think affects the way that you feel. It is real typical of kids to think in "never" terms. And as you said, "never" makes it feel much worse than it is. So one of the things that you and I need to do is keep our eyes open for those "nevers."

P: OK.

T: We need to stop for today. What do you think was helpful to you in what we just talked about?

P: Now I know how to deal with problems and all that. Try to make myself think not to say "never."

T: Not say "never." And realize that you have some choices in what you say to yourself. OK? Sometimes we don't realize that we choose what to say. We just do it automatically.

P: Uh huh.

T: But if you can see your choices you'll be more than halfway to making yourself feel better.

Example 3. In the following excerpt from a family session with a young girl and her mother, the therapist identifies for the patient's mother her tendency to think in dichotomous terms (all-or-nothing thinking) and the impact that such a cognitive error may have on her daughter.

Mom: We had kind of a bout last night. It was probably just exhaustion and different things, her not picking up her clothes, and I kind of unloaded on her last night. What came out is that she was saying to me that we're all too quickly telling her what she's done wrong, but we never tell her what she does right. So I need to be working on that, to try to be more complimentary about what she does than just what she does wrong.

T: Jessica, you learned to point this out? So you could tell your mom what she needed to do?

P: Yeah.

M: There had just been several things that happened over the day, and I let them all build up instead of taking care of each one of them at the time, which is something else I'm going to have to work on real hard too. I apologized to her, and I told her that I think it was more of my frustration than her behavior.

T: Jessica, how did you feel about what happened last night?

P: I just sat there and let her talk. She usually doesn't get that mad over something like that, it seems.

M: You know, I thought at least she's controlling it, and I'm the one going off the wall and I thought, "I'd better change my perspective here." It was flashing through my mind that I was the one being unreasonable. It hit me that I was unloading on her for something very simple, for what she'd done prior in the day.

T: OK. Well that's great. You noticed your own thought patterns too.

M: It's so easy to fall into the old trap and just unload and let all of your anger go on the other person.

T: Yeah. You could have easily said to yourself, "She never picks up her room. She always does this." Do you remember we talked about your daughter's "all-or-nothing" thinking? And it's easy to let yourself get fired up when you do that. But if your anger is unreasonable, that could have an impact on Jessica's depression.

M: Yeah. I realize I'm going to have to take a more balanced view.

Double-Standard Technique

The double-standard technique refers to the use of comparison between the patient's cognitions and those of someone else. The "other" may be a specific person known to the adolescent or a hypothetical person. Alternatively, the "other" may be a collective of people such as "people in general" or "most teenagers." The goal of comparison is to evaluate the reasonableness of the patient's automatic thoughts and beliefs, with differences between the cognitions of the patient and others being clues to potential problems in thinking style.

Example 1

An adolescent female tends to make self-deprecatory interpretations whenever she is disappointed in social interactions. The therapist encourages her to evaluate her automatic thoughts by comparing them to those she imagines a specific girlfriend would have in a situation similar to the one presented by the patient.

T: Suppose your friend Leah told someone that she liked him and hoped that maybe they could do something together, and the guy that she was talking to said, "Well, no. I like you, I think you're nice, but I don't really want to go out with you. I don't really want to have a date." How would Leah interpret that?

P: She wouldn't take offense from it. She'd just move on. Not like me.

T: Well what would her explanation be? How would she be different from you?

P: Well she wouldn't react like me. She wouldn't take that as "Oh, he doesn't like me," or "He thinks I must be the ugliest thing on the planet." She wouldn't really dwell on it; she just kind of moves on. She doesn't make assumptions about the worst.

Example 2

An attractive female adolescent has been struggling with depressogenic views about her physical appearance. In an attempt to have her modify her belief that she is ugly, the therapist first asks her to compare her self-criticisms to those of other people who would not make such a negative global evaluation of their physical appearance and then asks her to use the double-standard technique in collecting some empirical evidence for homework during the coming week.

P: And I guess one of the biggest things is instead of channeling my energy into hating myself, I started to channel it into liking myself better. Doing things so I'll like myself better.

T: Uh huh. Give me an example if you can.

P: If I think I'm fat I tell myself, "Well, if you think you're fat, that's fine, then go and do 20 sit-ups or something like that." I mean it may seem kind of silly, but that's a way for me to make myself feel better.

T: How does it make you feel better? What goes on inside your head that makes you feel better when you have a thought like that?

P: I used to get really down on myself and depressed and think, "I'm fat," and "I don't like the way I look," and then go eat a box of cookies. Instead of doing that, I can do something toward it, and I know that instead of just sitting there and saying, "I'm fat," I can do something about it.

T: OK, so that means you have a sense of control.

P: Yeah.

T: You're getting some sense of mastery or some power over your problem and that's the important thing. Is there anything about yourself physically that you like?

P: You had to ask that (*said jokingly*)! Well, no.

T: No? No redeeming qualities from your point of view?

P: They don't come to mind.

T: Is this something we should definitely be paying attention to?

P: Yeah.

T: How do you think many people would view themselves in terms of their physical appearance? Would they be happy with it or overjoyed with it?

P: I don't know. I suppose everybody thinks they have things that could be better, improved.

T: Uh huh. That's probably right. Would you like to check that out?

P: Uh huh.

T: You could do that for next time. Maybe I could ask you to check out with other people how they feel abut their own physical appearance. Do you see what I'm getting at?

P: That's actually a good idea.

T: Do you see what I'm getting at by doing that? What do you think I'm trying to get you to do there, to point out?

P: Uh, make me realize that people like things about themselves, but there are things that they don't like too.

Pro–Con Evaluation

Pro–con evaluation (similar to "cost–benefit" analysis; Burns, 1980) is a technique used to help the adolescent evaluate his cognitions by enumerating the advantages as well as the disadvantages of a particular situation. It is useful when the depressed patient appears to have adopted a particularly biased view, focusing primarily on the negative aspects of some circumstance. When the goal is to help the adolescent generate a more balanced interpretation, it is important that the therapist avoid focusing only on the more positive point of view because such a strategy may be interpreted as confrontational. In other words, the depressed adolescent may feel "unheard" and reject the positive side of the "pro–con" evaluation.

Example

A female high school student has revealed her ambivalence about the family's plans to move. Because the patient was somewhat ambivalent, the therapist chose to explore the potentially positive aspects of the move first. If the patient had been highly distressed about the move, asking her about the perceived disadvantages before exploring the possibility of any advantages might have been advisable.

P: I found out that we're moving for sure.

T: So how do you feel about that?

P: I'm kind of upset about it, I guess. I don't really know what to think.

T: Well, is there anything that you would categorize as positive about the move? Anything good about it?

P: I don't know for me, but I guess for my parents it's good because they're getting the big house they always wanted.

T: So you think the size of the house is attractive to them. Will a bigger house mean anything for you?

P: Yeah.

T: What?

P: More space.

T: How so? Will you get two bedrooms instead of one?

P: It's like three bedrooms. Compared to my bedroom now, it's like three times the size.

T: Does that make you feel better?

P: A bit. I'll have more room.

T: Will a bigger house give all of the family members more privacy? Or about the same?

P: I think more privacy.

T: Will that be useful for you or don't you really care?

P: I guess that doesn't really matter to me. But I can walk to school. It's only 2 minutes away.

T: Do you view that as an advantage to be able to walk to school, to be 2 minutes away?

P: Yes, because I don't have to take a bus for a half an hour or 45 minutes going to school.

T: What will you do with the time instead?

P: I'll be able to have breakfast in the morning.

T: OK, more time for breakfast. What else?

P: More time to get ready. Don't have to rush to the bus stop.

T: OK. Those certainly sound like some advantages, I agree. What things other than the particular house being bigger and the house being closer to school—is there anything else that's sort of an advantage for you with this move?

P: Not really.

T: OK. What about the disadvantages? How do you explain those?

P: Uh, not being able to see my friends again. Because when am I going to get time to visit with them?

T: OK. What else?

P: I think it's the whole point of changing schools again.

T: Another new school, uh huh. Anything else?

P: No. That's all.

T: OK. I'd like to understand these two disadvantages that you mentioned. The thing about starting a new school, how do you view that as a problem?

Sometimes it is useful to help the adolescent chart the advantages and disadvantages so that a concrete visual representation of a more balanced view is produced. Patients can also be encouraged to develop such charts at home to summarize the issues discussed in session or considered on their own after the session. The chart in Table 8.3 was developed by the therapist during the discussion with the patient above about the family move. Her homework for the next session was to attempt adding to the list of pros and cons in a balanced fashion.

Contradictory Evidence

The pursuit of contradictory evidence refers to the practice of examining factual information that contradicts the depressed adolescent's automatic thoughts or beliefs (Beck et al., 1979; Burns, 1980). The contradictory evidence can sometimes be generated by the patient himself in response to direct therapist request, for example, "Is there anything to suggest that you're not completely right in your thinking about that?" Alternatively, a series of therapist's questions may lead the patient to reveal contradictory evidence, which can then be identified for the adolescent.

Example

The patient in the following example feels insecure with friends and worries that they do not like him. He has revealed automatic thoughts such as "They don't want me," and seems to hold the belief that "I'm no fun." In the excerpt below, he related an incident from the previous week.

TABLE 8.3. Pro–Con Evaluation

Situation: Moving and changing schools	
Advantages	Disadvantages
My parents are happy.	I won't see my friends as often.
We get a bigger house.	I have to change schools.
My bedroom is a lot larger, so I'll have more room.	I will have to make new friends.
	The teachers won't know me.
Everyone will have more privacy.	I have to learn my way around the
I can walk to school.	school.
I will spend less time taking the bus.	My courses might be different.
I'll have time for breakfast in the morning.	
I'll have more time to get ready for school.	

P: Yeah, that's the way I felt. They weren't calling me, so I didn't know if they wanted me.

T: So you thought maybe they didn't really want you there. But you said you did call them anyway.

P: Yeah, I did.

T: How did it actually turn out?

P: When I called them the plan was to meet them in 10 minutes.

T: And did they mind telling you?

P: No.

T: So you didn't get any indication that anybody minded having you along?

P: No.

T: So the evidence says what about your initial thoughts?

P: I was jumping to wrong conclusions about them and me.

Operationalizing Beliefs

When a therapist wishes to use the technique of operationalization (Burns, 1980) to evaluate a belief, the patient is asked to state in concrete terms what he could observe that would verify the accuracy of the belief. Once a belief has been "translated" to a form that is potentially verifiable with empirical evidence, the therapist can help the adolescent evaluate it by considering the data available.

Example

A 15-year-old male's depression appears to be greatly exacerbated by his belief that he is stupid. In a previous session, he explained that he does not always understand what people are saying to him and stated that he is reluctant to ask questions that would clarify his confusion because the questions would publicly confirm that he is "dumb." A homework exercise was designed in which the adolescent would list the names of several people with whom he has contact during an average week. Beside each name on the list, he would record with a check mark each time he heard anyone ask a question.

T: Last time, you told me you thought an important part of your depression was that you felt silly or stupid because you sometimes didn't know things that other people knew. Sometimes you didn't ask any questions because you thought that was proof that you were stupid.

P: Uh huh.

T: (*noticing that the patient is holding his "homework"*) I see quite a few tick marks on your page there. Is this for the whole week or did you do it for a few days or what?

P: I did it for a week, on and off, because sometimes I'd forget it and try to remember how many questions each person asked.

T: OK. So it's not exactly every minute over the week. But it is for most of the time?

P: Uh huh.

T: And just glancing at it I can see that a lot of people were asking a lot of questions over that period of time. What were your thoughts when they were asking questions?

P: I would think they don't understand something so they are getting help.

T: So the fact that they didn't understand something meant that they needed help. Did it also mean to you that they were stupid, or just that they needed help?

P: Just that they needed help because there were a lot of smart people on the list asking questions.

T: Who on the list would you consider to be quite a smart person?

P: The teachers, and Tina is smart, and so is Paul. All of these except Rob are smart.

T: So even smart people ask quite a few questions. What does that say about your idea that if you ask a question it means you're stupid?

P: I was wrong.

T: Is that a good thing to learn?

P: Uh huh.

T: One of the things I notice looking at your chart is that other people ask more questions than you do. Do the people who are quite smart on your list ask more questions than you?

P: Uh huh.

T: I see your sister has a few more check marks than you, doesn't she? In your own words what do you think this helped you learn?

P: Well, just asking questions doesn't mean that you're stupid because everybody asks questions. My sister is smart and she asks a lot of questions.

T: What does that say about you?

P: I shouldn't be afraid to ask questions if I don't understand something. I'm not stupid for asking questions.

Logical Analysis

Logical analysis refers to the application of rules of logic to evaluate a belief. Through a series of questions, the therapist attempts to juxtapose two or more of the adolescent's assertions that may not be logically consistent. Alternatively, the therapist may attempt to demonstrate weaknesses in the adolescent's reasoning process that have led to an unjustified conclusion that appears to be depressogenic in nature. When attempted with younger adolescents, logical analysis may be a challenging proposition that requires the additional use of another technique such as the introduction of contradictory evidence. The speed at which logical analysis proceeds varies greatly with the cognitive development of the adolescent in question, as demonstrated by the case examples below.

Example 1

A 14-year-old male has learning disabilities and a history of school difficulties in addition to depression. In a discussion of the adolescent's sense of helplessness, he has revealed a strategy that the therapist believes is maladaptive because it is likely to result in continued experiences of failure, which will exacerbate the boy's depression. As the logical analysis progresses, the therapist meets with considerable reluctance on the part of the patient to take the therapist's reasoning into account.

P: Sometimes I think that if you don't expect it to happen, it will happen.

T: Now do you think that's realistic thinking or is that kind of magical?

P: It's realistic. I think the opposite of what I want.

T: So if you think the opposite of something, it happens? Is that right?

P: That's the way it's been for me.

T: So if you think, "I'm absolutely going to fail this exam," that's the way to guarantee passing it?

P: No. It might not work in some situations, but for most situations it works.

T: So you're telling me that most of the time the opposite of what you expect . . .

P: Happens.

T: . . . Happens. It that right? Most of the time are you pleasantly surprised or unpleasantly surprised?

P: Sometimes I'm unpleasantly surprised, and sometimes I'm pleasantly surprised. Depends on what the situations is.

T: Well you could do an experiment to test out this idea you've got. You said you have problems with exams, so if you really think that believing the opposite will get you what you want, you could test it out for a couple of weeks and see how it goes. Do you have a lot of faith in that method?

P: Yeah, I think I do.

T: Why haven't you used it then? Why haven't you done this on your own? Just really get it in your mind, "I'm not going to pass, I'm not going to pass," so that the opposite will happen?

P: That's what happens. I think I fill myself full of negative thoughts, and then the opposite of what I expect happens and then I'm pleasantly surprised.

T: But you haven't been pleasantly surprised in the area of passing exams too much.

P: I know (*said with disappointment*).

T: That's what you're telling me right? So at least with respect to school work and passing exams, your plan doesn't seem to be working real well.

P: I know.

T: Is that right?

P: Yeah. I guess it doesn't really work to think the opposite for school stuff.

T: What about for other stuff?

P: Maybe not there either.

Example 2

Logical analysis in the following example involves questioning the patient's basis for drawing the conclusion that she is in danger of becoming fat. The therapist pursues evaluation of the belief because the adolescent has previously expressed depressogenic views about her physical appearance that seem to contribute to her social withdrawal and isolation from peers.

P: I'm worried about getting fat.

T: Do you think you are fat now?

P: No.

T: But you think this might happen?

P: Yes, I'm worried about it.

T: How worried are you?

P: Very.

T: Very worried. Like 10 on the worry scale?

P: Probably about 9.

T: Have you ever been fat?

P: No.

T: Why do you think you'd get fat then?

P: I don't know. It's just a little fear I have.

T: Sounds like a pretty big fear. Do you think that the other women in your family are fat . . . are your sisters fat?

P: No.

T: Is your mom fat?

P: No.

T: So why would you be fat?

P: I don't know.

T: Fat uncles?

P: My dad's friend, we call him Uncle Jim. He's kind of on the chubby side.

T: But he's a family friend. He's not actually a relative.

P: He's more like an uncle to us than any of our other uncles.

T: Well, do you think you can catch fatness from him? He's just a family friend. I'm a bit puzzled. Sisters, mom, aunts, uncles, no one in your family is fat. Why would you get fat?

Example 3

A high-functioning 18-year-old understands her tendency to personalize problems and to blame herself for things that are not her responsibility. The therapist wishes to encourage evaluation of her belief that it is her duty to make other people happy regardless of the expense to herself. The logical analysis proceeds quickly, with the adolescent not only evaluating but apparently changing her belief in a short dialogue with the therapist.

P: The other night I went out with my friends. I gave him [boyfriend] the option to come, but he said, "No." It was bothering him for me to not be there with him. But I didn't try to make amends or anything and say, "OK, fine, there's your sad, puppy-dog eyes looking at me. I'm not going to go." I still stuck to going out.

T: Is there anyone else in the world who would have the same kind of power to influence you as a boyfriend? Have you ever been as concerned about the puppy-dog eyes or the sad feelings of anyone else?

P: Friends. I'm the kind of person who would sacrifice anything of myself, even if it meant keeping some things away from myself. Make it so that they're happier a little bit.

T: OK, so it's not just boyfriends. It's also friends you feel this way about.

P: For example, when my aunt phones me and says, "Can you baby-sit Saturday night?" And if I say, "No, I can't. I have plans." Then she says, "Oh." Then I'll give in. I'll say, "Fine."

T: And cancel your own plans? Why would you do that?

P: Just to make her happy. She sounds so sad.

T: But whose child is it?

P: Hers.

T: Whose responsibility is it to plan baby-sitting?

P: Hers.

T: And is it your duty to help her out every time she asks?

P: No. Probably it's up to me to stop myself if my aunt calls me next week. That thing we discussed about jumping to conclusions and personalization will stop me.

T: What will you stop yourself from thinking?

P: That it's my responsibility to make everyone else happy.

T: Is that something you've thought in the past?

P: Uh huh.

T: "It's your job." Do you think that's possible, to make everyone happy?

P: No.

T: So you were taking on the impossible task?

P: Uh huh. But I guess I can't do it. And it's not really up to me anyway.

Example 4

A 16-year-old with a tragically unstable family history has been making depressogenic predictions about her current friendships at school based on the belief that she never stays in one place more than a semester. The therapist wishes to evaluate the patient's belief that her life of instability will continue in the future as it has in the past because such a prediction could potentially lead to social withdrawal in order to avoid the anticipated loss of friendships at a later point in time. Rather than simply dismiss as illogical the patient's prediction of future events based on past events, the therapist undertakes a logical analysis by very carefully examining the various reasons for each residential move in the past, and the probability of their recurrence.

P: Every semester it seems I change to a different school. So I think, "What's the point in meeting people anyway?"

T: The last time you went to school, was it only for one semester?

P: Uh huh.

T: Where was it?

P: It was with my grandparents, and I went to school there for only one semester.

T: And why was it only one semester that time?

P: Because they sent me to live with my aunt. And I was only in that school for a semester too.

T: Why?

P: Because that was the semester I got really depressed and I went into the hospital. Then my cousins here in Wallaceburg took me from the hospital.

T: So you're telling me the last three semesters, it's been one semester in each of the schools? You also told me why that happened. When you were living with your grandparents you went to school only one semester because they sent you to live with an aunt. Of course, when a guardian changes, there's a chance you change schools. Is there any chance of you changing your guardian now?

P: Not really.

T: Have your cousins ever hinted that you're not going to be able to stay there and finish your school?

P: No.

T: Do you feel that's a secure home for you now?

P: Uh huh. Yes.

T: OK. So a change in school because of a change in guardian is unlikely now. Then you stayed with that aunt for one semester before you went to the hospital because you were quite depressed and suicidal. Do you feel that you're in that state of depression or suicidal now?

P: No.

T: Are you close to that state?

P: No.

T: What do you think is the risk of you sliding back to that point of suicidal ideation and depression?

P: Zero.

T: Not even 1%?

P: Well maybe 1%.

T: One percent?

P: But not serious, no.

T: You see, if you told me, Rebecca, that you were terribly depressed and you were starting to entertain ideas about suicide again, I would say you may be in your new school for only one semester because, if you're that depressed, you may have to go back to the hospital.

P: No way. I'm OK.

T: OK, last time your depression necessitated hospitalization and moving to your cousins', but now you're saying the likelihood of needing hospitalization is either 0% or 1%.

P: Zero.

T: Zero. So you don't have to worry about that reason for changing schools again. Now recently, you've moved because they sold a house and bought another one. Do you think they're likely to sell the new house after one semester?

P: Not after one semester but maybe after a year or something. They've already started talking about it.

T: So they're already talking about moving again?

P: Yeah, living in it for a few years and then selling it.

T: A few years or 1 year?

P: Well first they were talking about maybe 1 year, then maybe 2. They just don't know yet.

T: Since they don't know, it sounds to me like they might end up staying there for a few years. For all we know.

P: By that time I'll be out of high school and off to university or college or something.

T: Right. So for at least one semester it sounds like they are not going to be uprooting everybody.

P: No. That's true.

T: You said to me, "Every time I've gone to school in the past, it seems like I go for one semester, and then I move. And so I'm afraid that's going to happen again." But as I've examined the reasons for your moves in the past, none of them really seems to apply. I'm wondering if there's some other reason that you believe after one semester there will be another change?

P: No, I can't think of any.

Example 5

Logical analysis is also useful in family sessions to evaluate the potential inconsistencies in beliefs of various family members. In the following example, a 17-year-old male is helped to evaluate the coexistence of the two beliefs "I am independent," and "I need mom to solve my problems." Evaluation of these beliefs is pursued by the therapist because of the dilemma in which they place the patient and his mother, who are struggling with issues of individuation as a central aspect of the boy's depression.

P: I appreciate her [mother] worrying about my life and the mistakes I have made. I wouldn't want her to not worry about me. But sometimes I have to learn for myself. I have to be on my own. I guess it's kind of like being an adolescent or something and doing my own thing.

Mom: Except the mistakes do involve me. They actually bring me into it because I have had to get him out of the jams he gets into.

T: (*to mom*) Do you have to get him out of his jams?

M: Well I feel like I do. I guess I don't, but I don't know what he would do if I didn't.

T: (*to patient*) Does your mom have to get you out of the jams?

P: No, but she feels she has to. And sometimes I have really needed her help.

T: I think I just heard you say—tell me if I'm right, John—that you believe you are responsible enough to correct your own mistakes, that you want to be more independent, more on your own. How can you do that if your mom keeps stepping in and gets you out of those jams? It sounds like you have some mixed feelings about your mom. In other words, I hear you saying that you want to be more independent but you also appreciate the fact that she helps you out of jams. And I don't see how those can go together.

P: Maybe they don't. That's probably what my problem is. I do appreciate it when she helps me out, but she doesn't have to.

T: (*to patient*) What do you want her to do? Are you needing something different from your mom?

Time Projection

Time projection is a technique in which the usefulness of holding beliefs or continuing a pattern of automatic thoughts is evaluated by projecting the possible consequences of those cognitions over time. With some adolescents, the role of maladaptive cognition is more obvious if it can be related to concrete undesirable behavioral outcomes than if it is associated only with current emotional distress.

Example 1

A 14-year-old male's father has recently left the family home and is making no attempts to see the children. The patient has just told his family and the therapist that he isolates himself in his bedroom because he does not want to get close to anyone. Time projection is used to help him evaluate the usefulness of his belief that "Every time I get close to someone, they leave me." The therapist encouraged evaluation of this belief because continuing to hold it would likely engender further estrangement from the patient's father and increased social withdrawal.

T: One of the things that maybe is running through your head right now is, like you said earlier, "Every time I get close to someone they leave me, and then I hurt too much." So your solution for avoiding hurt seems to be "Don't get close to anybody." Is that kind of the way you think about it?

P: Yeah. I like my privacy.

T: Privacy is OK, but if you believe, "I'm not getting close to anybody because it's too painful," if that's how you think, how is that going to affect your relationships at home?

P: I might be afraid to get close to Sandy [brother] or Cindy [sister] or mom.

T: Right. Good. And if you think "It's too dangerous to get close to anybody," will you try to make contact with your dad?

P: Not if I think that way.

T: Your idea about "If I get close to someone, I'll get hurt," you might find isn't quite right all the time. And it seems like that belief might stop you from doing some things you want to. I get the feeling that you would like to see your dad. Is that right?

P: Yeah.

T: Is that something you want to do in real life or is it just something you think about?

P: Both. I really want to go see him and I think about him all the time.

T: If you continue to believe, "If I get close to someone, I'll just get hurt," what will happen down the road with seeing your dad?

P: I'd probably never see him because I'd be afraid to.

Example 2

A 16-year-old has revealed a series of automatic thoughts that interfere with his desire to pursue dating relationships with high school classmates. Time projection is used to evaluate the usefulness of the thoughts in relation to his goal of dating. The therapist pursues a discussion on dating not because dating per se is seen as the antidote for depression but because of the potential consequences of the patient's continuing to hold his maladaptive assumptions about his appearance, personality, and worth as a person.

T: You told me that the "assuming problem," as you called it, leads to all kinds of doubts. And we wrote down a whole bunch of doubts that you have. What do you think those doubts lead to?

P: Well I think that's about as far as it goes.

T: I think it goes farther. If you have doubts about your ability to get a date, how is the doubt going to affect your behavior?

P: Well I'm not going to go to dances or parties. I'm not going to bother trying.

T: So you're going to tell yourself, "Don't bother. Stop trying." Is that right?

P: Right. And I might think that even if I had one date, I'd never get a second one.

T: If you have doubts about a second date with the same person, then how's that going to affect your behavior?

P: Maybe I'll think that person likes someone else, would rather go out with them.

T: OK. But how would thinking that way influence what you might actually do?

P: I might not try to be nice on the first date because of assuming that what was the use of trying.

T: So if you assume something, then that can lead to a doubt about yourself that leads to your behavior: you don't bother, you don't try, right? And if you don't bother and don't try, then that leads to being alone.

P: Being lonely, being sad, feeling blue.

T: Feeling blue, right. You've got lots of words for how you end up feeling. And what you just did was demonstrate to both of us how your assumptions affect your mood. That's one of the really, really important parts of therapy that I'm going to do with you.

P: I've got to get out of this assuming thing.

T: And what if you don't?
P: I won't bother trying. I'll never have a date.

STEP V: CHANGING MALADAPTIVE AUTOMATIC
THOUGHTS AND BELIEFS

When exploration and evaluation of automatic thoughts and beliefs has revealed maladaptive cognitions, the goal of the therapist is to encourage cognitive change. The techniques discussed below are organized into two subgroups: those that address cognition directly and those that address cognition indirectly through behavioral interventions. Some of the techniques are primarily directed at changing maladaptive automatic thoughts, whereas others target change in maladaptive beliefs directly. Often the therapist will find it useful to employ a combination of techniques within one session, simultaneously intervening at the levels of both thought and belief.

Cognitive Techniques

Daily Record of Dysfunctional Thoughts

The daily record of dysfunctional thoughts (Beck et al., 1979) is a five- or six-column form used to record situations, distressing emotions that were initially experienced in response to the situations, automatic thoughts that occurred, rational responses to those automatic thoughts, and the emotional outcome after the rational response has been substituted for the automatic thoughts. When a sixth column is included, it is used to record the cognitive distortion(s) present in the maladaptive automatic thoughts. Although it is common to use a six-column chart with adult patients who are asked to keep daily records, it is usually not recommended for depressed adolescents. In general, adolescents quickly grow impatient with reviewing past events, especially if there is the additional requirement of recording them on paper. Furthermore, most adolescents will appear either overwhelmed or disinterested in the entire process by the time the therapist can complete an explanation of what is to be recorded in each of the five or six columns.

With an adolescent patient population, it is much more effective to request record keeping that is brief, focusing on only one or two components of the cognitive therapy model at a time. For example, recording an upsetting situation, rating the emotion, and noting automatic thoughts once a day for a week would be a realistic expectation for older patients well socialized into the model. If the first three columns of the dysfunctional thoughts daily record were completed as homework in this way, the therapist could continue to develop the remaining columns in session with the patient. More so than is the case with adults, adolescents will need repeated instruction in using the cognitive model, with demonstrations relevant to affect-laden issues during therapy sessions. With younger adolescents especially, more of the content of the daily record of dysfunctional thoughts is elicited during therapist–patient dialogue. In general, therapists working with adolescents must be prepared to rely more on in-session repetition than on self-guided discovery through homework assignments.

Table 8.4 is a dysfunctional thoughts daily record with all six columns completed. In the example shown, a young boy is upset about being denied the purchase of new jeans. The dialogue on which the six-column record was based appears in the following example.

Example. A 14-year-old male has reported being very angry the previous week but has not completed homework records of any kind. In conversation with him, the therapist addresses all six columns of the dysfunctional thoughts daily record, including identification of the cognitive distortion.

T: We've been talking about how what you think has a lot to do with how you feel. It's not so much the fact that you couldn't buy your new jeans that made you feel bad, right? It's what you thought about that made you feel bad. And you told me you were thinking, "We never have money, I never get anything." Does it make sense that those thoughts would make you feel bad?

P: Yeah.

T: What's the word in that thought that causes the trouble?

P: "Never."

T: Never. And what about "anything"? "I never get anything."

P: Well, I do get some things.

T: So by saying "never" and "anything," you are making things black and white. Right? All or none.

P: Yeah, I guess so.

T: What kind of thoughts could you have had that would not have made you feel quite so bad?

P: "I can just save my money and that way I could really go shop-

TABLE 8.4. Daily Record of Dysfunctional Thoughts

Situation	Emotion (rate 0–10)	Automatic thoughts	Thinking error	Rational response	Outcome
No money for new jeans	Angry—8 or 9	We never have money. I never get anything We don't make enough money. I don't get what I want.	Black-and-white thinking	I can save my money and then go shopping. Just give it some time and then we'll have more money. Maybe we can't do anything about it right now.	Angry—4 or 5
				I could save the money from my job delivering flyers. I just have to wait one more week until I get paid.	Angry—1 or 2

193

ping," or "Just give it time and maybe we can get some more, and then I'll have money and I can go shopping."

T: Right, so you have a situation where you need some stuff and you can't go get it. Right? Anybody would be a little bit unhappy in that situation.

P: I was sad because I hate not having any money, and I was angry because I don't like being without money, and I was frustrated because I get tired of it.

T: OK. Let's see if we can tease those things out. That might be helpful because sometimes kids feel a bunch of things and aren't sure what is related to what. And it's the thought that you have that probably decides to some extent what you feel. You were sad because . . . ?

P: Because I couldn't go shopping, and because we weren't making enough money.

T: Was that angry or sad?

P: I guess kind of angry.

T: Angry. OK. Let's start with anger, with 0 being not angry at all, and 10 being the angriest you've ever been. How would you rate your feeling yesterday when you were saying to yourself, "We don't make enough money; I don't get what I want."

P: About an 8 or a 9.

T: Eight or 9. OK.

P: Uh huh.

T: Now, where do you think you would be if you were saying to yourself the other things you just said to me, like, "I could save my money and get what I really want."

P: About 4 or 5. Because I'd be getting better but I'd still be kind of mad.

T: OK. What kind of thoughts do you think you could have to make the anger go even further down?

P: "Maybe we just can't do anything about it."

T: What, say that again?

P: "Maybe we just can't do anything about it." And "I guess I'll just give it time."

T: OK, good. "Give it time. That really is all you can do about it." How about reminding yourself that you have a job delivering flyers, so now it's more in your control? Do you think that would drive the anger down a little bit? Where do you think that would take it?

P: Maybe 1 or 2.

T: So then, you know in a sense you have a plan. You're thinking, "I just have to wait one more week until I get paid, and I'll have a little more money then." Right?

P: Uh huh.

T: And that would drive the anger all the way down to 1 or 2. Right?

Triple-Column Technique

The triple-column technique (Burns, 1980) refers to a subset of the dysfunctional thoughts daily record. The three columns that become the focus of attention include automatic thoughts, the distortion, and the rational response. As has been mentioned previously, adolescents are generally less inclined than their adult counterparts to complete written homework, so it is more common to use the triple-column technique orally in dialogue with the adolescent. In particular, adolescents seem to require the therapist's assistance to generate rational responses to maladaptive automatic thoughts. More so than will normally be the case with depressed adult patients, modeling and repetition will play a central role in changing the thoughts or beliefs of depressed adolescents using the triple-column technique.

A written example of the triple column technique is shown in Table 8.5. The contents of the three columns were derived from the therapist–patient dialogue, also reproduced below.

Example. A 17-year-old female was given the homework task of reading the definitions of 10 cognitive distortions commonly associated with depression. She was to monitor herself to see if any of them applied to her in the week before the next therapy session. The excerpt uses the triple-column technique to shift her thoughts about a family move scheduled to occur soon.

T: The 10 thinking styles that can be related to depression that we talked about last time, did you see yourself doing that this past week? Did you see yourself doing any of those?

P: Uh huh.

T: When?

P: I was just sort of thinking the worst yesterday. When I found out that we were moving for sure.

T: About the move, OK. So when you know that you are magnifying the worst, what can you do about that?

P: Catch myself and think of ways that it can be different.

T: So are you saying that you were thinking the worst about the school and the move and the change?

TABLE 8.5. Triple-Column Technique

Automatic thoughts	Thinking errors	Rational response
It's just terrible that we're moving.	Magnifying glass	It's not so bad. There's not really a lot of things to worry about.
Every time I go to school, we move again as soon as I make friends.	Jumping to conclusions (fortune telling)	It probably won't happen this time. It will probably last for a year or two.
I'm going to completely lose all the friends I've made.	All–nothing thinking (black–white thinking)	I won't lose them. I can see them or they can come see me. We can talk on the phone.
I won't be able to get registered in any of the classes I want.	Predicting the worst (fortune telling)	I can probably get some of my classes because I have a lot to choose from. The new school might have some new classes my old school doesn't have.

P: Uh huh. I was using binocular magnification.

T: How can you think about it differently now that we've talked?

P: Well, just say, "It's not so bad."

T: But if you were telling yourself why it's not so bad, what would you say?

P: "There's not really a lot of things to worry about," I guess.

T: OK, but which specific ideas of yours have changed?

P: The whole idea about friends, for one.

T: I made some notes initially on what you told me, so I'm going to give you your old idea, and you tell me how you think about it now. OK? One old thought was, "Every time I go to school, we move again as soon as I make friends."

P: It probably won't happen this time. It will probably last for a year or two.

T: Why would you say that?

P: Because, the way I see it, they're getting a new house and doing landscaping and everything, sort of looking to stay there for a few years I think.

T: OK. So you see how I gave you the old automatic thought, which was an example of jumping to conclusions, and you were able to come up with a more reasonable response in your own head that corrected the problem of predicting the worst. How about this one? The old thought, the automatic thought, "I'm going to completely lose all the friends I've made." What's the distortion?

P: "Completely" and "all."

T: What kind of error is that?

P: All-or-nothing thinking, like black and white.

T: Good. What would be more accurate than to think, "I'm going to completely lose all the friends I've made"?

P: "I can see them or they come see me. Call them on the phone."

T: Do you believe that?

P: Yes, it's possible. We like to talk on the phone, and I have a driver's license now so I could go see them sometimes.

T: What about "I won't be able to get registered in any of the classes I want"?

P: Predicting the worst again. I'm fortune telling about the future.

T: What would be better?

P: "I can probably get some of my classes because I have a lot to choose from," or maybe I could say, "The new school might have some new classes my old school doesn't have."

T: Good, good. Do you think it would be useful for you to practice this at home when you start feeling depressed?

Reframing and Relabeling

Reframing refers to the provision of a different context or frame of reference in which to view something that is contributing to the adolescent's distress. The real-life problem itself has not changed, but the therapist assists the patient to view it from a different perspective so that it no longer appears insurmountable. Relabeling refers to the practice of assigning a less catastrophic verbal tag to something that is causing the adolescent distress. A new label for an old problem can sometimes result in rapid amelioration of depression because the new label brings with it a host of connotative meanings that helps to address the previous constriction imposed by the old label.

Example 1. A 17-year-old, highly responsible and mature for his age, is severely depressed because he feels incompetent. Reframing is used to place "mistakes" in the context of "adolescent adventure" in an attempt to change his belief that mistakes are proof of his incompetence.

T: What gave you the courage to be a teenager?

P: I don't know. It happened one day, and then it just became easier and easier. I just started to fit in more. I really tried.

T: Well, let me ask you about the role of perfectionism. Did that interfere with your being a teenager?

P: I think so because when I set out to do something I'm going to do it well. At the same time, being a teenager is also making mistakes, goofing up. Especially when you're a teenager, that's when you're trying to explore and find out things. So that's one area I need to work on. I'm still trying to think it's OK to make mistakes, because it's not easy changing.

T: Are you practicing making mistakes?

P: I try.

T: You do? What mistakes have you tried to make?

P: Well, I don't purposely make mistakes. I can't do that.

T: I guess that's an example where we've made some headway in terms of helping you accept mistakes. But we haven't gone to the next stage in terms of helping you make a mistake.

P: Yeah.

T: You mentioned about being able to accept mistakes and that reminds me of the chapter that I gave you to read. How did that help you?

P: I still use it. There is no "perfect" so if you can be your own person, then that's perfect for you.

T: So you liked that? That appealed?

P: Yeah.

T: What other aspects appealed from that chapter?

P: Just making mistakes, because logically I need to make mistakes. The part about what's so bad if you make a mistake. In the book example, he was upset about a school assignment because he handed in the rough draft . . .

T: Yes.

P: . . . and then he made a list of the things that were going through his head and put down rational thoughts. That helps.

T: You said something a minute ago about being a teenager means exploring and making some mistakes. What was that?

P: Well, mistakes are normal if you think of them as signs that you're doing something new, adventuring in your life. If you never tried anything, you could probably avoid mistakes.

T: Good, that puts a whole new light on the idea of mistakes doesn't it?

P: Yeah, it helps.

Example 2. A 17-year-old male is diagnosed with attention-deficit hyperactivity disorder and learning disabilities in addition to depression. His difficulties at school appear to be a major source of maladaptive cognition about his intelligence, his worth as a son, and his future aspirations for a career. Relabeling is used to adjust the evaluation of himself as a "failure" to something less extreme, with more hope for remediation of the problem situation.

> T: Are you in fact a failure at school? Is school a write off?
> P: Sometimes I think so. Other times when I do get a good mark, I get a little hopeful I guess.
> T: So it's not in fact a failure in total.
> P: No.
> T: What's a better word then?
> P: Problem, I guess. School's a problem.
> T: Say it again.
> P: School is a problem for me.
> T: What's the difference between those words "failure" and "problem"?
> P: With failure, there's no hope. A problem can be solved.
> T: What do you think the impact on your mood could be by changing that definition from "failure" to a "problem"?
> P: Well, if it's a problem, I'll feel hopeful that maybe I can get a solution. So I guess I'll be more hopeful.

Positive Self-Statements

Positive self-statements are affirmations intended for oral rehearsal by the adolescent in situations that are likely to trigger depressogenic cognitions about "self." In using this technique, it is important that the patient avoid "parroting" positive statements about himself that are merely the opposite of negative automatic thoughts. The affirmations must be ones the adolescent believes in order to be effective, so the therapist will normally need to inquire about the degree of believability or confidence in the statement's truth.

Example. A 13-year-old with learning disabilities frequently is angry at himself when he has problems with his school work. The therapist helps him develop some self-statements for rehearsal when he anticipates feeling bad about his school performance.

T: What were you telling yourself when you got your assignment back this week?

P: I said things like, "Oh I'm so stupid, I should've been able to do this."

T: "I should've been able to do it. Why can't I do stuff? Why can't I do stuff right for once?" Is that right?

P: Yeah, I never get things right the first time. It's always wrong and I have to do it over again. And I get really mad.

T: So that pushes your anger up because of the things that you start to tell yourself.

P: Uh huh.

T: That make sense?

P: Yeah, if I didn't talk to myself I probably wouldn't get so mad.

T: But, Tony, the good thing about talking to yourself is you can choose what you say to yourself. What are some of the other things you say when you feel bad?

P: "I'm stupid. I should've been able to do it."

T: "I'm stupid. I should've been able to do it." And what else?

P: "Why can't I do this?"

T: And you know some of the most powerful ones that I bet you say a lot to yourself, "I'm dumb." "I'm stupid." That stuff is guaranteed to get you to a 10 on the anger scale. Right? Anybody saying that to himself would be very angry at himself. So what we need to think about is what script you can give yourself. We need to think of some things you can say to yourself instead.

P: Uh huh. I could say, "Well, I can do better. Next time I'll do better."

T: Or "Everybody makes . . ."

P: "Everybody makes mistakes sometimes."

T: Do you believe that next time you'll do better?

P: Well, maybe I will.

T: What could you say about yourself to make you less angry? Could you say something nice?

P: "I get most things right," or "I'm pretty good at sports."

T: OK. Good. Is it true that you get most things right? Or is it true that you get many things right?

P: For school work, many things. I could say that because it's true.

T: You said something else . . . you're pretty good at sports. What else?

P: "I try very hard. I'm a hard worker."

T: Great. What can you say to yourself when you are having trouble with your homework this week?

Reattribution

Reattribution (Beck et al., 1979) or "disattribution" (Burns, 1980) is a technique used when an adolescent's causal explanations for a particular negative situation are likely to worsen or prolong the depression. Internal, stable, or global attributions for negative events are the ones therapists should typically regard as the targets for intervention. Alternatively, the therapist should use reattribution with external, unstable, or specific attributions for positive events.

Example 1. A young patient has explained that he is very distressed by the fact that his separated parents often engage in heated arguments. In the excerpt below, he initially makes an internal attribution for the fighting that goes on between his parents; but, through discussion with the therapist, the attribution becomes external. As such, he is relieved of the self-blame he has been feeling.

T: That's kind of between the two of them [parents], isn't it? And somehow if the conflict is between the two of them, it makes you feel bad. Tell me how does that make sense?

P: I guess because it's about me.

T: They're fighting about child support, and it's to support you. Right? So explain to me why that should make you feel bad?

P: I don't know, because it's over me. I'm always getting involved in people's problems and mine.

T: OK. Now what I want to say to you is that, in any situation, your feeling bad or your feeling good is going to depend on what you say to yourself. Right?

P: Right.

T: So if your parents are fighting over something, what do you say to yourself to feel bad?

P: "They're fighting over me."

T: Uh huh. OK, and then you think about that and yeah, possibly true, it's true that they're fighting over you. What can you say to make yourself feel worse?

P: I just keep thinking that they were in this 'cause of me and maybe I think, "If I wasn't here they wouldn't fight."

T: OK. "It's all my fault. If I wasn't here they'd have nothing to fight about." Now what could you say to yourself to make you feel better?

P: "It's between them, and why should I put their problems on my back."

T: Right. Good, good, good. OK, what else can you say to yourself to make you feel better?

T: "They need to work it out between them. I don't need to be involved."

T: Good, good. OK. Somewhere you feel the pressure to get involved. Right? You feel like maybe you need to be more supportive to your mom when she's trying so hard. Because you said a little while ago she's always trying. Right? What about, "How they feel about each other has nothing to do with how they feel about me"?

P: I don't have anything to do with that. I didn't have anything to do with their hating each other.

T: Do you believe that?

P: Uh huh. Because, even if I wasn't here, they'd still hate each other.

T: You got it. You got it. OK. Was this helpful to you?

P: Uh huh. I'm going to stop sticking up for her and going against my dad. Now I think I can have a little power in what to do and say, "It's their problem, not mine."

T: What's going to give you the most power?

P: Just to keep saying, "It's not my problem."

Example 2. Reattribution will often be appropriate to use in family sessions either because the adolescent is making depressogenic attributions about himself, or because family members have causal explanations for particular situations that implicate the adolescent. Often, depressed adolescents struggle with internal attributions that lead to feelings of blame or shame, as in the following example. A young adolescent boy is the depressed patient. He appears to be making an internal attribution for an anticipated future circumstance. An older brother, who is also attending the family sessions, helps in the process of reattribution.

Brother: He [patient, his younger brother] thinks he's going to lose friends because of my past.

T: (*to patient*) Don [older brother] behaved in ways that were not good for him, or other people in the past. But Don is still Don. He chooses his behavior differently now. So I'm wanting to know what are the thoughts you have that make you so sad?

P: I don't like thinking about it. And when people talk about it, I feel sad.

T: If you lose friends because your brother behaved in ways that were not good for him some years ago, are those friends you want to keep around?

P: No, maybe not.

T: OK, that's one issue. The other issue is, do you see Don's past behavior as a reflection on you?

P: To some people it might be.

T: Some people think weird things. Are you going to be a victim of what they choose to think? Some people think your religious beliefs are things that determine whether you're worthy to be a friend or not. Are you going to buy that?

P: No.

T: Some people think that if your family is not wealthy, they don't want to associate with you. Do you want to buy that?

P: People already know that about me.

T: So then what do you want to do?

P: They forget about it and like me anyway.

T: Right. Some people think that if you're from a divorced home, they don't want to be your friend. You want to accept that?

P: No.

T: Some people think that if your brother behaved in ways that were not good for him 2 years ago, they don't want to be friends with you. Does that make sense?

P: I guess not.

T: Is his behavior from the past your responsibility?

P: No.

T: And if other people try to make it your responsibility, what will you think?

P: That it's up to him, not me.

T: Good, good. You're not going to take the blame for his behavior.

B: It boils down again that you have no control over what they think, so let it go. My life is my responsibility and not yours or any one else's.

Cognitive Rehearsal

Cognitive rehearsal (Beck et al., 1979; Burns, 1980) is a technique in which a thought process is practiced in the therapy session. Sometimes the rehearsal involves actual role play. Alternatively, the therapist will just talk the patient through the steps of a particular sequence. Because it relies on overt demonstration or detailed analysis of how to implement a change, rehearsal is particularly useful for younger adolescents

who have difficulty imagining themselves thinking any differently than
has they have in the past.

Example. A 13-year-old who lives with his father wants to see his
mother but has recently had an experience where his mother was unable to meet his request for visitation. The patient has explained that
when she said "No" the last time, his automatic thoughts included depressogenic ideas such as, "She doesn't love me anymore." The therapist
uses role play to demonstrate the technique of cognitive rehearsal and
how it could help change the maladaptive thought process.

T: Let me be you for a minute, OK? I'm just going to pretend I'm
you and that I've called your mom. And why don't you be your mom,
OK? Just for a demonstration. Here's what we'll do: I'm going to call
you, and I'm going to ask you if you can see me on Saturday. Since
you're going to be your mom, I'd like you to tell me something like,
"Oh gee, I'm sorry but that's not a good time," or however she'd say it.
So try to be like she would be and then I'm going to think out loud. I'm
just going to pretend I'm you and show you how maybe you can catch
yourself thinking harmful thoughts and change them to some other
ones.

P: OK.

T: (*pretending to ring the phone*) Ring, ring. (*pretending to speak in the
voice of patient*) "Hi, mom, this is Justin."

P: (*being mom*) "Oh hi, Justin. How are things going?"

T: "OK, I guess. Did you have a good business trip?"

P: "Uh huh. It was OK. I got lots done."

T: "Oh I was, um, I was sort of hoping maybe you could see me on
Saturday this weekend."

P: "I'm sorry, it's not a good day. I have to work."

T: "Oh, that's too bad." (*hanging up the phones*) (*returning to own voice
for a moment*) This is how you might be thinking: (*role playing the patient's
thought processes*) "Gee, mom can't see me on Saturday. I think she does-
n't want to see me. I think she doesn't like me anymore. . . . Wait a
minute, though. That first thought is pretty harmful. Maybe I can think
up some other explanations. Maybe there are some other reasons she
said no. For one, she said she had to work. I suppose that's reasonable;
she works on lots of Saturdays. I shouldn't feel too bad if she has to
work. Maybe she has to work on her new store. Well, that's a good reason. I know she needs to keep her boss happy to keep her job. I can't
really assume she doesn't want to see me, can I? Well, she didn't say
she didn't want to see me. She just said she couldn't see me on that Sat-

urday. Maybe she could see me some other time. When other people phone me, I can't always see them. Maybe that's her reason too. She used to like to see me in the past. I think that's a pretty good indication that she probably would see me in the future. I think I'm going to ask Mom when she'd like to see me or what a good time for her would be." (*returning to own voice*) We'll stop the pretending now. I was just trying to be you and talk out loud some of the ways that you could think about your mom. Just because she can't see you on Saturday doesn't mean your first thought is the right one. OK? Can you do that with yourself? Can you kind of talk to yourself that way?

P: Probably.

T: If you could talk to yourself, I don't mean you have to talk out loud, but if you could think to yourself that way, why do you think it might be good for you to do that?

P: Because it would make me think of more ideas for why she doesn't want to see me. I wouldn't think of all the bad reasons. I'd probably think of some good ones too.

T: And if you could think of some good reasons, what would that do to your feelings?

P: They'd feel better.

Stress Inoculation

Stress inoculation involves imagining or planning actual exposure to a situation likely to trigger maladaptive cognition so that the therapist and patient can anticipate and correct the automatic thoughts or challenge depressogenic beliefs. This technique is used when problematic situations are likely to reoccur, and the therapist wishes to do some preventive therapy. It is a particularly useful technique to employ when cognitive therapy for a particular adolescent is drawing to a close because it allows the therapist to check how well the patient is able to generalize from specific situations discussed in therapy to new or similar ones that have not yet occurred.

Example. The therapist has had several previous discussions with this 15-year-old male aimed at addressing maladaptive beliefs associated with the schema "people pleasing."

T: You said so far that wanting to be everybody's friend and wanting to stay out of trouble haven't been in conflict. Can you think of a situation where they might be?

P: If I get in with the wrong crowd or something and they try to get me to do something that I know I'm not supposed to do. But it wouldn't bother me. I wouldn't do it because I would realize they weren't the kind of friends I needed.

T: Could you walk away from those people and say, "I can't do this," and take the risk of not pleasing them?

P: Uh huh. I could do that.

T: Well, that's great. Then you're not a complete people pleaser.

P: Yeah.

T: Do you think that would be hard for you?

P: Maybe, but that's all I could do.

T: What if people didn't like you?

P: Well, it depends on who they were. If they were people whom I was friends with, then I'd think we weren't really good friends. I would say it wouldn't matter because if they didn't like me I probably didn't like them either.

T: Some people are not going to like you, no matter what. Is that what you're saying?

P: Some people don't like me, but it doesn't bother me.

T: It doesn't bother you?

P: No. I don't care.

T: So some of the things that could be problems about people pleasing are not problems for you. Right?

P: Right.

T: What would you say to yourself if you found yourself in a situation where you had to make a choice between having someone like you and staying out of trouble?

P: I'd stay out of trouble.

T: How would you do that? What would you say to yourself?

P: "I don't need to risk getting in trouble. It's not worth it."

T: Would there be a little voice that said, "But it's important to be liked"?

P: Yeah.

T: And what would you say to that voice?

P: "Shut up."

T: OK. What else would you say to that voice?

P: "I don't care. They might be my friends, but they're not true friends if they want me to do something that I'm not supposed to do."

T: How about, "These people are probably not worth having as friends"?

P: Yeah. They're not worth getting in trouble over.

Alternate Explanations

When therapists use alternate explanations (similar to "alternative solutions"; Beck et al., 1979) as a technique to help depressed adolescents evaluate their cognitions, potential explanations for past or future events are sought to augment the limited repertoire first generated by the depressed adolescents themselves. Depressed patients are more likely to make internal, stable, or global attributions for negative events that have occurred than are nondepressed people who have experienced similar occurrences. Also, depressed adolescents will often employ cognitive distortions that lead to catastrophic interpretations of past or future events. The goal of generating alternate explanations is to show the depressed adolescent that his first explanations may be overly biased.

Example 1. A 14-year-old male has a father who lives apart from the family and works out of town frequently. The therapist helps him to generate alternate explanations to evaluate his depressogenic automatic thought that something catastrophic has happened to his father.

T: When he wasn't home when you phoned this week, what did you think?

P: I started to get worried that something had happened to him.

T: What were you worried abut?

P: Well, since he is in construction, I thought that something happened with the dump truck or he broke his leg in a ditch or something.

T: Do you think there might be any other perfectly good explanations for him not being home that didn't involve some kind of injury?

P: He could've worked overtime.

T: Right. So maybe the job took longer than they thought, and he had to stay an extra 3 or 4 days or something like that. Yes. That would be one perfectly good explanation. Since it's winter time, can you think of any other explanations?

P: Well, his car wouldn't stall because he's kind of a backyard mechanic. He knows how to fix it so that wouldn't be the reason.

T: So it wouldn't be the mechanics of his car. Could it be the roads?

P: Not in this weather [unusually mild winter].

T: But, where he went in the north, is there any possibility that it would be climate or roads or a sudden blizzard, something like that?

P: I guess so.

T: So that might keep him where he's at. I suppose even mechanics sometimes have something happen to their car that they need parts for. Right?

P: Yeah. He could have had to order something.

T: So maybe that could be an explanation. What I'm looking for are some explanations other than the first one you came up with, the one where you think, "Oh he must be hurt." Remember the last time we talked about how sometimes the first explanation that comes to our mind is one that makes us depressed, or it's the scariest one?

P: Yeah.

T: Now what do you think of your first ideas about your dad not being home when you phoned?

P: I think that there might be other reasons.

Example 2. A male high school student is being taught to evaluate his self-deprecatory thoughts in response to being refused a date by a girl he had asked out from school. The generation of alternate explanations is aided by reference to a friend of the patient's who is predicted to react differently to the same situation (double-standard technique).

T: So you would predict that your friend John wouldn't dwell on it. That's what he wouldn't do. If I said to John, "Well, John, what explanations have you come up with for her refusal?" what things might John say?

P: Well, he might say that maybe there's a million reasons why a girl will say yes, and a million reasons why she would say no. So it could be a whole bunch of reasons why she'd say no.

T: So that's what John would start thinking, is that the girl said "no," but there might be lots of reasons that she said "no." If John went one step further and actually started coming up with explanations for himself, what would be some reasonable ones?

P: "Maybe she's seeing someone else," or "She doesn't have the time," or "She's too busy."

T: Good. And if John came up with those explanations, would that be a way of him putting himself down?

P: No.

T: So is he blaming himself?

P: No. He's just trying to find an explanation for why she said "no."

T: So he's generating in his own mind lots of perfectly good reasons that the girl might not want to go out with him. Do you think that might be a good strategy for you?

Contradictory Evidence

Contradictory evidence (like "examining and reality testing automatic thoughts"; Beck et al., 1979) is an effective way of changing automatic thoughts or beliefs if the evidence generated is given sufficient weight by the adolescent. To be most effective, the "evidence" sought to challenge maladaptive cognitions should be determined by the patient himself, although the therapist will often have to assist in the process of searching for contradictory evidence by making suggestions about the kind of data that would suffice.

Example 1. A 17-year-old had previously expressed some very negative views about his appearance. In the previous session, he and the therapist devised a homework exercise for him to test his belief that he was ugly. The therapist wishes to address this particular belief because it appears to be the basis of frequent thoughts that have hampered the patient's development of social relationships and is apparently contributing to increased self-derogation and social withdrawal.

T: Last week we talked about some negative views you have of yourself because you think you were ugly when you used to wear glasses. Did you do that experiment we talked about?

P: Yes. I showed the pictured to Sandy and he laughed at first. But he said he knows what kind of a person I am, and he likes me for who I am. So it wouldn't matter what I look like. The fact that I look really good today, now that I have contacts, it shouldn't really matter what I looked like all those years ago. That's just a picture of me, and I look different from that today. I know I shouldn't really worry about it.

T: He said all that?

P: Yeah.

T: And what was the value of doing that?

P: Well, I shouldn't be so down on myself just because of what I looked like 4 or 5 years ago. Just because I think people will laugh at me doesn't mean they necessarily will even if they look at a picture of what I looked like back then.

T: But he did laugh at the old picture.

P: Well, he did at first, but I don't mind because of who he is I guess.

T: Was it something about the quality of how he laughed?

P: It wasn't like a mocking laugh. It was like a warm laugh. It didn't bother me that he laughed.

T: When you think now, "What if other people saw the yearbook, or saw a picture of me back then?" how do you feel?

P: I'd still feel a bit embarrassed, but I could accept it more.

T: We talked about the scale of feelings last week. Where 100 is really uncomfortable and 0 is just fine, where would you rate yourself last week?

P: Ninety.

T: Ninety. OK, and where would you rate your discomfort now?

P: About a 60—50 or 60.

T: That's quite a drop.

P: Yeah. I do feel more comfortable with it, but still I wouldn't voluntarily show anyone pictures of myself. If it happened accidently, I'd probably feel really embarrassed and hide. But then it would be OK.

T: Would that be a normal level of embarrassment do you think?

P: I guess, yeah. I guess it's pretty normal.

T: OK. So what's the importance of doing that exercise?

P: Well, it makes me feel better about myself I guess. And I shouldn't be so down and hard on myself because I looked like that 5 years ago. It's not how I look today.

T: Was that more effective than your mom telling you you don't need to worry about it, that you look fine?

P: Yeah because I know my mom would say I look good if I had on brown pants and an orange sweater. Because I'm her son.

T: So checking that out for yourself was OK?

P: Yeah. It was helpful.

Example 2. The therapist asks a 16-year-old female to generate contradictory evidence in the session. The patient's belief that she is "basically stubborn" is thought to be maladaptive because it will inhibit her willingness to attempt making therapeutic changes.

T: I want you to convince me that you're not stubborn.

P: That is an extremely hard case.

T: That's another assumption.

P: Well, I know. I'm full of making assumptions about myself. I can't think of anything that makes me not stubborn.

T: OK, tell me things that you've done that have shown me you're not stubborn. If you're stubborn, you wouldn't change your beliefs, you wouldn't change your feelings, or you wouldn't change your actions.

P: Well, I guess you've got a point there. I have changed quite a few beliefs in the past. One of them a year ago was that I never wanted to get married, and now I do. And I never wanted children, so I guess I've changed my beliefs on that.

T: Some other beliefs you've changed?

P: Let's see, I don't believe suicide is the answer.

T: OK. Why not?

P: Because experiences I've had in the past year have taught me that there would be a lot missing out if I killed myself.

T: OK. Some other beliefs. I can think of a couple you've shared with me.

P: Anger is something I now consider OK, used properly, of course.

T: Yeah.

P: I'm quite good at analyzing myself actually. I'm now not afraid to analyze.

T: So you're not afraid of looking at yourself and understanding yourself better?

P: I now like myself.

T: You now like yourself. Lots of beliefs have changed.

P: Yeah.

T: And a belief in the last session about your desired profession. "It's being an actress or nothing. That's my last option." That's changed, right?

P: Well, it is almost the last option.

T: Almost the last option. But last week it was the last option. So you've had lots of beliefs that you've actually changed in the last while. And these are big things in people's lives about how they view themselves, their world around them, how they view their future.

P: I guess I have changed quite a bit.

T: Now, what would you say about your previous belief that you were a stubborn person, too stubborn to change?

P: I don't think I believe that anymore.

Example 3. The examination of contradictory evidence is also a useful technique for changing family beliefs. The young girl in the following example believes, as do other family members, that her father does not care about her or anyone else in the family. The belief is maladaptive because it appears to foster feelings of alienation in the patient and behaviors on the part of family members that make it even less likely that the father will continue to attempt any relationship with his daughter in the future. In a previous session, the family members (parents, patient, younger brother) had been asked to see whether or not there would be any evidence in the coming week to contradict their prevailing belief that father was uncaring and uninvolved. In the following excerpt, the family's evidence collected during the past week is reviewed.

T: Last time I said, "How about watching for the exceptions in your dad's behavior? If you expect him to be withdrawn and uninterested and negative and critical, watch for when he's not that way." Remember that? You take the mental filter off and look at things a different way. So I'm just wondering did anybody notice anything different?

Brother: Yeah, last night my dad came up to my room and he hugged me and kissed me and told me he was proud of me.

T: So your dad showed you he cared about you.

Mom: Bob's [husband] been concentrating really, really hard, and he's been doing great for the last couple of weeks. He has been less critical, and I think he's been trying to do things with the kids.

T: When have you seen him do things with the kids?

M: Even the disciplining of Carol [patient], the discussion. He was being a part of it. At least he was actively involved.

T: So you're seeing your husband interested and take a stand.

M: I think he's been trying harder with the kids. Yeah. He's being a lot less critical.

P: He bought steaks for us this week, because he knows I like to eat meat sometimes.

T: For you and him?

P: No, for the whole family.

T: So what do you think that means? Was he trying to show you that he thought about you?

P: Yeah, I think so. I wrote him a note.

Dad: I saw that.

T: What did you say in the note?

P: I said, "Thanks. Love, Carol."

T: Do you all think dad was behaving differently this week because he was being watched, or do you think he always does some things to show you he cares?

B: Well, I think he probably cares about us but doesn't show it.

P: I think he was just being better this week.

T: (*to patient*) What does it mean that your dad put in extra effort to behave differently this week then?

P: He wanted us to notice.

T: Why would he want you to notice?

P: So we would think differently about him.

T: Did it work?

P: So far. If it continues.

T: What do you think it means that your dad comes to therapy sessions and lets us all talk about him like this?

P: Well, I think he cares about the family and keeping us together.

T: What does that say about your previous belief that your dad didn't love you or care about you?

P: I think he does. Maybe he didn't try as hard before, or maybe we didn't notice things.

Distraction

Distraction (or "diversion"; Beck et al., 1979) is a technique used to prevent automatic thoughts by consciously focusing attention on something else. If the automatic thoughts can be prevented for a period of time, they will often extinguish because the association between certain situations and the thoughts will be disrupted. When the maladaptive thoughts no longer occur with the regularity they once did, a belief about oneself or certain circumstances is often changed indirectly.

Example. A 16-year-old has revealed that she holds depressogenic beliefs about her ability to do "normal" things like go shopping in a public place. Her negative self-image has fostered anxious cognitions and increasing avoidance of public places, which has in turn exacerbated her depression. By using the technique of distraction, the therapist hopes to demonstrate to the patient that she can, in fact, engage in activities thought to be impossible, thereby indirectly changing some of her depressogenic beliefs about herself.

P: I still don't know about going alone to the shopping mall. Like I said, I only went for 5 minutes to pick up a present.

T: You don't give yourself as much credit as I am giving you. Maybe we should talk about that. You said it was easy because you had a specific goal, to buy a present. So do you think you could do that again?

P: Uh huh. Sure.

T: What if you didn't have anything to buy? What if I just asked you to drive there and walk in and go to that exact same store for 30 seconds and leave?

P: I could do that if someone told me to go there as a test or something.

T: Well, could you do any test that someone asked you to do?

P: Um, it depends on the test. If I had to go in there and walk around for a couple of hours that might make me feel a little nervous. But that's how long my mom goes shopping, all day.

T: Would you like to be able to go to a shopping mall by yourself?

P: Yeah.

T: What kinds of things could you possibly do right now? Park and walk in?

P: I could go in. If I had a specific thing that I needed. I could probably go in and do it quick. Especially if I had an idea of where it was.

T: Why does that make it different, one specific thing as opposed to just window shopping?

P: Because I'm in there longer if I don't have something specific, I guess.

T: OK, what if you had 30 specific things to buy? You'd be in there a long time.

P: But I'd have a place to go, so it would be OK.

T: When we first talked about this you told me you avoided public places because you thought people were watching you. And so going into a shopping mall was hard just because you were on display. If you had 30 things to do on a list, you'd still be on display, right?

P: Right. But I'd probably be thinking about the things I was going to buy.

T: Oh, so you'd be distracted.

P: I wouldn't be thinking about the people because I'd think of my list.

T: Your mind would be on something else?

P: Uh huh.

T: OK. Could you use that technique to distract yourself at other times? Even if you were just browsing? Could you distract yourself in some way?

P: I don't know what way.

T: Well, you could count by 2's.

P: Yeah, but . . .

T: Or you could name all the objects you saw as you were walking.

P: I guess that might work, I don't know.

T: What I'm thinking about is using distraction to get you out of the habit of thinking that all the people in the mall would be looking at you.

P: Well, I guess that would work if I could keep my mind on something else.

T: What if you started by making a list of all the things you might like to browse for? Would that be enough distraction?

P: I could try it and see I guess. If it didn't work, I'd have to leave.

Thought Stopping

Thought stopping (Burns, 1980) is a technique recommended when the adolescent has repetitious depressogenic ideation that he feels unable to control. The technique involves two steps: first, doing some action to draw attention to the occurrence of the maladaptive ideation and, second, replacement of the maladaptive ideation with more adaptive self-talk.

Example. A 14-year-old male has experienced recurrent episodes of depression. Recently he presented for therapy complaining of extreme lethargy, with long periods of daydreaming in which his thoughts seemed "to get stuck." The therapist recommended thought stopping and substitution after identifying a couple of particularly repetitious thoughts.

T: When you find yourself sitting and doing nothing, is there anything that you're thinking about?

P: Not really. I sort of daydream and wonder about things.

T: Do you daydream about pleasant or unpleasant topics most often?

P: I just get confused. I don't know what to think.

T: Confused about what?

P: Everything. Mainly why I'm so sad.

T: What do you wonder about your sadness . . . can I call it your depression?

P: I don't know. Just how long it will last. And mostly why it always happens to me.

T: Do you answer yourself when you have those questions?

P: No. I just keep saying, "Why do I get depressed? Why me?" and stuff like that.

T: If you keep doing that for a while, what effect does it have on you?

P: I get even more depressed and lazy.

T: Can you make yourself do anything to get out of thinking those questions?

P: I wish I could, but I just get lazier and lazier.

T: How long does it take you to realize what you're doing when you get into that kind of thinking?

P: Who knows? It seems like I think the same thing hundreds of times over and over in my head.

T: What kinds of things are you saying to yourself over and over?

P: "Why do I get depressed? When will it go away?"

T: Are those the most common thoughts you have?

P: They're the ones I get stuck with. Because I can't answer them.

T: OK. Maybe we should focus on those to begin with. Part of the problem seems to be that you get trapped in the repetition without even knowing when it really started. Is that right?

P: Yeah. That's how it is.

T: Well, one thing that might be worth trying is to use kind of a silly reminder to be on guard for those ideas. That way you'll have a better chance of stopping them, just because you won't get into the cycle accidentally. Does that make sense?

P: I guess so. But what?

T: What about wearing a rubber band on your wrist to remind you to keep watch for the ideas? And then as soon as one of them occurs, flick the band a little to remind yourself that you need to snap out of those thoughts.

P: Could I wear two—like a red one for one idea and a blue one for the other idea?

T: Sure. That would remind you that you get stuck with two different thoughts. And you could flick the colored band that corresponded to the thought you had. Good. In addition, maybe you could use the rubber band to remind yourself to substitute something else instead.

P: Like what, though?

T: Well, what would be more useful to do than asking questions about "why" and "when" that are hard questions to answer?

P: Maybe doing something?

T: You mean getting up and being active?

P: Well, that wouldn't work in school because I'd get in trouble.

T: Right, there are some situations where you couldn't physically get up and become more active. So what could you think instead, as soon as one of those two ideas popped into your head?

P: I could think about what to do differently. And then if I was thinking about it, eventually I could do it.

T: Good. So you could say what to yourself?

P: "What can I do differently?"

T: Right. That would be a better thought. Would you be able to come up with some answers to that question?

P: Probably.

T: Or would you get just as stuck with it as with the other questions?

P: I think I would have some answers.

T: Why?

P: Because we talk about things to do in here. Like how to behave at home and stuff. And with my friends.

T: OK, good. I think you're probably right. It's easier to answer the question about what sorts of things you could do differently. How are you going to remember to ask yourself that question instead of the other ones?

P: I could write it down. And then if I forget, I could look it up.

T: Great idea. Is this something you want to try for the next little while?

P: Anything's better than those other thoughts.

T: Where will you get the two colored rubber bands?

P: My mom has a whole bunch in a drawer at home.

T: When do you want to begin?

P: As soon as I go home, I'll get them.

T: OK. Why don't you write the other question about what you can do differently down here, so you don't forget it (*offering a pencil and pad of paper*)?

TIC-TOC Technique

The TIC-TOC technique (Burns, 1980) contrasts "task-interfering cognitions" with "task-orienting cognitions" so that the adolescent becomes aware of the thoughts that decrease his motivation and can learn to substitute thoughts that will have the opposite effect. The technique is particularly useful when low motivation or procrastination is a problem. The primary goal of the technique is to change some of the cognitive obstacles to initiation or completion of a task.

Example. A 17-year-old male high school student has typically been an honors student. However, toward the end of 11th grade, his marks began to drop, and his interest in school appeared to be waning. His poor performance is, in itself, disappointing to him, and he is beginning to entertain negative thoughts about his future with respect to college and the law career he hopes to pursue. In conversation, the therapist discovers that a typical pattern is for the boy to initiate projects but to leave them unfinished. The therapist explores the cognitions that interfere with the patient's completion of school work and helps him to identify thoughts that would be more helpful in orienting him to the task at hand.

T: So, as I understand it, you eventually do get started at most assignments for school, but you have trouble finishing them. Is that right?

P: Exactly. I know I should do them and that I'm throwing away a good history in school if I don't, so that usually scares me into starting.

T: So, in part, you're telling yourself that you have the ability to do the work. Before you even start, are you expecting to finish the project, or do you have doubts about that?

P: Well, I always intend to finish it. I tell myself, "This time I'll just get it done." But more often than not, it doesn't work.

T: What happens instead?

P: Oh, I'll get distracted by something or decide to put it off just for a little while or while I take a break. I'll go watch TV and then never get back to the school work. I figure it won't work out the way I want anyway.

T: At what point do you get distracted and go do something else?

P: Well, things usually start off really well. I'm full of ideas for writing an English essay, for example. Then, after a few pages, I decide the organization should change a little, or I left out something that should have been said earlier, and then I think I need a break.

T: What else do you think at that point in time?

P: Oh, things like "Here we go again, an all-nighter," or "This is going to take about a dozen revisions."

T: If you were thinking that the job would take a couple of hours and only a couple of revisions, would you be more likely to return to the job after a short break?

P: Well, I probably wouldn't even take a break at that point. Because I'd still be quite hopeful of it going well.

T: What is your indication that something is or isn't going well?

P: Just how hard it is for me to write what I want to. Like last night, all I could think was that it wasn't sounding as good as I wanted.

T: Does the mark you get on an assignment have anything to do with how well you think something is going?

P: Well, sure. Because I'm used to getting all A's. So I can tell when my English teacher is going to make comments. I usually know the parts of an essay that she's going to say need a little more work to be really clear.

T: What do you say to yourself about the teachers' comments and your marks that might hinder you finishing the work you've begun?

P: I start making predictions.

T: Such as?

P: "This is the rough part. I'll lose a few marks here. She'll think the quality of my work is slipping. She'll wonder why I'm not doing as well as she knows I can from the past." Things like that.

T: How come those ideas didn't get in the way of finishing school work in the past?

P: I guess I just concentrated on different things. Like I didn't have this reputation as a good student to uphold. Whatever I did was what I did. No one would be disappointed.

T: What would happen now if you could tell yourself a similar thing? That you'd do what you could and that was enough?

P: Well, if I could do that, it would probably help.

T: Do you believe that "You can only do what you can do"?

P: It makes sense.

T: What if it meant you got slightly lower marks sometimes?

P: At this point, I suppose any mark would be better that none. After all, I'm now to the point of not even handing in a lot of things. So I end up with a 0.

T: OK. You've said some different things recently. Let me repeat some of your thoughts and see if you can distinguish a difference in them. What effect do you think these ideas have on your motivation to finish the task? "It's all mixed up. The organization is poor. Here's another all-nighter. This will take a dozen revisions. This is too hard. It won't work out anyway. This isn't good enough. My teacher will be disappointed."

P: Obviously, I feel like giving up. They just weigh me down.

T: Can you remember anything else that you said that would have the opposite effect?

P: The things like "I have lots of good ideas. Some mark is better than a 0."

T: How about: "I have the ability to do the work. This can be done in a couple of hours. Not too much revision is needed." Would they help or hinder you?

P: Yeah. I get your point.

T: How likely is it that you could start to substitute one set of ideas for the other that leads you to quit doing a task?

P: Well, it would take a conscious effort, I think.

T: Would the payoff be great enough for you to make that effort?

P: Yeah, I guess so. I could give it a try. I never really thought of it that way, like I had ideas that were killing my motivation to keep at it.

Behavioral Techniques

Activity Scheduling

Activity scheduling (Beck et al., 1979; Burns, 1980) is a technique that focuses on altering behavior as a way of changing maladaptive cognitions. The depressogenic automatic thoughts or beliefs typically concern the patients' views of themselves or their abilities to accomplish desired goals. Activity scheduling involves making a conscious plan of how the patient anticipates spending a fixed amount of time. The schedule may be done for a week at a time (e.g., "Weekly Activity Schedule"; Beck et al., 1979) or for shorter periods such as a day at a time (e.g., "Daily Activity Schedule"; Burns, 1980). Activities in which the patient wishes to engage are included on the schedule in blocks of planned time that can vary in length but typically begin with shorter periods such as an hour at a time.

Adolescents are often reluctant to consider an activity schedule because they do not wish to commit themselves to activities several hours or days in advance. As such, it is important for the therapist to explain the rationale for the technique so that adolescents understand that the plans need not be followed exactly. In fact, substituting an unplanned activity for a planned one, inserting extra activities, or adjusting the schedule in other ways would generally be considered even better than stringently following the tentative schedule originally designed. Of course, abandoning the schedule altogether and substituting extended periods of complete inactivity would not be viewed as therapeutic in most cases, since the goal of activity scheduling is usually to address problems such as lethargy or procrastination.

Example. A 16-year-old male does almost nothing but watch television. Although he says he wants to interact with school friends, pursue hobbies, or even get his homework done, he has been increasingly unable to motivate himself to take action toward these goals. His extreme inactivity concerns him, and the more he does nothing, the more negative his views about himself become. The following discussion occurs after the patient has explained that he had a "very depressing" weekend.

T: When did you get down on the weekend?
P: I think it was probably because I was procrastinating.
T: How do you think it affects your mood, procrastinating?
P: I know I feel irritated, annoyed, and angry.

T: If you wanted to feel less annoyed and irritated, would one way be to change your procrastination?

P: Uh huh. Yeah.

T: Why do you think you procrastinate? What gets in the way of doing things?

P: Because I'm low in self-esteem.

T: Help me understand. Low self-esteem has what effect on your motivation?

P: It kind of makes me feel like a failure. And I'll never be able to get anything done.

T: And when you think you won't get anything done, you don't bother trying so you procrastinate?

P: Yeah. I think, "What's the use?" Because I'm always a failure.

T: How are we going to make you feel like you can get things done?

P: I need some success.

T: You need some success, and then you'll start feeling like maybe you can succeed, is that what you're saying?

P: Yeah.

T: That's very good. One of the ways that I think you might get some success is to use an activity schedule. For example, when you get up, there are certain things that you know you have to do. Maybe go to a social class at 9:00, or have lunch at noon. Maybe doing homework with someone that night.

P: There isn't much that I really have to get done.

T: Well, for those few things that you think you really should get done, you can write them down beside the correct time on the schedule for the particular day. And in the other spaces where there's nothing scheduled, the idea is to write what you might like to accomplish, or what you might like to spend your time doing. Can you think of some things?

P: Maybe, but I don't feel like doing much of anything.

T: That's the problem though isn't it? So in the beginning, it might be best to write down what you think you would like to do if you had the energy to do it. For example, you've told me that you wish you could make yourself keep in contact with your friend Todd from school. One of the things could be to phone Todd. Another one might be to arrange to see Todd after school one day. So you would think about the things that might be good for you to do and then fill in the schedule. It's a way of giving yourself little successes through each day. Does that sound like something that would be worth trying for you?

P: Maybe.

T: What do you think makes you hesitate?

P: I don't know.

T: Is it dumb to schedule your day?

P: I don't really schedule my day that much.

T: I know you don't now. My idea was that if you tried to do that a little bit more, you would get yourself out of the procrastination problem.

P: I'm kind of a person who takes it one day at a time. I don't really think of something 2 days ahead.

T: Why couldn't you do the activity schedule just 1 day at a time?

P: I don't know.

T: Do you think it would work 1 day at a time?

P: Maybe.

T: What would be the problems if it didn't work?

P: I may be a little disappointed if it doesn't work out the way I planned.

T: What would be wrong with changing the plans?

P: Nothing.

T: OK. Then you wouldn't have to be disappointed, would you? Or are you the kind of person who makes a plan and has to stick with it no matter what?

P: No.

T: No, so you could change your plans. Good. Then would there still be problems with trying the activity schedule to see if it gets you over the procrastination problem?

P: I guess I could try it.

Mastery and Pleasure

This technique is designed to address an adolescent's depression by encouraging the pursuit of activities that will produce either a sense of accomplishment or enjoyment. It is particularly useful for patients whose depression is manifested in low motivation or withdrawal from activities that were previously found rewarding. For such purposes, the mastery and pleasure technique is often combined with activity scheduling (Beck et al., 1979). In other cases, the technique is a helpful way of addressing dichotomous thoughts about oneself or one's life by drawing attention to disregarded aspects of experience that are providing a sense of mastery or pleasure. Essentially, this technique involves helping the patient to rate activities on the degree of accomplishment felt when an activity is completed (mastery) or on the amount of enjoyment gained as a result of doing something (pleasure). The combination of mastery and pleasure is a useful one because it, in itself, helps to challenge the unrealistic idea that life should be "all fun" or, alternatively, that the only thing worth spending time on is "work to accomplish things."

Example. A 14-year-old who complained that life was "no fun" and "boring" spent most of her time alone in her room doing nothing. In a previous session, the therapist had introduced the technique of activity scheduling, and the patient had successfully increased the number of activities outside of her bedroom in the following week. Her mother seemed particularly pleased to have received some help with small chores such as loading the dishwasher after meals. During the family session below, the therapist added the mastery and pleasure technique to the activity scheduling.

T: (*to mom*) Overall, would you say Elizabeth [patient] spent as much time in her room alone this week?

Mom: Oh, no. I think it was an effort for her, but she did try to schedule one or two things each day. I even got her to help with the dishes after meals on a couple of occasions.

T: (*to patient*) What kinds of things did you write on your activity schedule that you actually did this week?

P: Nothing very exciting.

T: For example?

P: Help mom. Do some homework.

M: You also called a friend from school and had a talk.

P: Oh yeah. Rebecca.

T: Great! Did you call your friend only once, or more than that?

P: Just once. Another day, she came over after school.

T: Did she invite herself, or did you invite her?

P: Well, she asked if she could see our new dog, so I let her come.

T: Of all the things you did this week that you normally wouldn't have done if you stayed in your bedroom, what was the most fun?

P: Going to a movie with my brother [older and lives out of the home].

T: On a scale of 0 to 10, how much fun was that?

P: Is 10 the highest?

T: Yes. Ten is really a lot of fun.

P: About 8, I guess.

T: What about talking to your friend on the phone?

P: Maybe a 6.

T: Was having her come to visit your dog fun?

P: Yeah. We went for a long walk in the park with the dog. It was pretty good.

T: How good?

P: Maybe about a 7.

T: Your mom says you helped with the dishes. Do you like doing that?

P: No, not really. But she asked me to.

T: So what would you rate that for fun?

P: About 2.

T: If I asked you did you feel good for helping your mom, what would you say?

P: Yeah. I know she was tired after work all day. And I had the day off from school.

T: So it sounds like you felt good about accomplishing something, even if it wasn't exactly fun? Is that right?

P: I guess so. It's kind of like when I clean up my bedroom. It's tidier after.

T: Right. That's what I mean. Sometimes we do things that make us feel better just because they're useful or helpful to do for someone else or for ourselves. Maybe they're not the most fun in the world, but we feel good about getting them done.

P: Like homework too.

T: Exactly. Did you do any homework this week?

P: Once or twice. We had some arithmetic.

T: And how would you rate your feeling of accomplishment after you got it done, if 10 is feeling really good about doing it?

P: After the homework, about 6.

T: How about after helping with the dishes?

P: Well, about 5, I guess.

T: And cleaning up your room?

P: That was more because it was for me. About 7.

M: It was for me too. I'm tired of looking at her messy room. I had basically given up on it myself.

T: Do you think your daughter ever thought about the good feeling she got from accomplishing a clean room before?

M: Probably not. She just thought it was a drag.

T: (*to patient*) Is your mom right? That you didn't think cleaning your room was fun?

P: It's still not.

T: But you said you felt good about getting it done for another reason.

P: Right. But I never thought of that before.

T: If you keep realizing that some things can make you feel better because you got them done, even if they're not fun, do you think you might spend less time in your room doing nothing?

P: Probably.

T: What could you do this coming week that might be fun?

P: I haven't thought about it yet.

T: Take a guess?

P: Um . . . go roller-skating.

T: Great idea. Do you have a rink near you?

P: Yeah. There's one close to school.

T: Could you plan to do that with someone?

P: Maybe, I'll see.

T: OK, why don't you try to do that. What about some things that would make you feel better for accomplishing something? Can you think of anything like that for this week?

P: Maybe carry out the garbage.

T: Good. Anything else?

P: My mom might know.

M: Well, I've been wanting you to organize your books for a long time. That would be a good job.

P: Yeah, I guess.

T: Well, how about keeping track of the things you do other than sitting in your bedroom this week? You could use the same schedule as last time. Here's a blank one for you.

P: OK.

T: Then, beside each thing you write down, would you put an "F" for "fun" if you had fun doing it. And rate the amount of fun with a 0 to 10. OK?

P: I can do that.

T: And if something you do gives you a feeling of accomplishment even if it's not fun, then could you put down an "A" and rate it too? That way we can see how many things you're doing besides just sitting in your bedroom bored and doing nothing. And we'll see how much fun you're having and how much you're getting accomplished. Is that a good plan?

P: I think so. What if getting my books organized is fun *and* it gets something done?

T: Good question. Then you could put both an "F" and an "A" and rate them both. Good point. Lots of things in life might actually be both.

Antiprocrastination

Like the technique of activity scheduling, the antiprocrastination technique (Burns, 1980) is designed to address motivational problems. It is frequently used in combination with the TIC-TOC technique to challenge the cognitive distortions of fortune telling and mind reading. Adolescents seem particularly prone to procrastinate about tasks that are considered difficult or "work" rather than "fun." Sometimes, anxiety about performance plays a role in their lack of motivation. Other times, fear of rejection plays a role in the avoidance of initiating social interactions. The antiprocrastination technique addresses the negative predictions that depressed adolescents often make by encouraging a comparison of the anticipated difficulty or satisfaction with that actually experienced after the activity is undertaken.

Example. A 16-year-old was failing his school year because he rarely handed in assignments and often refused to study for exams. After some questioning by the therapist, he revealed that he intended to get the work done but "put if off" until it was too late to complete. The therapist addresses the procrastination problem because it seems to be directly related to the patient's depressogenic beliefs about himself as being "lazy" and "a failure," in addition to the obvious repercussions it is having on his chances of passing his grade in the current school year.

T: Once you actually get started on your homework or studying, does it seem like something you have trouble doing?

P: No. The problem is getting going. I just can't make myself get started.

T: Have you ever done your homework or studied for an exam?

P: Oh sure. But it's hard to get started. This year especially.

T: Let's focus on those times when you did actually get started, even though it was hard. How difficult was it really, now that you look back on it?

P: Well, afterward, I'm glad I did it. It wasn't really hard once I got going.

T: You say you're "glad" you did it. How come?

P: Well, it's satisfying to get something done that helps me in the long run. I know I'll be better off if my high school marks are decent. Otherwise, I won't even be able to consider college if I wanted to.

T: Satisfying. You mean you get a sense of satisfaction?

P: Yeah. And I know it's not that hard, really.

T: Do you tend to overestimate the difficulty before you get started?

P: I guess so. Now that I look back on the times I finished something.

T: When was the last time you did some homework? Do you remember?

P: A couple of weeks ago, maybe.

T: What was it?

P: A report for History class. On the Second World War.

T: If you had to try to estimate now how difficult you thought that would be before you got started, what would you say? Use a rating scale to tell me if you can.

P: Pretty tough. Maybe about 80% difficult.

T: And after you got the thing done? How difficult was it in actuality?

P: Better, of course. I always do that. Maybe about a 50%.

T: So in that case, it did seem like you overestimated the difficulty. Is that typical do you think?

P: Sure is.

T: Would I be guessing correctly if I thought you got a sense of satisfaction out of doing that report on the Second World War?

P: Oh, yeah. I felt really good about it. And I got a good mark too.

T: Would you have predicted that beforehand?

P: Not exactly. I didn't think about it.

T: If you could begin to think about the sense of satisfaction you'd get from doing your homework now, would that help you to get rid of the procrastination problem?

P: If I could remember to think about it, it might.

T: What about the difficulty you anticipate that doing homework assignments or studying will be?

P: I'd have to work on that too.

T: What if you were to keep track for a week? Like a study of yourself. Rate the difficulty and satisfaction before and after you do some homework. That sort of thing.

P: It might be worth a try.

New Roles or Behaviors

The development of new roles or behaviors for the adolescent is a technique used to change maladaptive cognitions by helping the patient observe something new about himself. The maladaptive target cognitions are often negative beliefs about himself, but changes in the adolescent's behavior may also serve to change his beliefs about interpersonal relationships, various problematic situations, or even predictions for the future. Because behaviors as well as cognitions usually depend on context, this technique is often used in family sessions with the depressed adolescent, where not only the roles of the patient but also the behaviors of family members may become the focus of discussion.

Example 1. A 14-year-old female acts impulsively when angry. The belief that she is a "bad person" and "out of control" seems to be contributing to her depression, so the therapist wishes to focus the patient's attention on new behaviors she might adopt to replace the impulsive acts of anger. Discussion of new behaviors during the session led to a collaborative homework assignment.

T: From our discussion today, are there a couple of major points that you remember as ways that you can cope with anger? What sticks out in your mind?

P: Well, like talking about it with people. Letting my feelings out more and stuff.

T: OK.

P: Don't procrastinate stuff as much or else you'll get stressed out.

T: OK. Anything else?

P: Um. When I do get angry, talk about it and stuff.

T: Uh huh.

P: Ask for help when I'm stressed out.

T: Good. Those are good things to cope with anger. I wrote them down as you were talking. The three major points that you took out of today were: (1) express feelings verbally, (2) ask for help when stressed, and (3) avoid procrastination. Because you know that not doing those helps make you more short-fused, right?

P: Yeah.

T: Shortens the fuse. So that's a really good beginning on a list for you to cope with anger. Maybe over the next couple of sessions we'll have things we can add to the list. Do you think you can try using these three coping strategies in the next week or so? (*Hands patient the list of three points.*)

P: Uh huh. And then when I do, should I mark it off on the chart?

T: Oh that's a really good idea! So when you use one could you put a tick mark down on the chart?

P: Sure.

T: We'll see which of these things you use the most. That's a great idea. Maybe you should keep the list in your jeans pocket or something.

P: Yeah. In my wallet.

T: Good idea. When you get feeling a little angry, take it out of your wallet, look at the list, then think, "Which one could I use?" Good idea.

P: So each of these things would be used in different situations?

T: Yes. They probably would be. Can you think of a situation where you need to use this one? (*Points to one of coping strategies on list.*)

P: With Sheila [patient's friend from school]?

T: Good. This one (*pointing to second strategy on the list*) you need to use with . . .

P: Mom and dad.

T: With your parents. Right. This one concerns what sort of stuff (*pointing to third strategy on the list*)?

P: School work and basically me.

T: OK. Right, so they do apply in different situations. And when you use them remember to put a tick beside that one on the list.

Example 2. An impulsive young patient feels bad about himself when he acts inappropriately. Prior to the discussion below, the adolescent has explained that he was able to control his temper on several occasions in the preceding week. The therapist initially asks what difference in thinking helped him achieve control but, in response to the patient's inability to detect cognitive change, the therapist quickly shifts the focus to behavioral change alone. In contrast with many changes, the new behavior involves the cessation of a previous action rather than the initiation of a new one.

T: What did you do to keep from having really angry thoughts that made you lose your temper?

P: I just try to control blowing up.

T: What do you say to yourself?

P: I don't say anything about it to myself. I just don't do it.

T: Well, OK. What you do is you stop. Right?

P: Yeah.

T: You stop and you think, instead of doing. Right. When I've asked you how you have done that, you've always said, "I just don't do it." And so instead of doing anything, you just stop and think. And that's your technique to keep from going to the top of the anger scale.

P: That's what I said. I just don't do it.

Example 3. The members of this 15-year-old female's family have a great deal of difficulty expressing displeasure with each other's behavior. For everyone in the family, anger either results in silent withdrawal or explodes into frightening, uncontrolled fits of rage. The adolescent's depression appears to be related to her inability to predict how people will behave, and she has expressed a sense of helplessness to predict not only her own but also the reactions of family members. The therapist discusses development of new "angry behaviors" with the family as a way of changing the patient's depressogenic cognitions about the circumstances in which she lives.

T: What do you think would happen if everybody could practice being angry? Let's say each of you decides, pretends to be angry even if you're not. If you were pretending to be angry, you would have the advantage of not being caught in a surprise moment. I know you don't want to do it for real, but what about pretending in the coming week?

Mom: I don't know. We suppress all this stuff, and then we let it go too far until eventually it explodes. But I'm afraid of a lot of anger, so I'm not really comfortable with you [husband] getting angry, you getting angry next week.

T: (*to mom*) Well, you see that's a problem for Mark [husband] though, because that sounds like you're saying he doesn't have the right to express his anger.

M: It's not that he doesn't have the right to express his anger, but I wonder if we could talk about things, if there's a better way to deal with anger than this physical stuff.

T: Of course there is.

M: And if he could just talk to me, so it doesn't have to get to that extreme anger thing, which is what I think Sandra [patient] does as well.

T: Well, I'd like to ask you to try acting in a different way this week. Could each one of you, at some time, without announcing this to the rest of the family, fake anger at some point? So it might be Saturday morning at breakfast that Sandra decides, "I am going to fake being really angry because someone's laundry is in the dryer" or because mom didn't have breakfast ready soon enough or something. And maybe it'll be Thursday night when Mark is going to really surprise you.

P: He gets angry, he just doesn't talk about it.

T: Your mom says he doesn't talk about it until it finally explodes. Is that how you see it?

P: Yeah, that's it too. He's like a bomb when he lets it go.

T: I'm not suggesting that any of you get angry for real. I want you to choose, without telling anybody, when you can act angrily. Because if you're acting, you're under control, and you will know the kinds of things to say in order to try and express your feelings with words.

P: Oh boy, an acting job.

T: So there should be three instances of a try at anger expressed, one from each of you. You know I don't mean you need to throw plates across the room or anything like that, because you're going to get angry under control.

Dad: I guess it's worth a try.

T: And as everyone gets more comfortable with acting angrily and knowing that anger can be controlled, then maybe it will be easier for Sandra to express anger in a controlled way. And eventually, maybe you can help her change her beliefs about how uncertain the behaviors of people in her house seem.

Successive Approximations

The use of successive approximations (like "graded-task assignments"; Beck et al., 1979) requires the therapist and the adolescent, working together, to develop a series of graduated steps leading to a desired behavioral change. Although behavioral change is the immediate target of intervention, the purpose of achieving the change is to alter maladaptive cognitions. The achievement of successive approximations to a goal provides several opportunities for reinforcing "success" and usually results in a gradual increase in self-efficacy for the adolescent. Because successive approximations require behavioral change toward a goal that the adolescent initially views as impossible, it is important for the series of partial steps toward the goal to be developed collaboratively. Each increment in the sequence must be large enough to demonstrate a new achievement but small enough to avoid failure. If failure to achieve behavioral change at some point in the series of successive approximations does occur, it is extremely important for the therapist to frame the "failure" as a problem with the size of the task rather than a problem with the patient's motivation or effort. In essence, the therapist must attempt to use reattribution to change what will typically be interpreted by the adolescent as his personal failure. Often, it is useful for the therapist to take responsibility for designing gradations that were inappropriately spaced for the patient in question.

Example. A 17-year-old male has feelings of extreme inadequacy. His negative view of himself is related to his belief that he cannot go anywhere or do anything without a friend's assistance. Although adolescence is normally a time of exaggerated feelings of need for the company of peers, the patient realizes that his dependency is excessive and interferes with his desires to engage in independent activities. Furthermore, arranging for the constant presence of someone else is becoming increasingly difficult, resulting in more constricted day-to-day experiences. The therapist wishes to address the patient's belief that he is unable to go places by himself because the more he sees himself as dependent on others, the more he feels inferior to his friend who can do what he cannot, and the more he restricts his activities.

   T: Could you plan sometime between now and the next time you see me to do something by yourself?
   P: Yeah. Probably, yeah (*sounding hesitant*).
   T: What wouldn't you want to do?
   P: Well, for example, going to the mall and looking by myself, for a nonspecific time.
   T: Is that something you would like to be able to do?
   P: Well, yeah. Kids from school hang around at the mall, and there's a video game store there that I like. Besides, sometimes I need to buy something.
   T: You mean you would have trouble just going in and wandering around? What about going back to that same shop you were already in with your friend last week? Just going there, walking to the shop and leaving. Can you do that?
   P: I can do that.
   T: Do you think you could step inside the shop and look around?
   P: Oh, I could step in and look around for a short time.
   T: You could do that?
   P: Yeah.
   T: That will be different from buying a shirt with your friend because you won't have anything specific to get, and you will be alone this time. So would you run in or walk?
   P: I don't know. I just have to wait till I'm there.
   T: But you'll do that?
   P: Yeah.
   T: Do you think that's worthwhile?
   P: Uh huh.
   T: What do you think you might learn by doing that?
   P: If I can go in there alone or not.
   T: What's the name of the shop where you bought your shirt?
   P: Howard's, I think.

T: Howard's. In what mall?

P: Um. I can't remember the name.

T: Do you remember exactly how to get there?

P: Oh, yeah.

T: So you'll go in and walk around the store, how long?

P: I don't know.

T: Five seconds?

P: It's a really small store.

T: Five seconds?

P: Sure.

T: That's not very long. Can you do 5?

P: Yeah. But I'm not going to go in there and just walk out in 5 seconds because people will think, "What the hell is he doing?" I'll pretend I'm looking around.

T: Good idea. So, shall we say 30 seconds at least? That's enough time to look around. At least 30 seconds.

P: Sure, I can do that.

T: What about 10 minutes?

P: That long? I don't know.

T: What about longer than 30 seconds but shorter than 10 minutes? What would be about the maximum that you think you could stand?

P: I don't know. Maybe a couple of minutes.

T: Two minutes. Would you be able to try that this week?

P: Yeah, I could do it for 2 minutes. Maybe longer, but I don't know until I get there.

T: Well, let's just start with 2 minutes then. That's probably long enough for a first time.

P: OK.

STEP VI: PROBLEM-SOLVING (OPTIONAL)

During the course of therapy with depressed adolescents, the therapist is constantly listening with a "third ear" for possible cognitive distortions evident in the automatic thoughts or beliefs that contribute to the emotional distress of the patient. However, the therapist must be careful not to assume that the patient's view of things is "distorted" and that the place to begin intervention is a "correction" of the distortion. To make a premature assumption about the effect of cognitive distortions is tantamount to "pathologizing" the patient when, in fact, their emotional distress might be a perfectly reasonable response to a truly "bad" situation. Once the therapist understands the nature of the automatic thoughts or beliefs associated with the depression, it is extremely important to devote sufficient time to the evaluation of those cognitions to determine whether they are realistic or distorted. By so doing, an appropriate decision can be made to proceed in therapy with changing the way the patient thinks about something or, alternatively, with changing the situation because a problem is evident. Sometimes a real problem exists, but the adolescent has also made cognitive errors in his interpretation of it, in which case both problem-solving and cognitive change are undertaken by the therapist.

Because of the adolescent's developmental stage, therapy will often involve problem-solving. In effect, the therapist addresses developmentally imposed cognitive "deficits" rather than cognitive "distortions," at least a proportion of the time. In addition to cognitive deficits, adolescents will frequently demonstrate social deficits relative to adults and will need assistance to negotiate interpersonal difficulties or to develop appropriate behaviors. By virtue of their developmental stage, adolescents are usually not independent of their families, and parents continue to exert considerable influence in some form or another. Thus, problem-solving will often require the involvement of the patient's parents in therapy.

Although the primary goal of this chapter describing "the middle phase of therapy" is to convey strategies for eliciting, evaluating, and changing maladaptive cognitions rather than to demonstrate various techniques for problem-solving, some examples of the latter will be presented because the therapist working with adolescents will seldom be able to avoid engaging in some discussion of real-life problems. The excerpts of dialogue presented below are not intended to represent a comprehensive review of problem solving strategies. Rather, their purpose is to demonstrate how some of the same techniques useful for changing cognitions can be adapted for changing problem situations.

Example 1: Problem-Solving with Spontaneous Role Play, Identification of Automatic Thoughts, Pro–Con Analysis, and Behavioral Homework

A 13-year-old who lives with his mother has explained that his mother will no longer allow him to see his father if her ex-husband continues to drink and drive with their son in the car. Because the patient's father apparently drinks frequently and excessively, the patient is upset about the fact that his mother's new rule will probably mean severe curtailment of his visits with his father. After enough discussion has occurred for the therapist to realize that the adolescent's distress is probably realistic, therapist and patient begin to address the problem of the father's drinking. In the excerpt that follows, note how the therapist assists in problem-solving by asking "leading questions" to guide the adolescent in his thinking. The excerpt also includes a section of spontaneous role play in which the therapist assumes the "voice" of the patient's father in order to give the patient some exposure to aggressive rapid-fire questioning and some practice in expressing himself orally with his dad.

T: I'm wondering if that is something we should talk about now, how to address these issues with your dad. Tell me this, if you were talking to him, what are the things that it would be important for him to know?

P: That I get upset when he drinks that much.

T: Right.

P: And I don't like the way he acts when I have friends with me.

T: You don't like the fact that he drinks that much. You don't like the way he acts when he's drunk.

P: Or when I have friends with me because he's always different and tries to show off instead of being himself.

T: What would be difficult about telling him he drinks too much?

P: I'm just afraid of what he would say.

T: And that might be?

P: Well, "If you can't handle it, then I guess you shouldn't be around me."

T: You're afraid he's going to say, "If you don't like me the way I am, goodbye." Well, that must put you in a terrible bind. If you feel the only alternative is either to say to him, "I don't want to endanger my life anymore by getting in the car with you when you're drunk," or, if you say that, then you take the risk that he'll say, "Bye."

P: Yeah.

T: So what are your choices then?

P: To either go ahead and tell him how I feel and if he says "goodbye" then I'll have to live with what he says, or not tell him and keep taking the risk.

T: Well, that's a difficult one. What could you do if he said, "You don't like me as I am. So you don't have to see me again"?

P: Well, I could tell him that there were other choices besides just saying "goodbye."

T: Good. You could say to him that there's some way other than that. OK. What could happen then?

P: Maybe he'd just talk about it, and he would try not to drink so much around me.

T: How could you talk to him about it that would make it more likely he would make some other choice?

P: Tell him that I do want to see him, but I just don't want to be around him if he drinks that much.

T: OK. So you could say to him, "I'm not saying this because I don't want to see you." What else could you say?

P: I don't know . . . I just can't think of anything else.

T: What would happen if, before you told him this, you shared with him the bind that you were in?

P: About not being able to go with him anymore?

T: About that horrible choice that either you not tell him something that really disturbs you, or, if you tell him, he's going to get so angry that he never wants to see you again.

P: He would probably say, "Tough, that's not true."

T: But do think that if he knew about the bind, he might be more able to listen to what you're saying?

P: Uh huh.

T: And not just get angry?

P: Uh huh. He might be mad but he wouldn't refuse to listen if he knew that. He wouldn't say that.

T: So you could share with him before you start this conversation, that this is hard for you to say because, on the one hand, you want to tell him what upsets you, but, on the other hand, you're afraid that if you do he'll never talk with you again. Or he won't want to be with you again? So that's one way to help him take another option.

P: OK.

T: What else could you do?

P: Maybe say, "This might make you mad, but it's the truth and I have to tell you." And tell him, and then he gets mad. But there's nothing I could do about it. 'Cause it would be the truth.

T: OK. And then just tell him what your bind is.

P: Uh huh.

T: What if he said, "Oh, you know I wasn't drunk, and you know I would never put you in that position"? Might he say something like that?

P: I would say, "Yes, you were drunk. I could tell by the way you were acting. You don't act that way when you haven't had too much to drink."

T: (*spontaneously adopting voice of father*) "Act what way?"

P: (*spontaneously responding to father's voice*) "Obnoxious and rude and only thinking about yourself."

T: "Well, if you don't like being around me, you don't need to be around me any more."

P: "That's not what I want."

T: "Well, what do you want?"

P: "I want to be with you, but I don't want you to drink so much around me."

T: "Well, if you love me, you would love me whether I was drunk or sober."

P: "I love you anyway, but I don't want to risk my life just because you're drunk."

T: "Did your mother tell you to say all these things to me?"

P: "No."

T: (*returning to own voice*) Is he likely to say that?

Later in the same session, the therapist identifies for the patient his dichotomous thinking style when he is generating possible solutions to the problem of his father's drinking.

T: What else could he [father] say that would be hard for you to handle?

P: "Well, I'm not going to change, so you'll have to live with it or else . . . I'm not going to quit drinking."

T: (*adopting voice of father*) "I'm not going to quit drinking and this has nothing to do with you. This is a decision that I make. I'm not going to quit drinking. Do you want to be with me, or do you not want to be with me?" (*returning to own voice*) What do you say if he says that?

P: "I don't want to be with you. The only way I'll be with you is if you stop drinking."

T: OK. Now that's a pretty tall order.

P: Or if he doesn't drink as much.

T: Good, good. "If you don't drink as much." Yeah. You need to try and get out of the tendency to think in all-or-nothing ways. You know what I mean? All or nothing. Either he can never drink or you can never be with him. Either he has to completely give up drinking, or he's totally irresponsible as a dad. Those are going to be things that I think are important. But you're doing a good job trying not to get into this all or nothing.

P: Uh huh.

T: What you have to be careful of is that when people get mad or when they get upset they do a lot of "all-or-nothing" reasoning. So, your dad might say, "Either you take me exactly as I am or you don't have me at all."

P: Uh huh. "I won't have you at all."

T: Well, I think you're wise if that's the only decision. But you said something else a little while ago, you said, "Dad, I think you have another choice that is somewhere in between what I would really like and what you would really like."

P: "You could not drink as much around me."

T: Yeah. Instead of "not drink at all" you could say "not drink as much around me." That gets out of the all-or-nothing choice.

After considerable discussion in the session about possible solutions to the problem of the patient's father's drinking, the therapist wants the adolescent to evaluate the potential course of action discussed. To guide the evaluative process, the therapist uses the technique of pro–con analysis, which leads the patient to consider the advantages and disadvantages of the proposed course of action versus maintaining the status quo.

T: Let's think through the advantages and disadvantages in a way that makes you feel like the worst that could happen if you talked to your dad is not as bad as the worst that could happen if you didn't do it. OK? What is the worst that could happen if you didn't tell him how you feel about his drinking when you are in the car?

P: I could go with him again, and he could get in a wreck, or he could hit me, or I don't know, something that I don't want.

T: What is the worst that could happen if you did tell him?

P: He could say that he wasn't going to change and that would be it. He wouldn't do anything about it.

T: Which is worse?

P: Me dying or him dying. 'Cause I could live with not being able to see him. It's not as bad as taking a risk of getting killed.

T: Are you sure?

P: Yeah.

T: OK. So you really have to be ready for the worst that could happen if you do this. That's pretty bad, but not as quite as bad as the worst thing that could happen if you didn't do it.

P: Right.

T: OK. What are the advantages of doing it, even if you don't get what you want?

P: I would've told him how I felt, and then he could think about it.

If he changed his mind, I would still be alive and he would still be alive. It's better than him changing his mind and me already being dead because of an accident. And it's better than me changing my mind about not telling him after it's too late because he's killed himself with drinking in the car.

T: That's really true. So even if he tells you, "If you don't like me as I am, see you later," the fact that you told him might make him think about it. And you said something important just now, "I'll still be here."

P: Right.

Finally, in the problem-solving session, the therapist helps the adolescent address the issue of translating ideas into action with his father. At this stage, the problem-solving involves two issues: first, how information will be communicated to the boy's father and, second, how the adolescent will remember to do the homework assignment agreed on by both him and the therapist.

T: So are you going to do this [have a conversation with dad about his drinking]?

P: I think I'll write him a letter.

T: OK. What are you going to say in the letter?

P: That I decided the only way that I will be with him is if he doesn't drink as much around me. I don't want him to say, "If you don't like me the way I am" . . . to have that idea that I don't want to be with him. But I don't want to take the risk of dying or getting killed in a car or in a truck.

T: So are you going to put in that letter everything we've been talking about?

P: Uh huh.

[Therapist and patient agree that the patient will prepare a draft copy of the letter and bring it to the next session so the therapist can help him revise it if necessary.]

T: Good idea. That will give you some ability to say exactly what you want. Also to think about what's the best way to present it so he might be more willing to hear it and give him a chance to think about it before he just reacts with anger.

P: Yeah. That's what I want.

T: Would it be helpful for you to get a call from my secretary sometime this week that reminds you about the letter? What day would be good?

P: Any day. It doesn't matter.

T: Let's see, today's Thursday. We meet again next Thursday.

P: It'll probably be better for me not to know when she's going to call.

T: So you just want her to call you sometime during the week to ask you if you've done it or to remind you to do it?

P: To remind me.

T: Why would it better to not know?

P: Well, it might be better because then I'll know that I should do it before she calls.

T: Well, you don't really have to do it before she calls unless you really want to. You could just use that call as a reminder to go ahead and do it. What do you usually do Wednesdays after school?

P: Nothing, come home.

T: You come home. There's no specific thing you have to do Wednesday after school?

P: No.

T: What time do you get home?

P: Around 4:30.

T: Four-thirty. Why don't you try and plan to do it Tuesday after school? Do you have something planned Tuesday after school?

P: No, nothing.

T: OK. What if she calls you at 4:30 on Tuesday? And then calls you again 4:30 on Wednesday? So then that way if you're reminded on Tuesday and somehow you don't get it done on Tuesday, you get re-minded again on Wednesday. Would that work?

P: Uh huh.

T: If you can suggest something better, that's how we'll do it.

P: No it's fine.

T: OK. Do you have an answering machine?

P: Yes we do.

T: So if she calls and you're not there she'll just leave a message on the machine that says, "Remember the letter for Thursday." Will you know what that means?

P: Uh huh.

Example 2: Problem-Solving Combined with Changing Maladaptive Cognitions

The following example concerns a 16-year-old male who has been diag-nosed with learning disabilities in addition to depression. Central to the patient's depression is his feeling that he is stupid because he has so much difficulty with school work. In addition to addressing the patient's maladaptive cognitions about his stupidity, the therapist devotes some time to the problem of studying for exams, which has been a recurrent difficulty for the patient, in part because of his attentional and learning problems.

T: You said it would be better to think of school as a problem rather than thinking you're stupid.

P: Yeah. Because if I think I'm stupid, I don't bother trying.

T: Well, good. So what are some solutions to the problem of school that you can think of?

P: Study habits.

T: What do you mean?

P: Well, I studied with Luke for my English exam. That works because he quizzes me because he had that course last semester, so he helped me with that.

T: Was that helpful?

P: Yeah, it was, because I have someone to prompt me and, if I forgot something, he'd give me hints.

T: You've picked up on that very well. You picked up on that here too. If you have somebody to prompt you, that really helps. That's a really important strategy for you. That's good.

P: For Science, I started to read over my notes by myself. But I got really overwhelmed. I was flipping through the pages and I thought, "There's so much here that I have to know." I just skimmed through my notes. I really didn't do a thorough job. For Religion, I just went over my notes; I haven't really done any serious studying for it.

T: Was that the course you were going to try to team up with somebody for?

P: Yeah. But he's kind of hard to get a hold of and my exam is tomorrow. So I don't know if I'm going to be able to do that. Luke said he'd help me and he could quiz me, and stuff, so I might do that tonight.

T: He has time to do that?

P: Uh huh.

T: And that's a helpful strategy?

P: Yeah.

T: Does it help you remember stuff better for an exam? Can you retain it better?

P: Yeah. If I explain it to someone, they'll ask me a question out loud. And I will say the answer.

T: So if you say it out loud, do you remember better?

P: Yeah.

T: OK. So prompting is good. Saying things out loud. Have you ever tried reading your notes into a tape recorder and playing it back to yourself?

P: No. That's a good idea.

In another session with the same adolescent, his parents are present and become involved in solving a problem along with the therapist and their son. The problem concerns a therapeutic homework task the patient and therapist had discussed the previous week. The therapist rehearses (orally) with the patient and his parents a way he might accomplish the task in the coming week.

T: You were going to get a book I recommended: *Feeling Good.* Did you do any reading in it?

P: I started reading a bit right after I got it, but then I didn't get very far.

T: What happened that you didn't get very far?

P: I started talking on the phone, and I never finished reading it.

T: That's kind of a long-standing problem when you sit down to learn something, isn't it?

P: Yeah.

T: You get on the phone and you never get back to what you were doing.

P: Also I thought, "I'll read some tomorrow." Like always, tomorrow comes and I say, "I'll do it the next day."

T: The part you did read, was it difficult or boring?

P: Well, the first part was a bit boring. But then I flipped through, and I saw some neat charts that looked interesting.

T: OK, the important part for you is going to be Chapter 11.

P: I'll read it. I will. I will.

T: I'm just trying to figure out what we need to do to help make it easier for you. Do you need to break tasks down?

P: No, I guess what I could do is put aside one night when my mother will read with me.

T: Good idea.

P: And not make any other plans. We'll sit in the living room together and . . .

Mom: Great idea, my favorite pastime, reading.

Dad: (*to son*) You know that's well intentioned but is it practical? After 15 minutes you're going to be champing at the bit to do something else.

P: No, no. Because when I'm reading, I can read for an extended period of time. If she's [mom] there and I have a question, I can ask, "What does this mean?"

T: Would you read out loud or what would you do?

P: Either one. Mom will usually read a magazine and I'll just read whatever I'm reading, and I'll ask questions if I don't understand.

T: What is a reasonable amount of reading for you in one evening?

P: Believe it or not, if I'm really interested in something, I can read a whole book in one night.

T: How about just Chapter 11?

P: Yeah, I could read that. If my mother's there, it'll motivate me I guess.

T: Is this something that could start a fight? [Therapist is aware of arguments in the past over patient's procrastination.]

P: No.

M: No, I'll make sure it doesn't. But I want you [patient] to follow through on that, OK? I want you, next Tuesday night, for example, to say, "This is what we're going to do. . . ." That's where I get frustrated. All of a sudden something better has come up.

P: Well, there's something better every day.

M: Yeah, every day there's something else.

T: Maybe that's the way it is when you're 16.

P: Well, I need somebody there working alongside of me.

T: Somebody to prompt you or ask you questions or just that sort of thing?

P: Yeah, it'll work better that way.

SELECTED READINGS

Beck AT, Rush, AJ, Shaw, BF, Emery G: *Cognitive Therapy of Depression.* New York, Guilford Press, 1979.

Burns DD: *Feeling Good: The New Mood Therapy.* New York, Signet, 1980.

CHAPTER NINE

The Final Phases of Cognitive Therapy: Obstacles and Aids to Termination

T. C. R. WILKES

GAYLE BELSHER

INTRODUCTION

Cognitive therapy is traditionally a short-term, symptom-focused collaborative psychotherapy. With adult patients, improvement in the biological, psychological, and social domains is generally followed by a shift in focus from maladaptive automatic thoughts or cognitive distortions to the underlying beliefs that may be contributing to a dysphoric mood. This revised focus on dysfunctional beliefs or "schemas" often characterizes the final phase of cognitive therapy and draws the adult patient's attention to areas of cognitive change that may be prophylactic against the recurrence of depression. With depressed adolescents, the final phase of cognitive therapy frequently deviates from the usual adult format in two significant ways. First, therapy with the younger population often involves the identification of dysfunctional beliefs earlier in the therapeutic process, during the initial and middle stages. Therefore, the termination of therapy may seem to occur rather abruptly in some cases. Second, some adolescents form very dependent relationships with the therapist, clinic, or hospital. In such cases, great skill is required to facilitate appropriate termination, particularly when separation from therapy acts as a metaphor for the age-specific developmental task of separation from the family and from infantile psychological beliefs or ambitions. For the adolescent, this "liberation" may be associated with transient behavioral and emotional disturbances not normally experienced by the adult patient.

This chapter reviews some of the obstacles to ending therapy with adolescent patients and some techniques useful for facilitating the termination process. In addition, some brief case examples will be presented to demonstrate the considerable variability in types of termination that cognitive therapists might anticipate when ending the therapeutic relationship with their adolescent patients. Beck often reminds his students that the "primed" mind will see potential opportunities or difficulties quickly. Similarly, therapists who begin therapy with an awareness of potential termination issues usually will not be surprised when problems arise later in the therapy process. Often, obstacles to termination with adolescent patients can be predicted when the initial case formulation is written. This ability to anticipate difficult terminations derives from the fact that in formulating a case, the therapist considers the relative contributions of the adolescent's temperament, learning style, personality, and phase of development on the idiosyncratic expression of the depression.

OBSTACLES TO TERMINATION

Inadequate Support Resources

If psychotherapy has been explicitly linked to the resolution of a problem or the completion of a certain number of sessions, the termination process is often self-fulfilling with the achievement of these goals. However, the resources of the family, school, and community, as well as the adolescent's own resources, also influence the termination of therapy. If these resources are perceived as inadequate in any way, demands for psychotherapy may increase. In such situations, the role of psychotherapy may change from relief of depressive symptoms and modification of depressogenic cognitions to "containment" and "parenting" of the adolescent during a period of psychological transformation. It is important to remember that many families attending clinics or hospitals will have limited psychological resources. They will be preoccupied with daily survival and will have little energy remaining to devote to the family "growth" or reorganization their adolescent may need. In these families, special efforts to establish adequate support resources within or outside the family unit will be necessary before terminating the therapeutic relationship.

When the adequacy of support resources is in question, the therapist may need to hold regular meetings with community agencies, the family, and the individual adolescent patient in order to clarify expectations or identify assumptions about the termination of therapy. A common parental assumption such as "I can't parent," may be reflected in thoughts such as "If he gets upset again, we won't be able to cope without the help of the hospital," or "We just don't have the time to look after him." Parental expectations of themselves may be reflected in thoughts such as "I want my relationship with my son/daughter to be better than the relationship I had with my parents," or "I'm not going to make the same mistakes my parents made with me." Such assumptions and expectations need to explored through meaningful inquiry before the therapist embarks on the termination process.

Misconceptions about "In-Depth" Therapy

The community, represented by the school, social service agencies, or the family, can hinder appropriate and timely termination of a therapeutic relationship if these parties adopt the position that "something more needs to be done for the adolescent, whether he wants it or not." Such a recommendation reflects the traditional developmental thinking of epigenesis, where change is viewed as a sequentially predictable process, and prior steps are seen to influence subsequent steps in a linear and progressive manner. One of the limitations of this model is that it overlooks the hierarchical reorganization that occurs during development. A model of change that includes the concept of hierarchical reorganization acknowledges that biological and psychological functions change over time, permitting new organizations that are not necessarily predictable or logical based on knowledge of a previous developmental stage. Thus, it is often the integration of new biological, intellectual, and emotional capacities that results in a new "state" of functioning, and this composite is greater than the sum of the individual parts. In short, it should be recognized that both continuous and discontinuous development are important contributors to change in the adolescent patient. As such, more therapy for longer periods of time is not necessarily the way to achieve more change or improvement in the adolescent patient (Watzlawick et al., 1974).

The process of discontinuous development can be illustrated by considering the case of a prepubertal 12-year-old boy who is entering a

3-year phase of development. At the end of this period, he is not just a bigger 12-year-old; rather, he is a postpubertal boy of 15 with new biological and psychological potentials. Just as with the metamorphosis from caterpillar to butterfly or tadpole to frog, both linear and hierarchical reorganization have occurred.

Sometimes social service agencies promote the belief that "in-depth therapy is needed to correct some deep psychological trauma," too readily communicating this opinion to parents or to the adolescent patient himself. Since adolescents referred for treatment of depression often will have endured profound emotional abuse or neglect, professionals, parents, or patients themselves may raise questions regarding "critical periods" in development and voice concerns about whether or not appropriate developmental milestones have occurred at the opportune times. Perhaps these concerns about time-limited windows of opportunity for growth and development arise in relation to the well-known work of ethologists such as Konrad Lorenz, who demonstrated the phenomenon of imprinting in his now famous geese. Or perhaps they arise against a background of experience held by pediatricians and child psychiatrists who are aware of optimal periods for the development of skills such as language and toilet training. Even adolescents themselves have been known to claim, "I'm not ready now," or "It's too late because the damage is done," when they are trying to negotiate the resolution of some emotional impasse.

In spite of the fact that it is impossible to undo the traumas that adolescents may have endured earlier in their lives, and although these traumas may have interfered with development during "optimal" time periods, cognitive therapists must remember that their patients are not simply the product of their past and present experiences. Fortunately, the adolescent's phenomenological field will be influenced by hierarchical levels of discontinuous development. A patient's emotional growth will have multiple determinants relating to the development of the physical, neurological, intellectual, and emotional systems (see Guidano and Liotti, 1983). As such, cognitive therapists need not necessarily know or understand the past in order to effect change in present emotions and behaviors. Despite pressure from well-meaning professional helping agencies that are recommending more prolonged introspection regarding the adolescent's past traumas, it is important for therapists to focus primarily on cognitive restructuring and coping strategies for the present and future. With some adolescents, pathological interpersonal behavior patterns can be reframed as age-appropriate actions accompanying the psychological transformation from child to adult, thereby allowing the therapist to focus on present solutions rather than past problems.

The Therapist's Own Role

Ironically perhaps, another obstacle to the termination of therapy may originate with the therapist himself. In the case of the family with limited resources, the therapist may rapidly become part of a "professional family" and may even become part of the problem by inadvertently reinforcing the patient's or family's feelings of inadequacy. Sometimes therapists are seduced by parents into treating them, resulting in a conflict of interest for all concerned and confusion about the goals (and therefore the termination) of therapy.

When depressed adolescents have borderline or narcissistic traits, therapists must remain cognizant of the patient's own psychological resources in order to avoid continuing with "more of the same" in the false hope of achieving a better resolution of problems. As in the case of the family with limited resources, the adolescent patient with limited resources may coerce the therapist into continuing his habit of being helpful, thereby unintentionally keeping the adolescent in a helpless role. For example, the therapist may selectively attend to dysphoric statements and self-deprecatory ideas, minimizing the adolescent's successes in the interpersonal, academic, and family domains.

With families or adolescents who entice the therapist into being overly helpful, it is usually productive to ask whether the patient will assist the therapist in "breaking the habit" of being too helpful. This request should be accompanied by an explanation of the reciprocity between the therapist's helpfulness and the patient's or family's helplessness. In essence, the therapist requests assistance in becoming less involved in the adolescent's world. This task is facilitated by focusing on competence, achievements, and behaviors that contradict the assumption that the adolescent or the family needs further help to become independent.

Finally, therapists themselves sometimes hold the belief that in-depth therapy is necessary. But it should be noted that this view may reflect a caregiver's personal agenda and not represent a truly collaborative approach with the adolescent patient. Frequent reviews of the cognitive case formulation and the goals for therapy that were established with the adolescent will assist the therapist in making decisions about the appropriate focus and length of therapy.

TECHNIQUES TO AID TERMINATION

Review Cognitive and Behavioral Change

After 10 or more sessions for the treatment of depression, termination efforts with the adolescent may be assisted by allocating two or three sessions to a review of therapeutic progress. In particular, it is useful to review with the patient and family the adolescent's previous cognitive domains, including the assumptions and beliefs that were contributing to the depression. These can be compared with present cognitive domains and the accompanying new beliefs and assumptions. In some cases, the termination process can be facilitated by outlining the cognitive formulation in a letter, which is sent to the adolescent and his family to be reviewed at home. The process of highlighting cognitive change is like giving the adolescent a ticket for the next stage of the developmental journey. However, the therapist must recognize that the progress and experience of this journey will depend on the adolescent's own efforts, conceptualizations, and determination. Although the therapist can prepare and guide the patient, the ultimate step into self-governing responsibility must be made by the adolescent himself.

The review of therapeutic progress can occur at several levels. For example, therapists might contrast "old" and "new" emotional responses or behaviors, "previous" and "current" automatic thoughts, the degree of influence that cognitive distortions held "then" and "now," or the "former" and "revised" assumptions and beliefs held by the adolescent. For younger adolescents, the review of therapeutic progress is best undertaken with reference to a specific situation. This strategy gives the patient a concrete example for the "before–after" comparison. Older adolescents who have developed better skills of generalization and abstract thought can often discuss their therapeutic gains without reference to a concrete example, much as an adult would. Toward the end of therapy, the opportunity for highlighting cognitive change will often present itself during a session, even if review was not specifically identified as an agenda item. Therapists should listen carefully for such opportunities and use them spontaneously. The examples presented below demonstrate the review of therapeutic progress.

Example 1

A young boy with learning disabilities is encouraged to contrast his current emotional and behavioral responses to a disappointing situation with those he would have exhibited before entering therapy. In addition, the therapist highlights for the adolescent the content of his automatic thoughts that contribute to his different emotional and behavioral reactions. Note the therapist's use of the "new–old" metaphor as it relates to the patient himself. The situation being discussed is a family move back to the boy's previous neighborhood.

T: When is the move going to be?

P: We were going to move May first, but now we can't. Now we're gonna move at the end of June when school is over. My dad wants me to stay there so I can get my testing done to see if I have a learning problem.

T: So was that switch hard for you, from May first to the end of school?

P: Yeah at first, because I was really excited, and I told my friends I was going to be able to move back to my old neighborhood. And now I'm not moving when I said. So I'm kind of mad, but whatever it takes (*shrug*).

T: OK, this is the new Matthew right? Tell me how you would have reacted to this 3 months ago? How would the old Matthew have reacted to the information that you're not going to move soon but you're probably going to move 2 months later?

P: I would've gotten mad, and I would've cried.

T: And what would the old you have thought to yourself?

P: That dad'll end up . . . he'll keep putting it off, and we won't move for a long time.

T: "He always does this," right? The old you also used to say, "Everything always goes wrong, nothing ever goes right for me."

P: Right. That's what I would have thought.

T: What are some more choice things you could have said to yourself?

P: Good or bad?

T: Bad.

P: "We'll end up not moving." The old me would say it won't happen.

T: OK. Now what did you actually say to yourself? How did the new Matthew react?

P: Well I thought that it'd probably be better for me to stay so I could get my testing done to see why I wasn't making good grades and stuff. And that's pretty much what I thought about.

T: So you said, "I'm not ecstatic about it, but maybe there are some advantages to staying"?

P: Yeah.

T: What else did the new Matthew say to yourself?

P: "I want to move because I don't want to stay here. It just keeps getting boringer and boringer. And now that I know I'm going to move, it's just making it worse to have to wait, because I'm excited. But I understand that we can't move now. So it would be better for me because I need to get my testing done. And we'd have to transfer me in the middle of the last 6 weeks of school."

T: So even with those advantages that you hadn't really thought of yourself, the fact that your dad brought them up made it much easier because the new Matthew has learned new ways to accept them. Right?

P: Yeah.

T: I mean it probably would be better in some ways if you could move right?

P: Uh huh.

T: It may be more fun. It was what you were looking forward to, but that's all it would be. It would just be a little better.

P: Uh huh.

T: And the old Matthew would've convinced himself that if he could not move May first, it would be the end of his chance for any happiness.

P: Right.

T: Do you see this change in yourself?

Example 2

A 17-year-old adolescent is encouraged to review the change in her beliefs about expressing anger. Unlike the previous example, in which a specific situation was used as the stimulus for discussing therapeutic progress, this dialogue occurs at a more abstract level. Note how the therapist elicits from the patient the nature of change in her beliefs and then restates the new belief for emphasis.

T: Has a sense of that changed now that you can express your anger? Or are you still scared you may hurt their feelings if you get angry?

P: I think I'm still scared I'll hurt their feelings.

T: But?

P: But I'm learning that I can't pussy foot around them, because the longer it builds up, eventually I will probably hurt their feelings a lot more.

T: How so?

P: Well, sometimes it feels like it's just going to explode. And I'm gonna say a lot of things that I might not even mean.

T: OK. So in some ways you're still scared that you can hurt their feelings. But how is it that you have come to the point where you can express your feelings now? That's actually something I haven't really understood from what you've said. In my mind it's not clear what really has changed.

P: Well, I'm realizing that I'm a human being and I have the right to my feelings.

T: Uh huh.

P: . . . So I feel that maybe they can take it more or that my feelings are hurting me . . . and why should I be hurting because it's not helping them if I'm unhappy.

T: Right. OK. So it's a sense that you're entitled to your feelings as well?

P: Yeah.

T: That's good. That's excellent. That's a big part of the change in you, from the belief that you had when you came in here, which was you had no right to say anything.

P: Yeah.

T: You've realized for yourself that it's important for you to acknowledge your own feelings and that you're just as entitled to your opinion and your feelings as anyone else.

P: Yes. That's been a big change for the better for me.

Challenge Dichotomous Thinking about Termination

It is important for the therapist to be aware of potential cognitive distortions about the termination of therapy. Depressed adolescents often display a marked proclivity for all-or-nothing thinking when issues of separation arise. For example, as the termination of therapy approaches, cognitive errors that were thought "always" to distort reality in the past may be dismissed by the adolescent as "never" playing a role anymore. Alternatively, an adolescent who described himself as "totally depressed" before therapy may claim that he is "totally happy" near the end of therapy. Or an adolescent who initially was convinced that he could never cope without the therapist later might conclude that he never again would benefit with therapy.

Therapists must challenge such primitive thinking with alternative mature thinking by using traditional cognitive techniques such as the cognitive continuum or reframing. Challenge of dichotomous thought regarding the termination of therapy is an important preventive measure against relapse because the adolescent will almost certainly experience periods of dysphoria after therapy has ended. If these experiences of negative emotion were interpreted by the adolescent as evidence that he was again "totally depressed," they could serve to discredit the gains made in therapy and contribute to a perceived sense of "failure." Socratic dialogue often allows the therapist to challenge dichotomous thought about termination and foster cognitive restructuring of the separation process. For example, it is useful to pose questions like "Is this really the end of our relationship or just the beginning of our new relationship where you are the one who decides when and what to talk about if you become depressed again?" The following examples demonstrate the therapist's awareness of the importance of challenging dichotomous thought as therapy nears its end.

Example 1

In the following dialogue, the patient is an 18-year-old adolescent whose perfectionistic demands of himself were a major focus throughout therapy. Note how the therapist reinforces the adolescent's shift away from dichotomous all-or-nothing thinking about his academic progress and future.

P: I think just my general outlook on life is improving. Instead of saying, "Oh, I need to kill myself," if something goes wrong, I try to force myself to say, "It's OK. Things are sometimes going to go wrong." Like I was talking to my mom last night and said, "I'm going to finish off this school year, you know. I'm going to do the best I can, but if I fail everything that's OK." It's all right because it's only to be expected with all the school I've missed. If I have to go back for 2 more years and get everything done and then go to university, that's OK with me.

T: OK. Good.

P: So instead of going, "Oh my gosh, what am I going to do? I don't have anything done on schedule. It's not perfect," I'm trying to be a little more relaxed about things.

T: The word I would use there is, correct my word if it's not helpful, is your expectations are more flexible.

P: Yes. Yes.

T: You're not quite so rigid. Now that's very important because that's what I call the difference between black-and-white thinking and realistic thinking. One minute it's looking rosy because you're going to be a physician and achieve your goals. The next minute you encounter some difficulty in school and life isn't worth living. So you've changed quite a bit on that dimension.

P: Yes. I'm definitely seeing that things don't have to be perfect or a catastrophe. There can be room in between.

Example 2

The following example concerns the same adolescent male presented in the dialogue above. Note how the therapist introduces a cognitive continuum to challenge the binary motif and assist the evaluation of change in the adolescent's adherence to a maladaptive schema.

T: Do you think you're getting to be master of your perfectionism or is perfectionism mastering you?

P: A bit of both. I think I'm getting more of a handle on it though.

T: Uh huh.

P: It's not ruining my life anymore.

T: Good. So when I first met you, perfectionism was ruining your life?

P: Most definitely.

T: So what percent would that be then?

P: Close to 100% I think.

T: And I think you told me your mood was about 1 out of 10 when I first met you. Now what would you say your mood is rated at?

P: I'd say it rates about 7 or 8.

T: OK. And perfectionism, in terms of control over you?

P: How much control it has over me?

T: Yeah. You were a 100% before, several weeks ago. Now what is it?

P: Maybe 60%.

T: So just 60% control? Good. That's an improvement then, and your mood seems to be improving too.

Heighten Awareness of Internalizing Cognitive Skills

The goal of cognitive therapy is to teach the therapeutic model to patients well enough that they can achieve independence from the therapist, applying the techniques of cognitive restructuring or problem-solving to difficult situations as they arise in their lives apart from therapy. Although adolescents may not be consciously aware of internalizing the cognitive strategies repeatedly employed in therapy with the guidance of the therapist, it is this process of internalization which enables them to terminate therapy successfully. Although the practice of setting an agenda for each session often results in the adolescent identifying problems whose surface content appears to be situation-specific, it is extremely important that the patient come to view therapy as an educational experience that will have general application in new and different situations. Thus, near the end of therapy, it will be important for therapists to heighten the adolescent's awareness of his internalization of new ideas and strategies for viewing himself, the world, and his future. Such an awareness can be fostered with questions such as "What part of the therapy will you carry around with you in your head to help you with any further difficulties you may run into in the future?" In some cases, the internalization process can be highlighted by relabeling a problematic cognition, such as in the example below.

Example

The following dialogue occurs after several weeks of therapy with a depressed and suicidal male adolescent. Note how the therapist uses a continuum to investigate change in the frequency of suicidal thoughts. Of particular note is the therapist's use of relabeling in an attempt to have the adolescent internalize his changed view of suicide as a "problem" rather than a "solution."

T: Do you remember your initial contract or therapeutic goal with me?

P: I think I said I needed to avoid something.

T: To avoid what?

P: Suicide.

T: Yes, that's right. Have you forgotten about it, or did that feeling get remote?

P: I wouldn't say it's remote. I'd be kidding myself if I said that because it's still there. But I don't think I'm a danger to myself anymore. If that does go through my head I correct it and go, "No, that's not right." I think of the positive. And so I think eventually, as time goes on, it will become remote. I hope.

T: Well, this is a very serious area, your safety. I know that we got the pills from you, the pills in your room. Do you have any others?

P: No, nothing.

T: And how often is this thought, "I might as well kill myself," coming into your head?

P: Every couple of days.

T: Every couple of days. When I first saw you, how often had it come up?

P: All the time.

T: So there's been a change in terms of the frequency? Has there been a change in terms of how you deal with it?

P: Oh yeah.

T: What are you able to say to yourself?

P: I can just turn it around. I can say, "No, there are a lot more options," and I don't pressure myself anymore. I try not to have the all-or-nothing kind of thinking.

T: So do you see suicide as a solution or do you see suicide as a problem?

P: Definitely a problem.

T: A problem. If you start to think suicide is a solution, will you call me, because that's really important?

P: Yes.

Cater to Personality Style

Throughout the course of therapy with a depressed adolescent, the therapist will learn much about the personality style of the individual. Some patients will appear highly dependent; and, as therapy nears its conclusion, these adolescents may make bids for a continued therapeutic relationship by raising new issues, by exaggerating the seriousness of a problem, or even by "inventing" topics of concern to them. Such actions by the adolescent are good opportunities for the therapist to review what has been learned in therapy, generalizing from specific situations discussed in the past to the new issues raised. Gradually, the therapist should shift the responsibility for application of cognitive techniques to the adolescent, by asking questions such as "What problem did we discuss a few sessions ago that sounds something like the one you're raising now?" or "Which one of those thinking errors we talked about could be getting you into emotional trouble with this situation?" Another useful strategy for the dependent patient is to ask the adolescent to adopt the role of therapist, imagining a friend or the therapist as a patient seeking advice. When terminating with dependent adolescents, consistent reinforcement for independent thinking will be especially important.

Adolescents with narcissistic traits also present a challenge to the termination process. These patients frequently have difficulty with authority figures, and, for them, termination of therapy may be perceived as an insult. Sometimes, they terminate the relationship with therapists in a passive-aggressive way by missing appointments. Dealing with such patients will be easier if the therapist remembers that control over the termination of a relationship is an age-appropriate issue that frequently arises in social contexts with adolescents. For example, it is not uncommon to hear an adolescent state, "I want to break up with my girlfriend before she breaks up with me," or "I didn't want to go to that party anyway." With a narcissistic adolescent, it is often useful for the therapist to engineer transfer of the decision-making about the final session to the patient. By so doing, the adolescent is invited to "reject" the therapist when therapeutic progress indicates that it is appropriate to terminate.

Therapists should be cognizant of the mode that each adolescent prefers for terminating relationships. One way of gaining this understanding is to ask the adolescent how he has ended relationships in the past. Do relationships end abruptly? Do idealized figures become devalued and denigrated, or are they merely denied and avoided? However, unlike the termination process in some models of psychotherapy, terminations in cognitive therapy would seldom involve extensive discussions about the patient's style of ending relationships and how that style was being replayed or should be changed in the current therapist–patient dynamic. More commonly, the therapist will simply cater to the adolescent's personality style, participating in whatever type of termination best suits the individual while the therapist meets the therapeutic goals of reviewing and reinforcing cognitive or behavioral change.

Utilize Metaphors

The power of metaphor can often be used effectively to reframe issues such as separation. For example, a new ship, after its construction in dry dock, is launched into untried waters but is always able to return to port for further refitting and refurbishing if necessary. Some adolescents are unable to comfortably and explicitly discuss termination, but they can discuss a metaphor for termination as represented by role models or public figures. For example, the sense of abandonment that Luke Skywalker felt upon the death of his teacher and guide, Obiwan Kanobi, may be a metaphor for all separation issues. With some adolescents, the world of sport can provide useful metaphors for psychological issues. For example, the behavior of Wayne Gretzky, an ice hockey player from the Edmonton Oilers who was transferred to the Los Angeles Kings, was able to help Bert, a 16-year-old with a passion for hockey who had been expelled from school for stealing. By observing Gretzky's public experience of grief and readjustment with his transfer from Canada to the United States, Bert was able to come to terms with his own pain of separation from his familiar school and way of life. Bert was able to accept that the end of things is normally painful but that this pain is not permanent. Rather, it is usually associated with a transition in one's life—the birth of a new stage, experience, or career (Campbell, 1973).

Therapists can select appropriate metaphors from whatever attracts an adolescent's interest in order to deal with the psychological issues of termination. Whether it be related to music, films, or sports, a metaphor allows discussion of the adolescent's conscious thoughts, underlying assumptions, expectations, and biases. His own personal script, story, or mythology can then be "rewritten" in a cocreated new story with new opportunities and potentials. The dilemma for many adolescents is the termination of one story, career, or life phase and the beginning of a new one involving a new identity, character, and potential. The idea that the adolescent is going through a transition between stories can help both the therapist and patient maintain a degree of psychological flexibility (see Viederman, 1983; Watzlawick et al., 1974).

Lengthen Interval between Sessions

It is recommended that the interval between sessions be lengthened as therapy progresses in order to promote a natural weaning process. School holidays and therapists' vacations are natural breaks that can foster "geographical cures." In these situations, it is important to arrange in advance a contingency plan for the family and adolescent to follow in case of relapse. This strategy can be combined with a stress inoculation test whereby the patient and family are asked to imagine the worst possible scenario and how they would cope with it. To assist the family's independence, a contract referring to the contingency plan can be written by the adolescent and his family (Beck et al., 1979).

CASE EXAMPLES

The ways therapy can terminate are almost as numerous as the individuals in therapy. Many factors influence the termination process, which must be designed specifically for each adolescent. Of paramount importance is consideration of the goals of therapy, including cognitive restructuring as well as problem-solving and symptom relief. And as mentioned previously, factors such as the individual's and family's resources and the adolescent's personality style must also be considered. To simplify the conceptualization of the final phase, we have identified four prototypes of termination and present a case example of each. Therapists should note, however, that individual cases will vary greatly and that none will replicate precisely the following examples.

The "Contracted and Timely" Termination

This type of termination occurs after a relatively short period of therapy that has focused largely on the dysfunctional behaviors or cognitions associated with the depression. The adolescent has typically been willing to participate in therapy, allowing the rapid formation of a good therapeutic relationship. In addition, parents have usually been cooperative in assisting the therapist by readily adopting the therapeutic model and helping the adolescent to apply it beyond the therapy sessions themselves. Patients with whom a contracted and timely termination is possible sometimes have psychiatric diagnoses other than depression, but these typically do not involve significant conduct disorders or major skill deficits. Nor would this type of termination normally be possible with adolescents who manifested significant Axis II personality traits. When the final phase of therapy is a contracted and timely one, the goals of therapy initially established with the adolescent have usually remained central throughout therapy and few, if any, major issues additional to them have been raised as the therapy progressed. In a contracted and timely termination, the therapist will usually have two or more sessions in which to employ a variety of the strategies discussed above as appropriate for the final phase of therapy.

Case Example

Mark was a 16-year-old who had no previous history of depression. He lived with his mother and a younger sister with whom he experienced considerable sibling rivalry, which caused him great frustration. In fact, Mark presented for therapy after a suicide attempt that apparently had been triggered by an argument with his younger sister, who had criticized his behavior. During the initial assessment, Mark's mother identified his increasing withdrawal as her primary concern, indicating that he was spending uncharacteristic amounts of time alone in his bedroom and was refusing invitations from friends with whom he had previously been quite active. A review of the family's history revealed that there had been several significant events in the 3 months preceding the onset of Mark's depression. First, Mark's grandfather had died suddenly. This was a man whom Mark admired greatly, and the family agreed that Mark was probably the favorite grandchild. Second, Mark's stepfather of 10 years had left the family home without warning and was living with another woman. Mark had idolized his stepfather and was particularly upset that the numerous hours they had spent together working on motorcycles, playing hockey, and practicing boxing in the basement had suddenly come to an end. Because Mark's mother worked rotating shifts, everyone agreed that her spouse had spent much more time with the children than did she and that his departure had resulted in a considerably more chaotic home life in addition to financial difficulties. Third, the family dog of 10 years had disappeared.

By the time the initial phase of therapy was complete, the therapist had hypothesized that Mark's depression was related to his interpretation of the losses he had suffered, preventing the normal resolution of a grief reaction. In particular, the therapist noted that the suddenness with which various relationships had terminated might be contributing to a sense of helplessness. In addition, the therapist hypothesized that a depressogenic view of himself, either because of self-blame or a sense of worthlessness, might be exacerbating Mark's depression and help to explain his recent suicide attempt. Since Mark's social withdrawal was notable, one of the goals of therapy was to reinstate his former level of social interaction with friends and his immediate family members. Mark, himself, wished to reinstate a relationship with his stepfather, so another goal of therapy was to explore the possibility and ways this might be accomplished.

During the middle phase of therapy, Mark's record keeping indicated that he was experiencing significant sadness, anxiety, and anger. Exploration of the precipitating situations for these emotions revealed that Mark experienced a variety of automatic thoughts with the common theme that he was stupid. Logical analysis and the examination of contradictory evidence were two of the techniques most useful in challenging his self-deprecatory ideation. In addition, many of Mark's cognitions were catastrophic in nature, and one of the cognitive distortions that appeared to play a significant role in his thinking was his tendency to predict the worst or engage in mind reading. The therapist found that the techniques of cognitive forecasting in combination with cognitive rehearsal and alternate explanations were particularly helpful in correcting the distortions.

Perhaps the most important revelation during the middle phase of therapy was Mark's belief that close relationships were to be avoided because they frequently ended in people leaving him. Considering the recent events in Mark's life, it was not surprising that he would draw such a conclusion. The adaptiveness of Mark's belief about close relationships was evaluated by using the technique of time projection. In addition, logical analysis concerning the belief as it applied to his stepfather, specifically, helped to clarify that the marital relationship had ended because of problems between his parents and not because of any difficulty between Mark and his stepfather.

At this point in therapy, Mark's mother was extremely helpful by reinforcing Mark's view of his relationship with his stepfather as a good one and by supporting Mark's desire to maintain contact with him. As this possibility was explored, it became apparent that Mark had little idea of how to go about achieving the desired goal of reinstating a relationship with his stepfather. Now the therapist shifted the primary focus of therapy from cognitive restructuring to problem-solving and used role play to address some skill deficiencies Mark exhibited. As new behaviors were learned, Mark's successful execution of them in relationship to his stepfather were occasionally hampered by his proclivity to jump to conclusions, predicting the worst of ambiguous situations. These distortions were systematically addressed as the therapist engineered a balanced focus on problem-solving and cognitive restructuring.

The final phase of therapy was probably indicated by Mark's initiation of contact with his stepfather. The cooperation of Mark's mother and stepfather in this regard helped Mark to challenge his belief that close relationships should be avoided. A change in this belief may have been responsible, in part, for improvement in Mark's social withdrawal. He reported joining the school soccer team and a science club. Mark's mother corroborated his reports of increased social involvement and stated that he appeared to hold a positive view of himself and to be generally happier. The other significant factor that played a role in Mark's recovery from depression and change in his social withdrawal was the skill development and problem-solving that had been undertaken in the context of his relationship with his stepfather. Once Mark knew how to contact and make arrangements with his stepfather, one might assume that he felt less stupid and helpless. In addition, because Mark was no longer required to be a passive wishful thinker about contact with his stepfather, he reported feeling free to pursue other activities rather than wait vigilantly in his bedroom hoping against odds that his stepfather would phone.

During the final phase of therapy in an effort to encourage Mark's awareness of internalizing the knowledge he had gained, the therapist repeatedly drew Mark's attention to his tendency to engage in catastrophic thinking about relationships. Together they reviewed the effect that a return to this catastrophic thinking style would have on his belief about the perceived risk involved in friendships or family relationships. The therapist combined review of Mark's cognitive and behavioral changes with stress inoculation by exploring hypothetical situations involving Mark's stepfather.

The final three sessions were spaced at intervals of about 3 weeks, and the last session, which had been planned in advance, included Mark's mother and younger sister. Because loss of relationships had been a central focus of Mark's therapy, the therapist was particularly concerned that Mark not view the termination of the therapeutic relationship in a negative way. Care was taken to ask Mark if there were other issues or problems he would like to address before therapy ended, but he repeatedly said his major problems had been addressed. The therapist asked Mark if he could be contacted by phone a few months in the future as a "check-up," and Mark readily agreed. The therapist's act of planning and initiating follow-up contact probably helped to address any catastrophic thoughts Mark may have entertained about the termination of therapy. Therapy terminated as scheduled, and the case was closed with no further contact from Mark or his mother.

At the follow-up contact, which occurred approximately 10 weeks after the last session, Mark's depression continued to be remitted, and he reported an active social life, including a relationship with his stepfather. Three months later, a second follow-up contact made by the therapist confirmed that Mark's therapeutic gains were being maintained. Interestingly, Mark returned some self-report questionnaires with a note stating that he appreciated the periodic checkups and would be quite willing to complete some more questionnaires in 6 or 8 months "if it was not too much trouble for [the therapist] to send them." Apparently, the therapist had been correct in anticipating that it would be important to challenge depressogenic cognition with respect to the termination of therapy.

The "Rushed" Termination

In the jargon of psychotherapy, this type of termination is probably best known as a "flight into health." A rushed termination is one the therapist may feel is somewhat premature but, nonetheless, agrees to because of the adolescent's insistence that he is no longer depressed and that problems identified as goals for therapy have been resolved. Although the therapist may have reservations about the prognosis for the adolescent's emotional well-being, to insist on continued therapy would risk alienating the patient and disrupting the collaborative relationship that is essential for therapeutic work. Unlike patients who drop out of therapy, those with a rushed termination have progressed through the initial phase of therapy and at least part of the middle phase, although it may be truncated prematurely, whereupon a greatly speeded final phase ensues. The extent of the speeding can be considerable, with the adolescent sometimes agreeing to only one final session in which to convince the therapist that he is no longer in need of therapy. Frequently, the harbinger of a rushed termination will be missed or canceled appointments following a positive turn of events in the adolescent's life. Adolescents with rushed terminations may represent a wide variety of psychiatric diagnoses in addition to depression, with the probable exceptions of dysthymia or dependent personality traits. Rushed terminations often occur when the parents have been difficult to engage in the therapy process; and, as such, the final sessions may, of necessity, include only the adolescent.

When ending therapy with an adolescent who rushes the termination, it is especially important for the therapist to approach the final session with an organized plan of strategies most likely to solidify the therapeutic gains made. In addition to reviewing cognitive and behavioral changes, special attention should be given to enhancing internalization with memorable "tags" or "catch words" and metaphors, if possible. Because there may be significant issues that were not fully addressed during the course of therapy and because the opportunity to examine the adolescent's generalization of cognitive techniques has been severely curtailed, the therapist may participate in a rushed termination somewhat reluctantly. When this is the case, caution must be exercised against the therapist's own fortune telling in predicting the worst for the adolescent and inadvertently communicating this message to the patient. However, since relapse may be a distinct possibility, a critical aspect of the rushed termination is challenging any black-and-white thinking the adolescent may have about "never" being depressed again or "never" needing therapy in the future.

Case Example

David was 18, the only child of parents who both worked in the family printing business. He had no history of depression but did report a sig-

nificant history of family distress, including severe conflict with his father and considerable marital strife between his parents. Although invited, David's father refused to attend the initial assessment, where it was
revealed that he had a lengthy history of his own untreated depression,
characterized by extreme moodiness and withdrawal. Shortly after therapy began, David moved out of the home to live with an aunt so he
could attend summer school because he had failed several courses in
the previous semester.

During the initial phase of therapy, David identified his lack of motivation for school and the hostility between himself and his father as
the central problems in his life. David portrayed his father as a selfish,
uncaring autocrat who made unfounded accusations about David's lack
of responsibility. David's mother elaborated on the father–son conflict
by explaining that both she and her husband were concerned about
David's constant requests for money and apparent unwillingness to assist in the family business in exchange for the financial favors his parents granted him. He did, in fact, drive a new car that his parents had
bought for him and continued to support with money for insurance and
gasoline. The therapist hypothesized that David's depression was related
to his perception of his parents as providers of material goods rather
than the love and attention he craved. In part, there seemed to be some
evidence to support this view, but the therapist remained cognizant of
the possibility of cognitive distortion on David's part. In particular, his
overly dramatic presentations in session led the therapist to entertain
hypotheses about the potential impact of dichotomous thinking, binocular vision, and overgeneralization on David's interpretations of life at
home. By the end of the initial phase of therapy, one of the goals that
had been established was to address David's motivational problems regarding summer school, since completion of the course work was essential for his eventual graduation and would help to demonstrate to his
parents that he could be responsible. An equally important goal was to
improve the relationship between David and his father.

During the middle phase of therapy, David's mood was erratic. Although it improved slightly when he moved in with his aunt, he quickly became overwhelmed with the task of attending school. Magnification of the difficulty of his course work appeared central to his sense of
futility, and the therapist used the TIC-TOC technique to address motivational problems with some success. When the 6-week summer-school
program ended, David had passed his courses and returned home. Then
he experienced a severe relapse. In fact, he refused to get out of bed for
several days, during which his parents (father included) presented for
therapy without him. The therapist employed the genogram probe tech-

nique to elicit some of David's father's beliefs about depression (his own as well as his son's), thereby successfully engaging the reluctant parent in the therapy session. Discussion with David's parents soon revealed that they lacked some parenting skills, in particular, the abilities to develop parental consensus about expectations for David and to enforce rules made for him. At this juncture, the therapist devoted some time to problem-solving and skill development with David's parents. David returned to therapy the next week and witnessed a heated debate between his parents about the degree to which each of them was or was not "spoiling" him. Just as his father was about to leave the session in a fury, the therapist introduced a spontaneous "experiment," which involved the collection of contradictory evidence to challenge their apparent belief that they would never agree on anything about their son. (The experiment involved having each parent write down the amount of money per month that would be reasonable to give David for various categories of expense. Amazingly, the parents agreed within $5 of one another, and the therapist related this "evidence" to their abilities to parent, in general.)

Almost immediately, David started canceling appointments. When the therapist tried to contact David, he discovered that David had moved into his own apartment with money borrowed from his parents. David's intention was to find a part-time job that would support his independent dwelling while continuing with school. His parents had apparently agreed to continue supporting his food and car expenses. In what was to become his next-to-last session, the therapist tried to address some of David's unrealistic expectations about his immediate future in light of his lingering reluctance to pursue employment or attend school. His procrastination now seemed more a function of unrealistically positive views of the recent changes in his life rather than the depression that had contributed to his lack of motivation previously. The techniques of logical analysis and time projection were employed to help David examine the probable consequences of his inaction. With the therapist's help, he developed an activity schedule, which included initiatives directed toward the goal of finding employment.

The middle phase of therapy abruptly became the final phase when David canceled another appointment, stating that he was no longer depressed and saw no need for continued therapeutic involvement. He did, however, agree to one final session 2 weeks hence. Because David's parents declined further involvement in his therapy, he attended the final session by himself. He had made some initial contacts with potential employers and continued to be excited about his new "independence." The issues with his father were dismissed as largely unimportant since he was no longer living in the same house. David's most significant cognitive change appeared to be the adoption of a new image for himself—one that involved work rather than school and the freedoms associated with his own apartment. Since David's "image" of independence would have to be supported by actions toward that end, the therapist chose to focus on a review of this particular cognitive change and the new behaviors that he had initiated, but would have to continue, in order to maintain the positive view of himself and his life.

Throughout therapy, David had tended to vacillate between extremes so, during the final session, the therapist was careful to address the possibility of dichotomous thought about terminating therapy. Specifically, he attempted to prepare David for the possibility of feeling discouraged at some time in the future and to caution him against interpreting setbacks in his plans as evidence that he was a "failure," "helpless," or "depressed beyond hope." Of course, the open invitation to return to therapy any time David felt he needed a "refresher" was extended. In addition, David agreed to let the therapist contact him for a phone "checkup" a few weeks later. Although the therapist was concerned about the possibility of David's relapse, the therapist's own negative predictions were successfully challenged by viewing David's termination of therapy as a process parallel to the developmentally appropriate autonomy he was achieving from his parents and home life.

At the time of follow-up approximately 2 months after the last session, David had quit school and was working part-time with hopes of increasing his weekly hours. He was still living in his own apartment and claimed to be coping well. His self-report questionnaire data indicated that his depression continued to be remitted.

The "Lingering" Termination

As the name suggests, a lingering termination is characterized by a lengthy, protracted process of ending the therapeutic relationship, seen especially when depressed adolescents have the comorbid diagnosis of posttraumatic stress disorder as a result of chronic abuse or neglect. This type of termination after a successful course of therapy should not be confused with the irregular pattern of missed or canceled appointments characteristic of patients who were never well-engaged in therapy at any point. Frequently, the initial and middle phases of therapy that precede a lingering termination have progressed at a "normal" rate, and improvement in the depressive symptoms has been noted after eight or

10 sessions. However, whenever the topic of terminating therapy is raised, adolescents may voice reluctance, often suggesting that their files remain open for a while longer "just in case they get depressed again." During the final phase of therapy in a lingering termination, sessions may be scheduled a few weeks or even a few months apart. With some adolescents, phone contact every 2 or 3 months eventually enables them to terminate the therapeutic relationship. Patients who indicate reluctance to terminate therapy are often adolescents whose histories would suggest that attachment issues are of paramount importance. When adolescents who have been abused or rejected by significant adults do succeed in establishing a trusting relationship with the therapist, they may be particularly likely to prefer a lingering termination. Rather than view the protracted termination as inappropriate catering to maladaptive dependent personality characteristics, therapists should attempt to view the recurrent "review" sessions as necessary repetitions of the cognitive therapy model and techniques in order to aid generalization across a variety of life situations for an adolescent whose life experiences have left him with limited self-efficacy.

When involved in a lingering termination, the therapist must exercise caution against the tendency to engage in disorganized or unfocused "chats" with the adolescent that exclude the strategies discussed as important for the final phase of therapy. Each session should include a purposeful review of the cognitive and behavioral changes the adolescent has made, stressing the ways in which these therapeutic gains can be internalized and applied to new situations or problems encountered.

Case Example

Karen was a 16-year-old who presented for therapy shortly after being discharged from a hospital psychiatric unit, where she had been admitted because of extreme suicidal ideation and unremitting depression. In addition to the depression, she endorsed sufficient anxious symptomatology during the assessment to diagnose posttraumatic stress disorder. Her history was a tragic one of abandonment by father, abuse by mother, abuse by grandparents who were guardians for a period of time, and several temporary guardianship placements with various relatives over the past 5 years. She had endured school changes with every residential move, so had fallen behind in her course work and had no close school friends. At the time of assessment, she was, in fact, not attending school so spent her days doing housework and preparing meals or babysitting for her aunt and uncle, who were the latest set of guardians. They did not understand why Karen should be depressed since they had provided such a "nice home" for her, and they attended the assessment somewhat reluctantly, expressing the view that Karen was exaggerating the extent of her depression in order to get attention.

During the initial phase of therapy, the therapist paid special attention to the development of a positive therapeutic relationship with Karen. Although Karen wanted to be in therapy, she had difficulty knowing what to discuss in sessions and relied on the therapist to suggest topics or guess at what might be troubling her. Karen's extensive history of rejection led the therapist to hypothesize that Karen's negative view of herself as unwanted and unlovable was central to the depression. In addition, Karen's experiences with primary caretakers had apparently taught her that the world was full of unreliable and even "mean" people. Her past experiences of neglect and abuse may have contributed to her heightened interpersonal sensitivity, which seemed to be one factor contributing to her short temper that was causing problems with her aunt and uncle. As such, one of the goals established for therapy was to explore how Karen might achieve a better relationship with her current guardians. Since Karen reported feeling especially depressed when she was bored and alone at home all day long while her aunt and uncle worked, another goal of therapy was to explore activities that would be reinforcing to Karen, including the possibility of returning to school.

During the middle phase of therapy, Karen found it particularly helpful to participate in cognitive replay with the therapist, who helped her identify the automatic thoughts associated with periods of anger and depression. When the therapist introduced Karen to the technique of identifying distortions, she immediately saw herself using binocular vision, predicting the future, and mind reading. Systematic use of logical analysis and the triple-column technique helped to correct the maladaptive automatic thoughts. In addition, a family session that included her aunt and uncle served to educate them about the symptoms of depression and anxiety; and it further helped to increase their limited understanding of adolescence since they had been thrust into the parental role with her rather suddenly and had only a preschool child of their own. Discussion about their intentions with respect to providing a permanent home for Karen helped her to address her fears about future residential moves and changes in school. As Karen began to feel more secure about her living arrangements, she expressed a desire to return to school, and plans were made with her guardians for this to occur the following semester. In the meantime, the therapist used the mastery and pleasure technique to help Karen discover activities that she found rewarding.

Her aunt's and uncle's passion for skiing helped Karen to keep physically active and develop a new skill that she enjoyed greatly. After returning to school, Karen quickly made some friends, and her mood continued to improve with the increase in academic and social activities. The one area that remained difficult was maintaining a good relationship with her aunt, who, the therapist discovered first-hand, was a difficult person, inclined to focus on the negative and to think in dichotomous black-and-white terms herself. Since her guardians were difficult to engage in therapy, a few individual sessions with Karen were devoted to problem-solving and the development of communication skills for use with her aunt. As Karen practiced them at home, she began to report less interpersonal tension.

By the eighth session, Karen's depression appeared to be in remission. Although she expressed no need for weekly sessions, she made an appointment 1 month hence. This was canceled and rescheduled by Karen, who continued to state that she wished to see the therapist. Four more sessions were held, approximately every second week. During these sessions, the therapist focused on reviewing the cognitive and behavioral changes that Karen thought were contributing to her improved mood. Although the therapist attempted to address Karen's dichotomous thinking about the end of therapy by explaining that a "closed" case could be reopened at any time that Karen felt necessary, she was adamant about keeping periodic contact with the therapist. The next session occurred 2 months later, and another 2 months after that. Each time, the therapist concentrated on increasing Karen's awareness of internalizing therapeutic gains.

Follow-up contact was made with Karen by telephone about 3 months after the last session. Her depression continued to be in full remission, and she declined the offer to schedule an appointment but appreciated the contact. In fact, she returned some self-report questionnaires with a note attached thanking the therapist for all the help she had received. A second follow-up phone call was made by the therapist 3 months later. Karen was well integrated into her new school and enjoyed an active social life. She reported a good home life and denied any depressive symptomatology. The therapist anticipated that a final phone contact would be made in 3 or 4 months' time and that Karen's beliefs about the termination of relationships would have undergone sufficient change by that time to allow closing the case, of course with the instruction that active psychotherapy would again be available in the future, if needed. Karen's termination is typical of the gradual detachment that some adolescents with posttraumatic stress disorder will require even after the successful resolution of the depression. With these adolescents, the termination of therapy can be experienced as a repetition of the emotional neglect they have endured for so long in the past. Their anxious attachment to the therapist seems to mimic their style of relating to other significant people and seems to be associated with the belief that "something bad will happen again" or with the automatic thought "I will be left alone without help again."

The "Shifting" Termination

Like the lingering termination, the shifting type of termination is also protracted, but for different reasons. In a shifting termination, the final phase of therapy involves a conscious change in the purpose of therapy from the original intent of treating the adolescent's depression. Typically, the initial and middle phases of therapy have resulted in amelioration of the depressive symptoms, and the final phase has included some review of the therapeutic gains the adolescent has made during therapy. But during the course of therapy, the therapist may have become aware of other issues that are thought to require ongoing therapeutic support. Hence, the final phase of therapy involves identification of these issues as the new focus of ongoing therapy contact. For example, depressed adolescents who also have learning disabilities or behavioral problems associated with the diagnosis of attention-deficit hyperactivity disorder may require ongoing therapy even after the depression has remitted. Additionally, adolescents who manifest significant skill deficits such as those associated with schizoid personality disorder may benefit from a shift in focus from the depression to other problems. The decision to continue therapy after the depressive symptoms have abated is often made because the adolescent's parents need continuing support, and the final phase of therapy in such cases would usually include them in all of the sessions.

A shifting termination should not be confused with one that is prolonged without focus or intent. Rather, it is one in which the therapist has made a conscious decision to shift the purpose of therapy from treatment of depression to something else, such as development of a behavioral management program to assist parents in addressing a particular problem their adolescent presents. In keeping with the collaborative nature of cognitive therapy, the decision to prolong therapy and adopt a new focus should be made with the adolescent and the parents. It should be clear to everyone that the depression is in remission, and a different problem is now being addressed in the therapy sessions. So that the final phase of a shifting termination does not last indefinitely, a clear contract should be established in which the number and frequency of sessions, as well as the goals of continued therapy, are discussed. Sometimes the final phase of a shifting termination will be primarily an educational exercise for the parents, who were previously unaware of any problems additional to the depression. Depending on the therapist and the treatment facility, it may be most appropriate for the therapist to work with the parents and adolescent to find an alternate treatment program that is more specialized in providing the kind of ongoing, perhaps long-term therapy the adolescent requires. For example, cognitive therapy may have addressed the depression in a relatively short period of individual and family sessions during which the therapist and parents became aware of other difficulties better addressed in an adolescent group-therapy program or a different school placement. In such a case, the final phase of cognitive therapy would involve a shift in focus from the depression to behavioral or social problems and where these might best be treated.

Case Example

Donna was a 14-year-old whose parents were well-educated professionals. Her younger brother was a socially and academically skilled honors student who often assumed the role of spokesperson for his older sister during therapy sessions. Early in her own educational career, Donna had been identified as a bright student, and teachers had encouraged her pursuit of independent study projects on somewhat esoteric topics. Over the past 2 years, however, Donna had demonstrated increasing difficulty with her school work, and her grades had dropped significantly. Her parents noted a marked lack of motivation and attributed the school problems to depression. In an attempt to find the most appropriate school setting for her, they had changed Donna's school twice in the past year, both recent placements being expensive private institutions with small classes and significant amounts of individualized instruction. Donna especially liked her current school, where the teachers knew her well and made minimal requirements for classroom participation with student colleagues who, she claimed, made fun of her because of her intelligence and "unusual" answers to questions in class.

During the initial phase of therapy, the therapist hypothesized that Donna's depression and lack of motivation might be related to her perceived inability to meet the high expectations of her parents and teachers, in spite of her intelligence. Furthermore, Donna's younger brother provided a constant point of comparison in which Donna would likely experience second-rate status, also threatening her self-esteem. Rather than compete and lose, perhaps Donna had adopted the strategy of withdrawing from the perceived competition with her younger brother by not bothering to try at all. It was also hypothesized that because Donna viewed herself as having superior intellectual abilities, she felt estranged from other students her own age and interpreted their normal adolescent teasing as criticism. Based on the concerns of her parents, one of the goals identified for therapy was to address Donna's lack of motivation for doing school work. Donna herself expressed a desire to explore how she might engage in more rewarding activities involving same-aged peers.

During the middle phase of therapy, the therapist attempted to address Donna's motivational problems with cognitive interventions such as the TIC-TOC technique, but the efforts were without much success. However, some family sessions, which explored beliefs about the importance of education, revealed some maladaptive ideas Donna held about her school performance. Because her current school placement, which she liked greatly, had occurred largely as a result of failing grades, Donna had reasoned that improving her school performance might endanger her continued attendance at the current school, which she knew was a financial burden to the family. Thus, it seemed that the special privilege conferred on Donna (attending the private school) was itself serving to reinforce her continued refusal to do homework or study for exams. The therapist's original hypothesis about the reasons for Donna's lack of motivation were revised to include the new information.

In family sessions, which all members attended, it became increasingly evident that Donna's parents and brother were unaware of the extent to which they compensated for her inappropriate behaviors and lack of understanding subtleties in social interaction. The therapist drew attention to this fact by engaging the parents in a discussion of expectations for Donna as compared to those they would hold for other 14-year-old students. The result was revelation of another parental belief that they, as parents, were fully responsible for the well-being and success of their children. The adaptiveness of this parental belief was evaluated using the techniques of time projection and pro–con analysis. In the end, Donna's parents decided that their overprotectiveness and overcompensation were interfering with Donna's own experience of success or failure based on her own efforts. The therapist used extensive modeling to demonstrate for Donna's parents some appropriate ways of interacting with her to challenge her somewhat bizarre interpersonal mannerisms and behaviors. At this point, the therapy included remediation of skill deficits (Donna's and her parents) as well as remediation of the depression. As Donna's social behaviors became the focus of therapy, the therapist used the technique of activity scheduling in an attempt to have Donna increase her social contact with school peers and experience pleasant rewarding activities while simultaneously gathering contradictory evidence with which to challenge the belief that other kids did not like her because she was intelligent.

Throughout the middle phase of therapy, the therapist experienced relatively little success with cognitive techniques employed with Donna herself. Although intelligence, per se, did not seem to be the problem, Donna did exhibit significant difficulty following the therapist's logic, staying on topic, or even seeing the relevance of concrete examples used to explore issues. As such, both the therapist and Donna's parents began to adopt more behavioral than cognitive interventions in an attempt to ameliorate Donna's depressive symptoms and change her inappropriate behaviors. In contrast to Donna, her parents readily understood the cognitive therapy model and used the techniques to address their own maladaptive cognitions about various issues such as parenting and education.

In the final phase of therapy, a careful review of Donna's depressive symptomatology was undertaken. Her mood was less depressed. In addition, her school performance had improved somewhat, probably in response to a clarification by her parents of the contingencies operative with respect to decisions about her future school placement. There was also some moderate improvement in Donna's attempts to socialize with peers. Although her reasoning abilities and social behaviors remained immature and/or inappropriate, she no longer met criteria for depression. As such, the therapist began to consider termination. However, since the majority of Donna's sessions had included her parents, the therapist had become aware of their relative naivete about "normal" adolescent development, their relative paucity of skill in dealing with Donna's apparent cognitive and social deficits, and their constant accommodation of her behavior. A shifting termination was marked by the therapist's explicit review of Donna's depression, the consensus by everyone that it was no longer her primary difficulty, and the definition of a new focus for the final phase of therapy. The therapist agreed to prolong the termination with regular monthly sessions to review Donna's and her parents' progress in establishing new behaviors that would encourage Donna's development of appropriate independence and peer socialization. It was anticipated that about six sessions over a period of 6 or 8 months would characterize the final phase of this shifting termination.

SELECTED READINGS

Beck AT, Rush AJ, Shaw BF, Emery G: *Cognitive Therapy of Depression*. New York, Guilford Press, 1979.

Burns DD: *Feeling Good*. New York, William Morrow, 1980.

Campbell J: *The Hero with a Thousand Faces*. Princeton, Bollinger Series, 1973.

Guidano VF, Liotti G: *Cognitive Processes and Emotional Disorders*. New York, Guilford Press, 1983.

Tomm K: One perspective on the Milan systemic approach. *Journal of Marital and Family Therapy* 1984; 10:253–271.

Viederman M: The psycho-dynamic life narrative: A psychotherapeutic intervention useful in crisis situations. *Psychiatry* 1983; 3:236–246.

Watzlawick P, Weakland JH, Fisch R: *Change*. New York, Norton, 1974.

PART IV

Comorbidity in
Depressed Adolescents

CHAPTER TEN

Cognitive Therapy with Depressed, Substance-Abusing Teenagers

ANTHONY NOWELS

INTRODUCTION

Depressed teenagers who also abuse drugs present a complex and diffi-cult array of problems for all therapists. The combination is extremely common, yet "dual-diagnosed" patients continue to create conflicts in both addictionology and psychiatry, with particular disagreement over issues of biological treatment (medication) for target symptoms and is-sues of "responsibility" for behavior when suffering from a psychiatric illness. Successful treatment occurs when symptoms are *simultaneously* viewed from an illness model and a recovery or "12-step" approach. A therapist using cognitive-behavioral approaches with concomitant chemical dependency treatment must be conversant with substance abuse issues; potential areas of conflict; and the differential perception and use of goals, tasks, prescriptions, and patient logs by the different treating systems.

Since it is common for such dual treatment to occur in an inpatient residential setting (see Chapter 13), the cognitive therapist may antici-pate working with a unique treatment team whose members have some significant philosophical differences, if not conflicts (see Table 10.1).

Cognitive therapy offers several advantages: it can be applied con-currently with recovery-oriented interventions, especially in its "cother-apy" orientation; between-session tasks can continually remind the ado-

TABLE 10.1. Philosophical Differences

Psychiatrically oriented cognitive therapist	Chemical dependency orientation
Goals is to resolve illness or symptoms	Goal is to establish "recovery"
Comfortable with medication	Demands abstinence
M.D. usually in charge	Team of equals
Reduce discomfort	Confront to establish "responsibility"
Program individualized to patient	Patient adapts to program

lescent of the goals of therapy; and mutually established goals can help to cement the therapeutic alliance. Yet, the cognitive therapist must ensure that the necessary therapeutic tasks are carried out, while at the same time he promotes recovery.

COMBINING RECOVERY AND COGNITIVE THERAPY

The cognitive therapist *must* support the recovery process and reframe portions of the recovery within the cognitive philosophy. Substantial anecdotal data suggest that any approach, however well intentioned, that fails to support recovery concepts will ultimately be self-defeating. Yet, attacks on negative self-image in the service of "responsibility," hostile group confrontations, and intense negative peer activities within the recovery model will frequently appear to conflict with cognitive restructuring goals. Substance abuse in adolescents is probably one of the most difficult arenas for all mental health therapists and frequently requires some dichotomizing of the "substance-abusing identity" from other self-constructs.

The concept of a "personal recovery" is derived from a cognitive process whereby the teenager designs, with the cognitive therapist, a unique set of daily behaviors and responsibilities aimed at maintaining that recovery. The process is usually written by the patient in detail, is goal-oriented, takes one day at a time, may be frequently modified, and is usually congruent with a 12-step program. The family and other potential "enablers" in the environment must be included.

The sequence of treatment steps (not to be confused with the 12 steps) can be organized in many patterns, but the example of one "outline for personal recovery" in Table 10.2 should be helpful. The use of the personal recovery outline in treatment will be different for each patient. Just the process of creating the outline is a large portion of the

TABLE 10.12. Outline for Personal Recovery

---

1. Manage each day without chemical support.
2. Maintain my therapy, including medication.
3. Not crave drugs or alcohol I may see at school, at home, or with peers.
4. Plan my life—school, fun, and friends—without chemicals.
5. Not get depressed without drugs.
6. Attend my meetings and keep in touch with my sponsor.
7. Learn to get "high on life."
8. Take good care of myself—diet, exercise.
9. Educate my family, friends, teachers, and even my doctors about being "enablers."
10. Give up the myths about myself and my family.

---

therapy. Some therapists may want to use a preestablished "starting" outline with which each patient begins and then modifies to suit his own needs.

One of the most important differences in working with substance-abusing teenagers is that the cognitive therapist must scrupulously guard against becoming an enabler for the patient. In the wish to be helpful or to reduce pain or suffering, the therapist can easily and inadvertently excuse drug-related behaviors or diminish responsibility. The therapist must often walk a difficult "tightrope" between responsibility and illness, between confrontation and nurturing. Sometimes strategies and tasks will have to be employed *sequentially* to avoid conflicting goals.

Close communication with substance abuse counselors and sponsors is absolutely essential to carry out a coordinated approach. Those implementing the substance abuse component of treatment *must* understand some of the depressive "illness" concepts and be prepared to support treatment for that component of illness, even pharmacotherapy, should medication prove to be necessary. An example of such treatment will help clarify the important issues.

Dawn was a 16-year-old high school junior whose grades had plummeted during the 6 months prior to treatment. She had "lost" many of her friends, quit the cheerleading squad, and had severe crying spells brought on by self-deprecatory feelings. Minor marijuana abuse had blossomed into almost daily smoking of joints and escalating weekend use of cocaine. Dawn's parents were divorced, her mother had remarried, and Dawn felt that her new stepfather was taking most of her mother's attention.

Dawn enjoyed the therapy process, filled out copious logs, and worked hard to avoid the painful depressive feelings. She was initially much more concerned with her depression, whereas her family was more interested in treatment of her cocaine abuse.

At the beginning Dawn wrote:

"My emotional illnesses deal with anger, depression, and low self-esteem. The reasons why I feel these things are because I expect perfection from myself and from everyone around me. I have to be perfect in everything I do so that I'm noticed in all activities. I want to be the one and only concern in everybody's life. I have to be special. . . . I don't know how I got this fairy-tale way of thinking about life, but it's there and there's nothing I can do about it. I still sometimes catch myself daydreaming about what someone should do or should say, but I can deal with it now. I know that I cannot change how other people feel, and I cannot make somebody feel close to me. I know that people cannot live their lives to make me happy and serene. It's up to me to do that."

Dawn's ideas about herself emerged in the first week as treatment encouraged self-exploration and objective definition of the problems. It was important for Dawn to hear that things could be different, that she could feel better. The strategy employed was primarily to have her question the assumptions she had about herself, especially those related to her feelings of rejection from her parents.

By the third week, Dawn wrote:

"Before, I never expressed my needs; I figured if that person loved me, or cared about me, they would know exactly what I need. People are not mind readers. Now I can find ways of having my needs met. . . . In relationships, I have to be very careful. I am very needy and sometimes, just to feel like I'm special, I'll hook up with people who are bad for me. I always settled for less than I deserved because I felt I was unworthy of anything good. I honestly don't know what caused me to feel these things. One thing I did a lot was to try to make myself feel better. I didn't think I had anything in myself so I would give myself ego boosts about things I did have. For example, I'm thinner than her, I'm prettier than her, I have a nicer car than she does, and therefore I am better than her. But then I felt inferior to people who were thinner, prettier, or had a (God forbid) nicer car than I. Because I expect so much from others, I get angry really easily when someone I like does something not perfect. Because I'm needy I like a lot of attention and a lot of compliments."

As the depressive feelings and self-attacks subsided, Dawn began to explore other behaviors and feelings and wrote for the first time about drug use as a problem:

"I think that when I expect perfection I am disappointed. Since I am disappointed I try to be perfect. It's like a cycle. I then feel guilty that I'm not perfect and I try to cover my feelings of guilt by trying to excel in everything I do. It's really a sick way of doing things. I'm really one screwed up person when I think about it. But I know that there are people out there with the same feelings as mine. There have to be or there wouldn't be these kinds of groups. . . . When I become happy with myself, I won't need other people constantly praising me to feel good. I guess my ultimate goal is to be able to love myself the way that I so much want other people to love me. I want to be happy and meet my full potential. I know it will not be easy but I think I can do it, and I think one day in the near future I am going to be very happy and very content without having to use other people or chemicals to feel good."

This patient used the logs as an extension of the therapy process and her own thinking. She reread them frequently and used them during sessions to provide examples and to organize her thoughts.

When she brought her "chemicals" into therapy, some of her depression and self-"putdowns" recurred. She used these feelings as evidence of how fragile her improvement was but also began to explore her drug abuse for the first time. The overall sequence and timing were critical to a successful outcome.

ONE MODEL FOR COGNITIVE THERAPY COMBINED WITH SUBSTANCE ABUSE TREATMENT

Cognitive methods can be combined with chemical dependency treatment in an infinite number of ways. This model demonstrates just one example.

The entire program is organized around a 12-step sequence interwoven with cognitive-behavioral approaches. To simplify the process, the 12-step program is subdivided into four phases:

Phase 1—Surrender
  1. Admit powerlessness
  2. Seek help from higher power
  3. Decide to turn life around

Phase 2—Therapy
   4. Personal moral inventory
   5. Admit wrongs to "God" and others
   6. Prepare for "God" to help
   7. Ask "God" to remove defects
Phase 3—Relationship
   8. List those who have been harmed
   9. Make direct amends
Phase 4—Maintenance
   10. Continue personal inventory
   11. Seek wisdom to deal with life
   12. Carry message to others

The phases represent progress in treatment and include completion of both the 12 steps and cognitive tasks.

Phase 1, "surrender," includes attention to steps 1, 2, and 3, but also to the completion of an autobiography; acceptance of writing complete, meaningful daily logs; participation in therapy; and the prepartion of a written statement, completed with the family, as to why hospitalization occurred—what emotional and chemical dependency problems existed.

Phase 2, "therapy," addresses steps 4, 5, 6, and 7 while the patient continues to complete daily logs. The patient has to pass a drug information test in school and complete a written treatment plan outlining how his personal recovery will occur.

Phase 3, "relationships," includes steps 8 and 9, completion of daily logs, and the family's preparation of a written plan for accepting the patient home. The patient has to teach a class on substance abuse to peers. The cognitive therapist and patient have to create and prepare to implement the written outpatient plan.

Phase 4, "maintenance," usually occurs on an outpatient, follow-up basis for 1 year.

Throughout the program, the patient has to attend daily Narcotics Anonymous/Alcoholics Anonymous meetings and participate meaningfully in individual, family, and group therapy.

The program also maintains the usual "psychiatric level system" based on the patient's behavior and offering privileges in exchange for evidence of responsibility and progress. The levels are maintained as elsewhere in the hospital, except that a patient's level cannot differ from his phase by more than one. So a patient can never move to level three until he has successfully achieved Phase 2, and a "drop" to level one (i.e., for violent behavior) will necessitate a drop to and *repeat* of Phase 2.

The details of the program are not so important as the concept that cognitive therapy can be successfully interwoven with chemical dependency interventions to provide a very structured and operationalizable system of inpatient "dual diagnosis" treatment.

Substance-abusing adolescents will frequently lie about their drug use and include the therapist within the ongoing manipulative process that so commonly occurs in this arena. The therapist must maintain healthy skepticism regarding the accuracy of drug-related and other behavioral information, yet he must constantly support the patient's recovery without condemnation should the patient relapse during treatment. It is the patient's identification with the therapist's own assessments and refusal to "give up" that ultimately serves as a model for the patient's recovery.

Jessica, a 17-year-old, had been treated in two previous chemical dependency inpatient programs and rapidly relapsed after each discharge. She used alcohol, marijuana, and cocaine almost constantly; and her family had essentially "given up." She was admitted to the dual-diagnosis program, where staff described her as an "angry bitch" who constantly cursed them out, creating strong negative countertransference feelings.

She wrote this first log July 29, some 3 weeks into treatment:

"Today sucks. I'm pissed off at a lot of people. Someone took a tape and gum out of my cube and no one will admit to it. Fuck that shit. I'm pissed off about the way things are dealt with around here. I'm pissed off that no one will confront me about Billy. Whoever made the accusations owes me a big-time apology, and they don't even have the balls to confront me. My dad's pissed off because of all the shit, and he's telling me to tell everyone to get fucked. I'm pissed off because I know I could manipulate my mom into getting me out of here if I got pissed enough but I don't want to do that. I want to be here because I want to work out all of my shit, but I hate dealing with all the bullshit everyone puts on me. I'm tired of being disappointed because of unfulfilled promises. And I'm especially pissed about assholes who talk shit to me when they don't know a damn thing about me. One good thing is that my mom brought me some new tapes."

She wrote logs constantly after that, shocking some staff with the rage, hostility, and the language she employed. Three long-term meetings were essentially devoted solely to her—where staff expressed their very negative feelings and thoughts that she was "hopeless." A variety of staff strategies were developed, including support for each other when they felt attacked, reframing Jessica's cursing as pushing others away, and pointing out how the treatment team *and* staff had replicated the family system. Staff were required to carefully review Jessica's lengthy logs with her daily.

The August 5 log came only 1 week later:

> "Today I really learned something about myself. During group today I got really upset with someone because of something they did. Then that person said that they didn't think they had done anything wrong, and they didn't care about anyone in that group. I became pretty tearful because I cannot even imagine not caring about the other people here. You'd have to be sick. Really sick. There's a lot of caring, loving kids here who I am going to miss big time, and this guy could actually sit there and say, 'I don't care.' After the group I had time to think about it, and I realized that the reason I got so emotional over it was because that's exactly how I used to be. I could openly say I didn't care about anyone but myself—now I care for lots of people. I guess seeing him reminded me of how pathetic and sick I was. My parents have been telling me how much I've changed and I could never see it. Now I do. I guess it just takes assholes to make me realize how much I've grown. I'm very happy!" [A happy face was drawn on the entry log.]

The tears that began August 5 successfully made Jessica a patient to the staff and treatment team. It was crucial for them to be aware of her depression in order to tolerate her vitriolic attacks and to nurture her; yet she would never reveal those vulnerable feelings (except in logs) until she was cared for. Her logs and treatment team meetings broke the impasse.

The final log entry occurred on August 18, the day before discharge.

> "Today was super-duper fantastic! (1) level four, phase three, (2) Anthony came and visited me on a grounds pass for an hour, (3) Dawn and Rhandi called me! I had a fantastic day. I'm still shocked that I got level four. I didn't think I really did much but I guess I did something right. I have gotten real used to writing these logs! I'm not looking forward to my goodbye group at all. I was hoping to get out of it. For some reason, goodbyes have always been like rejection to me. But that's OK. It's not like I'll never see anyone here ever again. This is going to sound so screwed, but I'm so glad I came here. Before Grant, I was sad all of the time. Everyone and everything made me cry. I

would cry for no reason at all. I had no goals, no hopes, and no love. I figured that's the way life was, and I would feel like that until I died. In the last 7 weeks, I have real goals, good feelings, and I'm generally happy. My mom keeps telling me that every time she sees me, I'm more like myself. And, I'm happy with myself."

It should be clear that the therapeutic philosophy, evaluation, and most interventions are similar to those usually conducted in cognitive therapy for other depressed adolescents. The therapeutic tasks of log-keeping, essays, and exploration of the past, present, and future self blend extremely well with substance use management. The cognitive therapist should feel comfortable using strategies and techniques that take into account those self-constructs that include substance use behaviors. Compulsive self-stimulating thrill-seeking behaviors are a particularly frequent accompaniment with these patients and are target symptoms from both the substance use and depression (suicidal behavior) points of view. Extremely detailed and accurate logs in this area can be enormously helpful in pointing out to teenagers how their behaviors emerge from their depression and the assumptions they make about their future and present selves. Another example will help illustrate these problems.

Cindy was a 14-year-old extremely bright eighth grader whose total rejection of school and parental controls had the family in chaos. She had recently discovered that her father was not her biological parent (her mother had had an affair), was associating with teen gang members instead of attending school, and had begun using a variety of street drugs as well as alcohol. Her overt behavior was manic-like in intensity, with pressured speech and frequent joking in the service of discounting the value of everything.

In the initial evaluation session, Cindy at first cried and expressed overwhelming feelings of hopelessness but then became mute. In joint meetings with her mother, she was described as having uncontrollable rages and as lying constantly.

In an attempt to avoid replication of the family's intrusive style, the strategy employed in subsequent sessions was primarily aimed at helping create a nonthreatening cotherapy alliance.

For the first several meetings, Cindy continued to be mute but communicated effectively, although indirectly, through histrionic facial expressions and eye-rolling. She would nod or shake her head in response to issues that were probably important to her and, in that fashion, the mutual goals were established: to be liked by others; to control her anger; to avoid anxiety and pain during sessions.

Cindy refused to keep her own logs, instead permitting a brief assessment at the beginning of each session, so that logs were kept for her by the therapist as part of the patient record. She occasionally asked to review these during sessions.

The process of conducting these sessions included "going public" with the therapist's thoughts and feelings, allowing her to see how ideas about her emerged from her behavior, how feelings could be surmised from behavior, and how even simple events could be understood in multiple ways. Cindy particularly enjoyed the idea of multiple points of view and probably first began communicating openly by discussing the options she had in understanding her parents and peers.

However, she strongly resisted ideas *applied to her*, becoming mute again. She would accept alternatives if attributed to others, and then she could internally apply them to herself. It proved to be extremely important that the therapist not directly suggest changes in Cindy's assumptions or beliefs but leave her free to apply them to herself after she experienced them with others. The need for this process may well have reflected an identity so fragile that direct alternatives were painfully destructive.

Cindy was able to verbalize how she was victimized by others whose friendships she sought—drinking, getting "high," and cutting school in order to be liked. "That's me. That's what I'm like," she said.

Confronting those self-assumptions and suggesting alternatives was the essence of Cindy's treatment. Doing it indirectly without evoking her mute behavior was the art.

Cindy found "recovery" a difficult process. Although she enjoyed reading about the 12 steps, AA meetings were threatening for her. She minimized or entirely denied her drug and alcohol problems and would withdraw or reply, "That's stupid," to provocative questions by her peers. She engaged her therapist in a "campaign" to excuse her from meetings. Instead, recovery became a portion of the initial assessment period that still began each session and defined Cindy's logs and objective data base.

The first step was the *first step*—that Cindy had to accept the problem as hers and acknowledge her powerlessness. The process of Cindy's taking recovery as her own task was gradual. She went from being mute, to making angry denials, followed by hesitant admissions, to defining major alcohol and drug use. Her ability to progress in this manner emerged from repetitive, nonjudgmental explorations of how her life was being negatively affected by drugs. She eventually reported feeling that no one could like her or accept her if they knew the extent of how "bad" she was. Yet, she also reported how drugs were her only mechanism for feeling good inside. As she said this, she repeated several times, "Now that's sick," and she discussed for the first time her need to get away from drugs. *Recovery* had finally begun some 8 weeks into treatment.

Cindy began to notice how her anger emerged whenever she felt rejected or unloved by a significant other. She reported how hard others had to work to get to be her friend—how hard therapy had to be with her.

CONCLUSION

Treatment of depressed, substance-abusing teenagers is *very* difficult. Concepts of time appear particularly distorted with this group of adolescents, perhaps in part even supported by direct effects of abusable drugs. Because of this, more frequent sessions, especially during certain critical periods (relapse problems, family system problems, school and peer stress problems) may be necessary. Long-term success rates, if measured by complete remission and total abstinence, are low. Objective verification by specific research of the success of cognitive therapy is not yet available. However, cognitive methods appear to be extremely helpful, both as a treatment strategy for individual therapy and as an organizing philosophy for treatment systems, usually on an inpatient basis.

SELECTED READINGS

Bry BH, Conboy C, Bisgay K: Decreasing drug use and school failure: Long term effects of targeted family problem solving training. *Child and Family Behavior Therapy* 1986; 8:43–59.

Szapocznik J, Perez-Vidal A, Brickman AL, Foote FH, Santisteban D, Hervis O, Kurtimes WM: Engaging adolescent drug users and their families in treatment. *Journal of Consulting and Clinical Psychology* 1988; 56:552–557.

CHAPTER ELEVEN

Special Issues Related to Sexual Victimization

ELLEN FRANK

INTRODUCTION

Among the special issues that the cognitive therapist working with adolescent girls may need to address is that of sexual victimization. Although males can also be victims of sexual abuse, adolescent boys with such histories are seen relatively infrequently in treatment settings focusing on depressive symptomatology. There are two relatively distinct types of sexual victimization that adolescent girls may have experienced: rape and incest. These two types of victimization produce quite different psychological sequelae (with some overlap in the area of loss of self-esteem) and require different approaches to treatment. Both require special assessment techniques.

ASSESSMENT OF RAPE-TRAUMA SYNDROME

Whereas some adolescents will spontaneously report sexual victimization, many will not. It is the therapist's task to inquire about these issues in an appropriate way, at the appropriate time. In our experience, rape is a much less complicated therapeutic problem, requiring far fewer special assessment and treatment skills, than the problem of incest. Typically, rape can be asked about quite directly, with patients often being relieved to talk about their experience to a nonjudgmental person who is not frightened by what he is being told. The therapist needs to understand the specifics of the assault: Was the assailant a stranger or someone known to the patient? Was a weapon involved? Had the patient believed herself to be in a safe situation, or did she feel she was taking a risk by being where she was at the time of the assault? Was the patient or the assailant intoxicated? What kinds of sexual acts were involved? Was the patient beaten or tortured? Did she attempt to defend herself? If so, how? If not, what went into the decision not to do so, or was she simply unable to do so? Did she experience "frozen fright"? What went through her mind just before, during, and after the assault?

Once the therapist has a clear picture of what transpired, it is important to get a sense of the kinds of difficulties the patient has experienced as a result of the assault and how they relate to her depressive syndrome. Are all of the symptoms she is experiencing a result of the assault? Does she now present with posttraumatic symptoms (flashbacks, nightmares, exaggerated startle response) superimposed on her depressive syndrome? In our experience, many adolescents assert that the rape was "no big deal" and cope, sometimes quite effectively, by throwing themselves back into their normal routine. In such cases, it is especially important to be certain that the patient is not experiencing posttraumatic symptoms.

The therapist will also want to know who has been told about the assault and what their reaction has been. Have significant others been supportive or have they blamed the patient? Has the assault resulted in increased (and unreasonable) restrictions on the adolescent? Is she now in a control battle with her parents? Has the assault been reported to the police? If so, what have the patient's experiences with the police been like? Is a rape crisis center involved? If so, it is important that the therapist and the rape crisis advocate communicate in order to clarify their goals in implementing their respective interventions with the adolescent and to be certain that these goals do not conflict.

The Therapeutic Alliance

Another consideration in working with the adolescent rape victim is how the therapist should position himself or herself with respect to the therapeutic alliance. Whereas work with the depressed adolescent who has not been victimized usually necessitates an alliance with the parents as well as with the adolescent, work with the adolescent rape victim may require an alliance that is more clearly with the patient, especially if her family has been unsupportive of her in the aftermath of the assault. Thus, while in treating the depressed adolescent, the therapist may give relatively fewer choices to the patient than might be the case with an adult, in treating the adolescent rape victim, the issues of choice (such as control) are often paramount. It is often helpful to give the patient as much control over the treatment process as seems reasonable, especially following the kind of loss of control that rape represents.

Intervening with the Patient's Social Network

One of the strongest predictors of poor outcome following sexual assault is the presence of one or more important social network members who are overtly or covertly unsupportive of the victim. This lack of support can take the form of overt blame: "If you hadn't had on that obscene outfit, this never would have happened," or "What can you expect with the kinds of friends you have?" Or the unsupportive stance can be more subtle: the father or brother who flinches when the victim goes to hug him, implying that she is now "damaged goods"; the mother who is too caught up in her own self-blame to be able to listen to what her daughter is feeling. Clearly, when an adolescent patient reports these kinds of responses from important network members, the therapist needs to work with these individuals as well as with the patient herself if that is at all possible.

The problem of unsupportive or overtly taunting peers is a more difficult therapeutic problem. If an entire class is involved, sometimes working with the classroom teacher can be helpful, especially if the patient was not a problem student prior to the assault and the teacher is reasonably supportive and psychologically sophisticated. Often, however, the problem of unsupportive or taunting peers must be handled in the therapy through efforts to ameliorate the patient's reaction to the behavior of her peers.

Treatment Intervention with the Adolescent Rape Victim

Cognitive therapy as originally described by Beck et al. (1979) fits extremely well with the therapeutic needs of the adolescent who has experienced a rape victimization. A skilled therapist from any of the healing professions (psychiatry, psychology, social work, or nursing) can be trained to conduct cognitive therapy with the adolescent rape victim. Its mechanisms of change are made explicit from the outset of treatment, and each treatment session is intended to reinforce the patient's understanding of how the treatment works. The essence of the change sought as a result of cognitive therapy is increased control (in particular, of cognitive processes), a goal entirely consistent with our perception of the needs of rape victims.

A rape victim is likely to focus on exaggerated perceptions of her inadequacy, powerlessness, and incompetence, and on such thoughts as "Being raped was my own fault," or "I'm worthless now that I've been raped." Cognitive therapy techniques are designed to help patients identify and test the reality of such distorted and dysfunctional beliefs. The three steps in treatment progress from concrete to abstract interpretations of the problem (the steps described here overlap with several of the "steps" defined in Chapter 8 as part of the middle phase of therapy; the reader should not be confused by this slight difference in terminology). Group I cognitive techniques challenge maladaptive thinking with homework tasks that change behavior and encourage novel thinking about specific situations and behaviors. Homework includes (1) a weekly activity schedule on which the patient rates the amount of mastery or pleasure she got from the activities listed in her log, and (2) graded task assignments through which the patient undertakes a series of tasks to reach a goal she considers difficult or impossible (for example, going out alone).

Beck and colleagues (Beck et al., 1979) argue that experiences that give a distressed individual a sense of mastery or pleasure reduce discomfort and automatic negative thoughts. Guided by responses to the activity schedule, graded-task assignments may also be designed to increase the sheer level of activity, to upgrade the quality of activity, or to enable a gradual approach to situations or tasks avoided since the assault. Early in treatment, the weekly activity schedule is also used to identify situations that elicit automatic negative thoughts. This technique is helpful when patients have difficulty identifying and recording automatic negative thoughts. Both during the explanation of the rationale for cognitive therapy and during the early treatment sessions, the therapist listens carefully for statements that have the characteristics of an automatic negative thought. These statements typically include an absolute such as "always," "never," "only," or "none," and are usually statements about the patient herself, her world, or her future. "My parents will never trust me again" would be a classic example. The therapist labels these statements as automatic thoughts and explains how the patient can record when they occur, along with the situations that elicited them and the feelings that result, on the daily record of automatic negative thoughts.

In the second treatment step (Group II cognitive techniques), therapist and patient work together to identify the cognitive distortion that gave rise to the automatic thought and to construct a rational, adaptive response. For example, Susan, a recent rape victim, found herself talking with a boy in her class whom she believed knew about the assault. She immediately thought, "Kenny is disappointed and upset with me. He will never think good of me again." The feelings she recorded in association with that thought were "anger" and "depression." In the therapy session, the therapist might ask Susan to examine the evidence that (1) Kenny is disappointed or upset now, and (2) even if he is currently upset, that this necessarily means he will never alter that view. If Susan pointed to a look on Kenny's face as evidence of his disappointment, the therapist would question the meaning of the evidence, asking her to offer alternative explanations such as "He was having a bad day," or "He was worried about an exam." If Kenny clearly was disappointed with Susan, the therapist would question the permanence of his current feelings by asking the patient to recall times when Kenny or other people were upset with her and got over it. The therapist would then ask Susan to formulate an adaptive response to this particular situation such as "Kenny is obviously upset about something. It's probably the math test he just got back," or "Kenny is disappointed that I got into the situation I did last weekend, but I know he'll get over it in a few days. He always does." Susan would then be asked to reevaluate her depressed and angry feelings about Kenny in light of her new view of the situation. Invariably, reevaluation produces positive feelings to the formerly distressing situation. A patient, in formulating adaptive responses, is asked to explore a variety of rational views of a situation and to choose the view that promotes the best feelings for her. Patients are not encouraged to formulate belief systems based on lies. A belief whose accuracy cannot be proven is retained as long as it can be considered a reasonable possibility.

Some patients eventually go on to the third phase of treatment (Group III cognitive techniques), in which they explore their basic assumptions about the world. Beck (Beck et al., 1979) argued that certain beliefs predispose individuals to depression and anxiety. Basic assumptions are common themes that unify a patient's automatic negative thoughts; basic assumptions are resistant to change perhaps because each one is supported by numerous automatic thoughts. In the group of rape victims we have worked with, young women have reported assumptions such as "I can't live without love," "If someone disagrees with me, it means he doesn't like me," and "My value as a person depends on what others think of me." When faulty basic assumptions are replaced with realistic attitudes (e.g., "It is more pleasant to be loved, but I can live without love," or "If people disagree with me, it simply means they have a different view of the topic or situation; it says nothing about what they think of me as a person"), the patient is able to improve her view of herself, the world, and the future. This new attitude facilitates positive thought and action in a variety of circumstances. The exploration of basic assumptions is particularly important in the rape victim with a past or concurrent major depression, since the rape-related negative cognitions are often supported by long-standing basic assumptions.

ASSESSMENT AND TREATMENT OF INCEST VICTIMIZATION

The assessment and treatment of incest victimization in depressed adolescents represents a much more complicated process than the assessment and treatment of rape victimization. When we write about incest victimization here, we employ a relatively broad definition of the term. As Finkelhor (1979) points out, anthropologists have one view of what constitutes incest, the criminal justice system another, and mental health professionals yet a third. Psychological definitions of incest were developed when it was discovered that sexual activity between relatives who are not too closely related to marry, or even with surrogate or quasi relatives, frequently has psychological effects that are indistinguishable from sexual relations between those who would be barred from marriage (Courtois and Watts, 1982). For the purposes of his research, Finkelhor defines incest as "sexual contact between family members, including not just intercourse, but also mutual masturbation, hand–genital or oral–genital contact, sexual fondling, exhibition, and even sexual propositioning." Curtois and Watts expand the definition to include all instances in which the female child should rightfully have been able to expect warmth or protection and sexual distance from the person who engages in sexual behavior with her. It is this expanded definition that we use in the sections that follow.

Incest, even defined in this way, was once thought to be a highly uncommon event; however, recent empirical studies suggest otherwise. In a study of a random sample of 930 women in San Francisco, Russell (1983) found that 16% reported at least one experience of intrafamilial abuse before the age of 18, and 12% reported such abuse before the age of 14. A series of studies of college students (Alexander and Lupfer, 1987; Finkelhor, 1979; Sedney and Brooks, 1984), each involving at least 300 students, consistently found that between 13% and 19% of young women reported a sexual experience with a family member while growing up.

Surveys of clinical populations tend to yield considerably higher rates. Beck and van der Kolk (1987) found that 46% of a group of chronically institutionalized, actively psychotic women reported histories of childhood incest. Other investigators (Hartman et al., 1987; Rosenfeld, 1979; Spencer, 1978) reported rates as high as 32–33% in general outpatient case loads, suggesting a strong link between childhood sexual abuse and adult psychological distress.

The clinical problem of incest victimization may present itself in at least two ways in depressed adolescents. Some patients may report or give the clinician reason to believe that they have experienced victimization at an earlier point in time; however, they give no indication that the victimization is ongoing. Another group of patients will report that the incest victimization is either currently ongoing or just recently ended. These scenarios represent two different therapeutic challenges in working with the adolescent.

In the case of ongoing abuse, a variety of reporting requirements and consequent involvement of other agencies (such as child protective services) will often complicate and set limits on what the therapist can do. Often in such cases the child may be removed from the home, sometimes precluding ongoing treatment. In the case of a report of or the suspicion of earlier victimization, if the therapist is assured that abuse is no longer ongoing, the therapeutic work can proceed in terms of helping the patient to address the psychological sequelae of this earlier victimization.

Setting the Treatment Contract

In our experience, early childhood incest victimization results in a large number of psychological sequelae affecting multiple domains in the young woman's life. These problems cannot all be addressed in a single short-term therapy contract. Indeed, the most typical pattern seems to be one in which the patient enters treatment, is able to maintain a relatively good level of adherence to the treatment contract for a period of time, and then appears to need a "break" from therapy, returning at some later time to work on additional issues. Multiple short-term contracts with planned or unplanned breaks in treatment seem to be a reasonable way to work with this population. Having said this, it should be pointed out that, in working with adolescents who have experienced a sexual victimization in childhood and who are coming in and out of treatment and at the same time experiencing relatively rapid developmental changes, the therapy may differ considerably each time the patient returns to treatment.

Coping Skills and Developmental States

In working with the adolescent incest survivor, the therapist needs to consider both the developmental stage at which the incest occurred and the developmental stage at which the patient currently finds herself. Coping strategies that may have been appropriate at the time of the victimization or shortly thereafter often become decreasingly age-appropriate as the incest survivor matures. However, the tension between her coping mechanisms and her own expectations of herself and how she should behave may become greater and greater as time goes on.

Assessment of Incest Victimization

A number of nonspecific indicators may suggest the probability of sexual victimization in adolescence. Many of these overlap with symptoms of depression and with symptoms of borderline personality disorder. Complicating the picture is the fact that some adolescents will actually have access to very clear memories of their incest victimization, whereas others will have only vague recollections or impressions. Still others will have no memories of sexual abuse; however, the symptom pattern is so strikingly like that of those who do remember the victimization that the therapist's index of suspicion will remain high. Among the symptoms frequently observed in this population are sleep disturbance, social withdrawal, sexual acting-out, free-floating anxiety, and/or anxiety specifically related to heterosexual activities or to specific men in the family. Incest survivors often also display limited capacity for trust and closeness in their heterosexual relationships. A frequent problem is fear of or unwillingness to permit a physical examination. As in adult incest survivors, substance abuse and self-mutilation are common. In our experience, a report of absolutely no memories before an age at which most children have some memories (e.g., age 7, not age 2) or no memories for a fixed period of time (e.g., second and third grade) should greatly increase the therapist's index of suspicion that incest victimization has taken place.

Using Cognitive Therapy Techniques with This Population

The primary therapeutic issues with incest victims are those of guilt, blame, and responsibility with respect to the incest itself and issues of self-esteem and personal value as a result of the incest. Cognitive therapy provides strategies and tactics that are especially effective in working with these issues. The dialectic of cogntive therapy permits the therapist to examine the cognitions the patient is experiencing with respect to feelings of guilt for participation in the incest, self-blame for participation and/or failure to stop the incest, and her feelings of responsibility for permitting the incest to start and/or failing to make it stop. Much more difficult to deal with are the cognitions the victim may have with respect to the perpetrator. In our experience, these feelings are often highly ambivalent, particularly in those cases where no violence was involved, where little pain was experienced, and where the victim was made to feel "special." Once the incest victimization ended, the parent, sibling, or other relatives responsible for victimizing the patient may have continued an otherwise appropriate and even loving relationship with her. It is around these strong feelings of ambivalence and attempts to resolve them that therapy often becomes the most complicated, and it is during work on these issues that the patient most often seems to need a "break" from treatment. Giving the patient permission to hold ambivalent feelings and acknowledging how difficult a state of ambivalence is to maintain may be the most the therapist can do at this point.

In general, efforts to normalize the patient's responses and behaviors—to make her feel less "crazy" and to help her see that her responses are appropriate for someone of the age at which she was victimized (if not appropriate for someone at her current age)—can provide enormous relief of distress and anxiety for this population. This can be especially true with respect to self-mutilitating behavior. Helping the patient to understand the many and varied reasons she may be engaging in such behaviors (e.g., a desire to make herself unattractive, a release of self-blame through "just punishment," an attempt to see whether she is capable of feeling) can be facilitated by understanding the cognitions that accompanied the self-mutilitating behavior. Once these cognitions are understood, alternative behaviors can be found that are both less physically and less emotionally damaging.

Finally, and perhaps most important, is to keep the focus as much as possible on the problems the patient is experiencing in the present as a result of the incest rather than on what happened or may have happened in the past. No amount of cognitive therapy (or any other kind of therapy, for that matter) can ever make what the perpetrator did right. Going back endlessly to these distressing events in an attempt to "work through" what can never be worked through often makes incest survivors worse and sometimes appears to increase the likelihood of dissociation. By emphasizing the patient's current reality and encouraging the most positive view possible of that reality, much can be accomplished to decrease depressive symptoms and enhance self-esteem. The therapist should keep in mind, however, that goals for short-term results with adolescent incest survivors may need to be more modest and that recurrences are common. Leaving the door open for a return to treatment at any time is essential.

SELECTED READINGS

Alexander PC, Lupfer SL: Family characteristics and long-term consequences associated with sexual abuse. *Archives of General Psychiatry* 1987; 16:235–245.

Beck AT, Rush AJ, Shaw BF, Emery G: *Cognitive Therapy of Depression.* New York, Guilford Press, 1979.

Beck JC, van der Kolk B: Reports of childhood incest and current behavior of chronically hospitalized psychotic women. *American Journal of Psychiatry* 1987; 144:1474–1476.

Courtois CA, Watts DL: Counseling adult women who experienced incest in childhood or adolescence. *Personnel and Guidance Journal* 1982; 60:275–279.

Finkelhor D: *Sexually Victimized Children.* New York, Free Press, 1979.

Hartman M, Finn SE, Leon GR: Sexual abuse experiences in a clinical population: Comparisons of familial and non-familial abuse. *Psychotherapy* 1987; 24:154–159.

Rosenfeld AA: Incidence of a history of incest among 18 female psychiatric patients. *American Journal of Psychiatry* 1979; 136:791–795.

Russell D: The incidence and prevalence of intrafamilial and extrafamilial sexual abuse of female children. *Child Abuse and Neglect* 1983; 7:133–146.

Sedney MA, Brooks B: Factors associated with a history of childhood sexual experience in a nonclinical female population. *Journal of the American Academy of Child Psychiatry* 1984; 23:215–218.

Spencer J: Father daughter incest. *Child Welfare* 1978; 57:581–590.

CHAPTER TWELVE

Cognitive Therapy with Affectively Ill, Suicidal Adolescents

DAVID A. BRENT

MIRIAM S. LERNER

INTRODUCTION

Despite numerous investigations into the correlates of suicidality among adolescents (for review, see Brent and Kolko, 1990), there is currently little consensus regarding the therapeutic approach to the suicidal adolescent. However, there is growing theoretical and empirical support for the use of cognitive therapy in the treatment of suicidal adolescents with affective illness (Wilkes and Rush, 1988). This chapter reviews the association between suicidality and affective illness; describes the factors that predispose to suicidality among affectively ill adolescents, with a particular emphasis on domains amenable to cognitive approaches; elucidates a clinical approach to the affectively ill suicidal adolescent; and discusses the indications and contraindications for cognitive therapy.

AFFECTIVE ILLNESS AND SUICIDALITY IN ADOLESCENTS

The proportion of adolescent suicide attempters with affective illness ranges from 33% in community surveys (Velez and Cohen, 1988) to 50–80% in clinically referred samples (Brent et al., 1986; Carlson and Cantwell, 1982; Pfeffer et al., 1988; Robbins and Alessi, 1985). According to two psychological autopsy studies, at least 60% of adolescent suicide victims had a lifetime history of affective illness (Brent et al., 1988; Shafii et al., 1988). Moreover, depression confers an eightfold risk for suicide among adolescent girls and a 49-fold risk for suicide among comparably aged boys (Shaffer, 1988). Previous suicidality is also a significant risk factor for completed suicide. Estimates of the prevalence of previous suicidality among completers range from 44% to 80% (Brent et al., 1988; Shafii et al., 1988), and a prior suicide attempt confers a nine- and 23-fold risk for completed suicide among adolescent girls and boys, respectively (Shaffer, 1988). Therefore, the identification of effective treatments for affectively ill, suicidal adolescents is a key element in prevention of youthful suicide and suicidal behavior.

Nosologic characteristics associated with suicidality in affectively ill adolescents include affective illness with nonaffective comorbidity (especially substance abuse), double depression, earlier age of onset, and longer duration of illness (Brent et al., 1990b; Myers et al., 1991; Ryan et al., 1987). Specific psychological characteristics appear to be associated with suicidality among youths, including cognitive distortion, hopelessness, and lack of assertiveness (Asarnow et al., 1987; Brent et al., 1986, 1990b; Kazdin et al., 1983; Myers et al., 1991; Ryan et al., 1987; Topol and Reznikoff, 1982). Finally, exposure to familial suicidality, family discord, family violence, and abuse, both physical and sexual, are associated with suicidality in children and adolescents (Brent et al., 1990b; Kosky et al., 1986; Hibbard et al., 1988; Taylor and Stansfeld, 1984a, 1984b). These findings suggest that early and aggressive treatment of affectively ill youngsters, targeting cognitive distortion, hopelessness, lack of assertiveness, and family discord, may be helpful in the amelioration of suicidality (Brent and Kolko, 1990).

THEORETICAL AND EMPIRICAL SUPPORT FOR THE USE OF COGNITIVE THERAPY IN SUICIDAL ADOLESCENTS

Cognitive therapy has the following features that make it particularly applicable to the treatment of suicidal adolescents. First, hopelessness is the domain most closely associated with attempted and completed suicide (Beck et al., 1985; Hawton et al., 1982), and cognitive therapy directly targets hopelessness. Second, cognitive therapy requires continuous assessment throughout treatment, thereby mandating that the clinician maintain a vigilant attitude toward depression and suicidality. Third, the active nature of cognitive therapy makes it particularly appropriate for this population. Depressed patients can become indecisive, inert, and not forthcoming with critical clinical information, such as suicidality. By actively pursuing a shared agenda, the cognitive therapist can help the depressed patient stay focused on the goals of treatment. Fourth, the cognitive therapist promotes the values of collaborative empiricism (Beck et al., 1979). The collaborative effort inherent to cognitive therapy necessitates input from the adolescent, thereby providing a sense of control and autonomy. Given that most adolescents do not request treatment and are somewhat distrustful of adult authority, collaborative empiricism allows the therapist to build trust and rapport and, at the same time, fosters self-reliance on the part of the adolescent. Finally, cognitive therapy emphasizes coping strategies that can be applied to stressful circumstances in the future. Given that depression and suicidality are likely to be recurrent (Kovacs et al., 1984a, 1984b) and that those adolescents with early onset and chronic depression are more likely to become suicidal (Brent et al., 1990b; Ryan et al., 1987), it follows that cognitive therapy may be particularly appropriate to help adolescents vulnerable to recurrent depression successfully deal with stressful situations and dysphoria in the future.

In adults, cognitive therapy has been shown to be more effective than antidepressants with respect to two outcomes relevant to the prevention of suicide: amelioration of hopelessness and the prevention of depressive relapse (Kovacs et al., 1981; Rush et al., 1977, 1982). And previous case studies have attested to the feasibility and potential efficacy of cognitive therapy in the treatment of suicidal, affectively ill adolescents (Bedrosian and Epstein, 1984; Trautman and Rotherman-Borus, 1988; Wilkes and Rush, 1988). Cognitive therapy has also been shown to be more effective than no treatment, although equal in efficacy to relaxation therapy in the relief of depressive symptomatology among nonreferred but symptomatically depressed high school students (Reynolds and Coates, 1986). In the open treatment application of cognitive therapy to clinically referred, affectively ill suicidal adolescents, we were able to demonstrate significant remission rates for both depressive symptoms and suicidality, which are maintained 9 months after termination of treatment (Brent DA and Boylan MB, unpublished data). In this open study, we were able to demonstrate that, by use of the Cognitive Therapy Rating Scale (CTRS; Vallis et al., 1986), cognitive therapy could be delivered along accepted lines to an adolescent population. A controlled study with older adolescents (ages 18–22) showed that cognitively oriented problem-solving group treatment (Clum et al., 1979) was more effective than a supportive treatment group in relieving depression and suicidality both at the termination of treatment and at 3-month follow-up (Lerner and Clum, 1990). Finally, Lewinsohn and

Clarke (1990) demonstrated that a cognitive therapy group was superior to a wait-list condition in ameliorating depression in depressed high school students, and that these gains were sustained upon longitudinal follow-up.

A CLINICAL APPROACH TO THE
SUICIDAL ADOLESCENT

Assessment

The first step in the treatment of suicidal adolescents is a careful assessment of the patient and family. In this way, the therapist can develop a treatment plan that considers all of the critical issues presented by suicidal patients. When this information is available at the outset, decisions regarding the need for hospitalization, the appropriateness of cognitive therapy, and the need for alternative or additional modalities such as pharmacotherapy can be made with greater confidence. A thorough assessment includes (1) psychiatric symptomatology, (2) suicidality, (3) cognitive style, (4) social competency, and (5) family environment.

Psychiatric Symptomatology

Psychiatric symptomatolgy is best assessed by interviewing both the adolescent and parent(s) about the adolescent's symptoms. One useful approach is to use a semistructured interview such as the K-SADS (Schedule for Affective Disorders and Schizophrenia for School-Age Children, Present Episode Version; Chambers et al., 1985; Orvaschel et al., 1982). Both past and current disorder should be assessed.

Suicidality

The most critical feature of the initial interview is the establishment of the degree of suicidal intent. This can be inferred from the intent (using the Beck Intent Scale; Beck et al., 1974) and lethality of a recent suicide attempt (using the Risk Rescue Rating; Weisman and Worden, 1972) or from subsequent persistence of suicidal ideation with a concrete plan, pervasive hopelessness, and a persistent, active wish to die. Patients who have these features and cannot promise to keep themselves safe should be considered for hospitalization, even if they must be committed involuntarily.

Other aspects of suicidal behavior that are important to ascertain are onset, chronicity, and relationship to other psychiatric symptoms and syndromes. For example, a chronically depressed patient may have had an exacerbation of suicidality following abuse of marijuana. Therefore, it is not the depression alone, but the comorbidity with substance abuse, that must be addressed acutely.

It is also critical to ascertain the nature of the precipitant (if any) to the suicidality. The most frequent precipitants are interpersonal discord, loss, or personal humiliation (Shaffer, 1974; Shaffer et al., 1988; Brent et al., 1988). Reconstructing the external and internal (within the patient's mind) sequences of events linking the precipitant to the suicidal event can provide helpful clues to the type of thinking that led the patient to consider suicide. For example, if the precipitant for a suicide attempt was a fight with a boyfriend, the internal sequence of events may have been "Without him I'm nothing; I might as well be dead."

Motivation is also a crucial aspect of the suicidal episode. Many adolescents who engage in suicidal behavior actually do not wish to die but instead may wish to gain attention, induce guilt, or express anger to another person. The choice of such an indirect route for the expression of negative affect suggests deficits in communication skills and interpersonal effectiveness that will require amelioration if the suicidality is to remit. It is also important to identify the affect associated with the suicidality. Frequently, the adolescent suicide attempter is angry rather than depressed at the time of the attempt; thus, the management of anger and the accompanying impulsivity will be an important component of treatment.

Two other important aspects of suicidality should also be assessed. One is whether the patient is modeling his behavior after some other suicidal person to whom he has been exposed. If so, steps should be taken to understand and diminish the appeal of this model to the patient. The other concern relates to the availability in the household of lethal agents for suicide, particularly firearms. Firearms should be removed from the homes of suicidal patients; merely securing them is not adequate (Brent et al., 1987, 1988).

Cognitive Style

This can be ascertained by discussion or by pencil-and-paper assessments such as the Automatic Thoughts Questionnaire (ATQ; Hollon and Kendall, 1980), Beck Hopelessness Scale (BHS; Beck et al., 1974), Beck Depression Inventory (BDI; Beck et al., 1961), or the Cognitive Negative Errors Questionnaire (CNEQ; Leitenberg et al., 1986). From these sources of information, one can learn whether the patient persistently engages in cognitive distortions, such as overgeneralization, dichotomous thinking, or personalization, and whether the person is pervasively hopeless. This information is critical to the formulation of a treatment plan in cognitive therapy because the basis of cognitive therapy is that the identification and modification of distortions will result in an improvement in depressive symptomatology.

Social Competency

The ultimate harbinger of the success of any psychiatric intervention is the level of social competency attained by the patient. There are three arenas of social competency for most adolescents: school (academic and behavioral), peers, and family (this will be discussed under "family environment"). Frequently, difficulties in one of these areas may precipitate suicidality, and sometimes the psychiatric problems that predispose to suicidality may also have an impact on social competency.

With regard to school, it is important to establish whether expectations are appropriate, that is, whether the patient and family expect too much academically relative to the patient's ability. On the one hand, stress may result from an inappropriate class placement. On the other, the patient's grades may have declined because he has had difficulty concentrating. In this case, ameliorating the concentration difficulties is likely to result in improved performance.

Problems with peers may relate to discord stemming from poor negotiation skills. Also, many patients harbor feelings of rejection, which may have their origin in poor self-esteem, unrealistic expectations, and a tendency to overpersonalize situations. Patients may also report isolation, which may stem from actual difficulties in initiating and sustaining friendships or from a distortion of reality (i.e., they may actually have friends but, while depressed, may feel they do not). All of these types of interpersonal problems are potential targets for treatment. However, it is important to differentiate distortions about ability (e.g., a popular student who *feels* unpopular) from actual skill deficits (a socially unskilled person who actually has few friends).

Family Environment

An understanding of the family environment is critical to the treatment of suicidal patients because parent–child discord is one of the most important precipitants for suicidal behavior (Brent et al, 1988; Hibbard et al., 1988; Kosky et al., 1986). The components of assessment include a history of any disruptions of relationship with either parent, the presence of discord or abuse (parent–child or interparental), and the degree of support and warmth in family relationships. Significant disruption in the parent–child relationship (such as divorce or death) may lead a patient to be consumed with anger, to conclude that he was unworthy, or to believe he may even have contributed to the disruption.

Discord is a frequent precipitant of suicidal behavior and may need to be addressed in family sessions in which a "truce" is negotiated. However, sometimes the amount of discord at home is so great that it is difficult for the patient to benefit from any amount of cognitive treatment. In this case, parents are invited in, and a list of expectations from both parents and child are solicited, with the aim being the negotiation of a viable behavioral contract. It is important to stress that what is being sought is not a solution to all interpersonal problems but simply agreements on the key problem(s) and a truce to abstain from discord in other potentially conflictual areas. It is helpful to rehearse with both parents and child how such a contract can be maintained. Active abuse usually precludes cognitive treatment and always requires legal action through children and youth services and more of a family systems and case-management approach. Another family problem stems from parents' inability or unwillingness to provide the kind of support a child may want. In these cases, it is important to help the patient adjust his expectations and learn other appropriate ways of gaining the support and affection he requires.

Another difficulty may be that the parents may view the child's depression as "manipulation" or "weakness." *Depression: A Survival Manual for Families* (Poling, 1988), a psychoeducational manual about depression that has been developed especially for parents, is given to parents at the time of the initial contact and then discussed in subsequent meetings with parents. Recent evaluation of this psychoeducational approach provides support for its acceptability and efficacy (Brent et al., 1993).

Finally, one should try to obtain diagnostic information about each parent; if either has untreated psychopathology, he or she should be referred for treatment. If a parent is depressed, he or she may be irritable, which, in turn, may contribute to discord within the home. Also, if a parent is suicidal, he or she may function as a model for the suicidal adolescent. One of the tasks of the clinician working with the parents of adolescent depressed patients is the referral of psychiatrically ill parents for clinical evaluation and treatment. Steps should also be taken to estimate the degree to which the parent makes suicidal threats in the presence of the patient and the familial response to these threats. Parents are instructed not to discuss suicidal feelings in front of the child and not to visibly reinforce this behavior.

Parents may also function as auxiliary therapists by providing a support net to the patient, for example, monitoring medication compliance, noting a recurrence in symptoms of depression, or even aiding the patient in practicing assertiveness or monitoring cognitive distortions. However, it is best to avoid involving parents as auxiliary therapists if they are also involved in a highly conflictual relationship with the patient.

Initial Clinical Decisions and Interventions

Obtain a No-Suicide Contract

As part of the assessment, the patient should be asked to make a no-suicide contract. This means that the patient promises not to hurt himself and that, if he feels suicidal, then he will notify a parent, another adult in authority, or the therapist (Brent and Kolko, 1990). The patient will then be led through the events precipitating the current episode of suicidality, and alternative methods of coping with the same stressors that initially precipitated the suicidality will be suggested. These steps can be written down on a business card for the patient to refer to in times of stress. The parents are also a party to this contract, and the procedure for involuntary commitment should be reviewed with them.

Decide Whether Treatment Should Be Inpatient or Outpatient

Psychiatric hospitalization is indicated for patients who, unless monitored in a structured and protective environment, are judged to be in imminent danger of suicide or suicidal behavior. Patients who are preoccupied with death, who show evidence of a suicide plan and have intent to carry it out, and who have made suicide attempts of high intent or of extremely high lethality are best treated on an inpatient unit. Furthermore, those patients whose psychiatric illnesses preclude outpatient treatment, such as those with active substance abuse, psychosis, and unstable (rapidly cycling or mixed state) bipolar disorder, are best initially stabilized in an inpatient facility. Other relative indications for hospitalization include a chaotic family that is unlikely to be able to sustain outpatient treatment and a history of previous suicide attempts with failure to follow through with outpatient treatment.

One helpful clinical tool in the decision to hospitalize the patient rests on the clinician's judgment of the patient's ability to keep a no-suicide contract. The no-suicide contract is not fool-proof but is a measure of the therapeutic alliance and should be viewed within the context of other clinical risk factors. If the patient and family can agree to the contract and there are no clinical contraindications (e.g., psychosis, active substance abuse, unstable bipolar disorder), then treatment can proceed on an outpatient basis.

The patient may oppose psychiatric hospitalization; if a no-suicide contract cannot be obtained and/or the patient has a dangerous constellation of risk factors, then the therapist should seek an involuntary commitment. One exception to this recommendation is when both the patient and the family are adamantly opposed to hospitalization. In this case, the clinician must weigh the need of the patient for immediate protection against the possibility that commitment may alienate both the patient and family against subsequent psychiatric care. Unless the patient is at immediate suicidal risk, the clinician may be better off trying to arrange for frequent outpatient monitoring of the patient, while maintaining a strong alliance with the family.

Hospitalization is at best a temporary respite from suicidality. The risk of suicide and suicidal behavior is greatest in the time immediately after discharge from the hospital. Therefore, linkage between inpatient and outpatient programs is essential, as is a clear postdischarge follow-up plan, so that treatment and monitoring of suicidal risk can continue uninterrupted after discharge from the hospital.

Evaluate Possible Contraindications for Cognitive Therapy

Patients with bipolar disorder or psychotic depression are best treated somatically, although cognitive techniques may be a useful adjunct. Similarly, patients with severe eating disorders, accompanied by nutritional problems, require refeeding before psychosocial issues can be addressed. Patients with substance abuse must be detoxified before treatment with cognitive therapy can be successful, and one must continue the ex-substance abuser in some supportive work such as Alcoholics Anonymous (AA) or Narcotics Anonymous (NA) in order to maintain abstinence. Also, if the patient is cognitively limited, either developmentally or as the result of depression, progress with cognitive treatment alone may be slow and difficult. Finally, families in crisis, particularly those with interparental or parent–child physical or sexual abuse, will probably require a family-oriented approach because the abuse issue tends to override other psychotherapeutic issues. However, a history of abuse is not incompatible with a cognitive approach; in fact, the distortions accompanying such traumatic events ("I deserved it; I'm dirty; I'm unworthy") are quite compatible with cognitive therapy.

Decide Whether Pharmacotherapy Is Indicated

Cognitive and pharmacotherapeutic approaches are not incompatible, and some tentative evidence suggests their synergy in the treatment of depression (e.g., Blackburn et al., 1981). However, as in most clinical interventions, it is best to add one intervention at a time, in order to ascertain the additive efficacy of each separate intervention. Pharmacotherapy is absolutely indicated for patients with psychotic depression or mania. Patients with a history of hypomania but who present without the classic hypersomnic, hyperphagic depression may be treated cognitively, but those with major depression and a frank history of mania should definitely receive pharmacotherapy. In adolescent patients with other types of affective illness, no compelling evidence yet suggests the efficacy of antidepressants (Ryan and Puig-Antich, 1986; Ryan, 1990; Kramer and Feiguine, 1981; Geller et al., 1989). However, antidepressants are recommended if the patient makes no progress symptomatically after 4 to 6 weeks or if fatigue, sleep, and concentration difficulties interfere with the patient's ability to grasp and apply the model. Use of selective serotonin reuptake inhibitors (SSRIs) is recommended over tricyclic antidepressants because the risk of fatal overdose is much less with SSRIs (Kapur and Mann, 1992).

Begin Socialization and Education with the Patient and Family

The process of educating and socializing the adolescent and family to treatment begins with the initial feedback session to the family. Assuming the adolescent is appropriate for cognitive therapy, the basic principles of the approach should be explained to both the adolescent and the family. Feedback on the adolescent's evaluation should also be provided to the family. This feedback should include (1) a summary of the diagnostic findings, (2) a discussion of the factors that seem to have contributed to suicidality, and (3) discussion of the no-suicide contract. Ground rules should be set about the structure of the sessions, setting (or canceling) appointments, contacting the therapist between sessions, and confidentiality. Both the adolescent and parents should be encouraged to call between sessions for any concerns about suicidality or other serious psychopathology (possibility of psychosis, substance abuse, homicidal thoughts or behavior). A back-up number (such as a psychiatric emergency room) should be provided in case the adolescent or parents need consultation when the therapist is unavailable. As noted previously, the parents should be educated about the removal of firearms from the household.

Set Ground Rules for Confidentiality

Absolute confidentiality should not be promised to the adolescent. Instead, the patient must understand that serious issues (such as suicidality) that necessitate an abrupt change in treatment plan must be shared with the parents. Also, parents have a right to know, in a general sense, the therapeutic goals and progress toward those goals in treatment. However, parents should not expect the therapist to give them a "blow-by-blow" discussion of therapy sessions. Also, if the parents call during the week between sessions, the general nature of the call should be shared with the patient, if clinically indicated.

Establish Treatment Goals

The establishment of goals is a critical part of the treatment contract, and the goals of treatment and their rationale should be reviewed with the family. These goals should be as empirically defined as possible to minimize ambiguity about the goals and their achievement. For example, an ambiguous goal would be for a depressed patient to "feel better." An unambiguous goal for that same patient is behaviorally defined as "I want to be able to concentrate on my school work better and improve my grades."

AN OVERVIEW OF THE APPLICATION OF COGNITIVE THERAPY WITH AFFECTIVELY ILL, SUICIDAL ADOLESCENTS

Establishing Trust and Rapport

An integral part of all treatment modalities is the establishment of trust and rapport with the suicidal patient. When working with adolescents, trust is important for a number of reasons. Adolescents do not usually present for treatment on their own behalf. Rather, parents or school personnel are often the referring parties for adolescents. The mental health clinic and the role of a therapist may also be unfamiliar to an adolescent. Given the referral process, the adolescent may perceive the therapist to be an ally of the parent or the school. The adolescent's general suspicion of adults increases his mistrust of the therapist. Thus, building trust and rapport is an essential part of therapy with adolescents; without it, all therapeutic interventions will fail.

A number of strategies can help to create such a bond of mutual confidence. For example, the therapist should be honest about the limits of confidentiality, as noted earlier; treat the adolescent with respect and as an independent person, capable of his own independent actions and opinions, as much as possible; and work collaboratively with the adolescent to formulate goals for treatment. Since the foundation of cognitive therapy is that of collaborative empiricism, building rapport will also be facilitated by soliciting the patient's feedback and ideas about each aspect of therapy. One example of how rapport can be facilitated is through the agenda. In essence, the therapist and patient mutually establish the priorities for a particular session. Any interventions that the therapist undertakes should be explained to the patient. If homework is assigned, the therapist should explain why it is being assigned and how the patient is expected to benefit. Furthermore, the patient's thoughts about this intervention should be solicited. In this way, the patient has input into every aspect of treatment.

Review of Presenting Problems and Therapeutic Goals

Patients who are not yet socialized to cognitive therapy tend to generate vague and nonspecific goals such as "I want to feel better." One therapeutic response to this fuzzy goal is "If you were not depressed, what would you be doing differently?" Once the patient has operationalized the problem, then patient and therapist can mutually assess whether or not this problem stems from a skill deficit or is related to a cognitive distortion.

In the formulation of a treatment plan for suicidal adolescents, it is important to include knowledge of the precipitant and motivation for the suicidal episode, as well as the patient's affect at the time of the episode and his degree of suicidal intent. For example, if a patient became suicidal in response to interpersonal rejection, it will be important to assess the meaning of rejection and the affects and behaviors usually triggered by such an event. Often the motivation for engaging in suicidal behavior is other than to die, such as to gain attention or to induce guilt in another person. For such patients, one goal of treatment should be the acquisition and consistent utilization of direct communication skills.

At the time of the suicidal episode, the patient may have been overwhelmed by strong affect, typically dysphoria or anger. If this is a typical pattern, then treatment must focus on ways to help the patient to prevent strong affect from subverting appropriate problem-solving, generally by teaching methods of affect regulation (e.g., anger control, relaxation techniques) and problem-solving (see section on "impulsivity and problem-solving"). Finally, knowledge of the suicidal intent, or the degree to which the patient wants to die, contributes to formulation of the treatment plan. A patient with high suicidal intent is likely to be hopeless, and hopelessness must always take a high therapeutic priority because of such a patient's potential lethality.

Targeting Hopelessness

For suicidal adolescents, hopelessness is often pervasive, extending to many areas of the teen's life. By the time the adolescent comes to therapy, he may believe that therapy or any other intervention will be of little use. Thus, an important initial step in cognitive therapy with suicidal adolescents is to decrease the hopelessness, especially about the potential efficacy of treatment. It is vital early on in treatment to get an understanding of the patient's assumptions, concerns, and expectations of treatment because, if a patient feels hopeless about treatment, the likelihood for drop-out is high.

Behavioral Techniques

Behavioral techniques must take priority over cognitive interventions in severely depressed patients. In these types of patients, the first goal of the therapist is getting them moving and motivated enough to begin to try to change their thinking patterns. Parents may be able to help implement these behavioral techniques in severely depressed adolescents. In such patients, it may be helpful to find out exactly what activities are in the patient's weekly schedule. The patient should simply fill out a weekly schedule and rate each activity on a scale of 1 to 10, according to the level of mastery and pleasure he experiences from participating in that activity. For some patients who claim to "do and enjoy nothing," an examination of this schedule may reveal significant cognitive distortions (e.g., they actually may be engaged in a lot of activities). Alternatively, the patient may truly be inert, in which case the therapist can help the patient to set behavioral goals for the subsequent week aimed at helping him to become more active. For example, activities such as shopping, having lunch with friends, and cleaning the house are much more incompatible with depressive rumination than lying in bed and watching television.

To help the more inert patient, the therapist may need to resort to the techniques of graded-task assignment, cognitive rehearsal, or role reversal. In graded-task assignment, the patient may be instructed to complete only the first step in a series of tasks. For example, if the patient wants to have a dinner party but cannot get out to shop or plan a menu, the first step might be shopping for supper for the family or just picking menus that appeal to the patient. Cognitive rehearsal is a method whereby the patient imagines performing a task and, in doing so, identifies the roadblocks that may interfere with task performance and prepares in advance to overcome them. Role playing with the therapist may facilitate the identification of roadblocks and their successful management. Another useful role playing technique is role reversal wherein the patient may play the role of the "nemesis." For example, to return to the case of the reluctant shopper, the patient may perceive the checkout person as disapproving; yet, when this patient reverses roles, he may discover that the checkout person is too detached to really care about any given customer.

Socialization to Cognitive Therapy

As in any type of treatment, it is important to educate the patient about the therapeutic interventions and explain their rationale. Because of the collaborative empirical approach of cognitive therapy, the socialization phase is particularly important. The sooner the patient is adequately socialized, the sooner he can function as an equal partner to the therapist in therapy. Socialization is largely a psychoeducational process. Aside from orienting the patient to the types of things that go on in treatment (e.g., weekly sessions of about an hour, procedure for emergencies), the critical aspect of socialization is to get the patient to think in terms of the cognitive model. Often, reading materials will be helpful (e.g., Boylan, 1990), with a didactic presentation of the cognitive model by the therapist for emphasis. It is useful to ask patients to check off portions of this reading material that seem to pertain particularly to their own situations.

The foundation of cognitive therapy is the concept of the *cognitive triad:* a negative view of the self, the world, and the future. After presenting this information, it is helpful to ask the patient if he has evidence to test the extent to which his views of self, the world, or the future are negative. To demonstrate how this theoretical concept relates to the patient's depression, it is helpful to illustrate the interrelationship among thoughts, affects, and behaviors. This framework then allows for the introduction of the concepts of automatic thoughts and the errors in cognition that depressed patients frequently make: selective abstraction, personalization, overgeneralization, dichotomous thinking, and catastrophization. As a further illustration, it is important to explain to the patient that by identifying and recording these automatic thoughts, he will be able to alter them by examining the evidence for and against holding such beliefs as true.

The therapist should look for every opportunity to reinforce the concept of the cognitive model. For example, if the patient notes that his teacher yelled at him, and he felt down the rest of the week because he felt that he was a dummy, this incident offers an opportunity to emphasize the relationship between thought and affect. Moreover, if cognitive distortion is involved in this interchange, it is important to show how some of the patient's errors in thinking were related to his subsequent low mood, and that this outcome is precisely what cognitive therapy would predict.

While the therapist is trying to engage and socialize, and perhaps even "convert" the patient to the point of the view of the cognitive model, he should also be eliciting any negative thoughts the patient might have about the model, treatment, and therapist. For example, patients may feel that this model is too simplistic and may add that they have tried such approaches in the past without symptomatic relief. This response, in itself, may be an example of dichotomous thinking (e.g., something either works or it does not). Other patients may be partially socialized to alternative models such as psychodynamic treatment, the biological view of depression, or family treatment. Again, it may be helpful to point out that it is possible to hold more than one view simultaneously about as complicated and heterogeneous a disorder as depression.

Identification of the Downward Spiral of Events, Thoughts, Feelings, and Behaviors

Hopelessness and thoughts about suicide are usually endpoints in a chain of thoughts, feelings, and behaviors. Helping adolescents identify their own individual thoughts, feelings, and behaviors can help them feel less out-of-control and begin to circumvent the downward spiral. For example, when a depressed suicidal adolescent experienced rejection by her boyfriend, her initial thoughts were "I'm not good enough"; her initial feelings were ones of hurt, and her initial behavior was to withdraw from social situations. In turn, her thoughts became "Nobody likes me." She felt sad and began to avoid all contact with friends. Eventually, she came to believe that if no one liked her, life was not worth living; then she considered suicide as an option. Once this patient was able to identify the thoughts, feelings, and behaviors that led to suicidal thoughts and actions, she gained a sense of control over her hopelessness and depression. This control can mark the beginning of working collaboratively with the adolescent to discover possible treatment goals. The identification of thoughts and behaviors that lead to hopelessness can be used throughout therapy as different situations provoke different response cascades. For adolescents, it is particularly important to attend to affective shifts during the sessions in order to illustrate the relationship between their thoughts, feelings, and behavior in the here and now.

Modification of Behaviors and Cognitions

The next step in cognitive therapy is to help the adolescent modify cognitions and behaviors to interrupt this downward, depressive spiral. As noted above, behavioral interventions may be warranted early in therapy, especially if the adolescent is experiencing significant impairment in activity level or degree of social involvement with the onset of depression.

Cognitive modification can be more difficult with adolescents than adults, depending on the adolescent's ability to think abstractly. The ability to consider multiple perspectives varies greatly in adolescents as a function of their variability in cognitive development. Rather than *challenging* the rationality of a cognition, it may be more productive to have an adolescent test the reality of a cognition. For example, to return to the adolescent who experienced rejection from her boyfriend, she may examine the reality of her thought "Nobody likes me," by recontacting friends and observing their responses. It may or may not be true that none of her friends like her. If it is not true, she will be able to disprove her negative thoughts and begin new behaviors that lead to a reduction in depression. If it is true that none of her friends like her, then the adolescent and therapist can work together to determine how to renew friendships or make new friends. Thus, testing the reality of the cognition is the first step in confronting the extent to which it represents a distortion.

   With an adolescent who is more capable of abstract thought, challenging the logic of the thinking can lead to cognitive modification. For example, one adolescent felt suicidal whenever he received a failing grade. Examining his chain of thinking revealed that he believed a failing grade meant he would flunk out of school, never go to college, never get a job, and therefore be a failure in life and to his father. The therapist examined the reality of each of these cognitions with the adolescent. Progress was slow, and the adolescent continued to feel suicidal. The therapist reported a turning point in the therapy when the therapist asked him if an "F" was worth killing himself over. The adolescent smiled with realization of the absurdity of this proposition and was able to begin to reexamine the reality of the other thoughts in this downward chain of thinking.

   It is important to solicit feedback from the patient during the session and encourage him to summarize frequently so as to monitor the degree to which the concepts of cognitive therapy are being assimilated. Moreover, it is helpful to use concrete examples to illustrate specific concepts in order to be certain that the therapist and adolescent are tracking the same issues. Targeting "hot" cognitions that arise from material in the session is one of the best assurances that the adolescent will grasp the model. One can get a clue that the adolescent is experiencing "hot" cognitions by shifts in affect (from happy to sad, engaged to bored, anxious to relieved, etc.). When one observes affective shifts, it is critical to ask the adolescent, "What's going on?"

Targeting Dichotomous Thinking

One type of cognitive distortion commonly found among depressed suicidal adolescents is dichotomous thinking (Brent et al., 1990b). Some research has documented the rigid thinking of suicidal individuals (Clum et al., 1979; Schotte and Clum, 1987). For example, when asked to generate solutions to a problem, suicidal individuals offer fewer solutions than nonsuicidal individuals (Schotte and Clum, 1987). Black-and-white thinking is also indicated by statements implying that something or someone is "all bad" or "all good." For example, a suicidal young man believed he had to be a straight "A" student to be considered a success. When he failed to meet this goal, he perceived himself as a total failure. Several techniques for working with dichotomous thinking are as follows.

Juxtaposition

A successful technique developed by Linehan et al. (1991) for working with the dichotomous thinking of borderline suicidal adults is the juxtaposition of dialectical opposites. For example, if an adolescent discusses the difficulty with being too dependent on his parents, the therapist might raise questions concerning the difficulty with being too independent. Again, the usefulness of this technique would depend on the youth's level of cognitive development.

Examination of the Grey Areas

Another technique to target black-and-white thinking is to examine the gradations of reality between the extremes. For example, if an adolescent believes she is acceptable to her friends only if she is beautiful, the therapist can explore with her the concept of beauty as a continuum. In the case of the young man who believed success meant straight A's, an examination of a varied notion of success might be helpful. Empirical methods may be used to enhance this exercise, like having an adolescent look at his environment to identify different types of success or beauty.

Looking at the Advantages and Disadvantages

Sometimes patients will adhere to a particularly dysfunctional cognition. In this case, if disputation, gradation, and other techniques fail, it may be helpful to ask the patient to look at the advantages and disadvantages of holding such a point of view. This exercise may help the patient prepare to let go of this particular cognition.

Impulsivity and Problem-Solving

The cognitive model of depression often presupposes a psychomotorically retarded, emotionally blunted adult who, if nothing else, will not engage in any risky behavior or make any major life decisions within the course of the first few sessions. This picture is in sharp contrast with the labile impulsivity and poor problem-solving that characterize many depressed, suicidal adolescents. A broader array of cognitive and behavioral techniques, while certainly consistent with the overall cognitive framework, is required to work with more impulsive patients (Lerner and Clum, 1990). The main indication for invoking interventions that target impulsivity is when the impulsivity, or the problems stemming from it, appears to be clinically paramount. For example, a depressed adolescent girl got into verbal battles with teachers and pupils at school and was continually getting suspended. A three-step approach proved useful. First, she was encouraged to subject these events to behavioral analysis: antecedents, behavior, consequences. Second, she was encouraged to look more carefully at the process by which she lost control. Third, she was taught to ask the five problem-solving questions: (1) What is the problem? (2) What are the alternative solutions? (3) What are the consequences of each alternative? (4) What is the best solution? (5) How did I do?

Relaxation techniques, self-statements, and written reminders may be helpful in slowing the impulsive adolescent down enough to reevaluate the consequences of a potentially self-damaging impulsive act. An additional technique for the impulsive, anger-prone adolescent is the use of the "feeling thermometer" (Rotheram, 1987). This technique links physiological signs of distress to intensity of feelings and helps to alert the adolescent to the need to "cool down" before he is so overwhelmed by negative emotion that all newly learned coping mechanisms are suspended. A key role of the therapist is to help the adolescent become an observer of his situation so that he can focus in on the problem, generate alternatives, and examine the consequences (Lerner and Clum, 1990; D'Zurilla and Goldfried, 1971). Practicing this skill may help reduce depression and suicidality (Lerner and Clum, 1990).

SUMMARY

In assessing for suicidality in depressed adolescents, the crucial question is the degree of lethality, that is, the likelihood of a suicide attempt. Lethality can be examined by inquiring about present suicidal ideation and suicidal intent associated with recent suicide attempts. Assessment of thoughts, feelings, and behaviors associated with suicidality, as well as motivation for suicide, lays the groundwork for treatment. The cognitive model is a collaborative way of conducting therapy with teens. Cogntive therapy allows the therapist and adolescent to identify and modify cognitions and behaviors associated with depression and suicidality. Careful assessment, establishment of trust and rapport, and implementation of cognitive therapy are likely to prove effective for the reduction of depression and suicidality in affectively disordered teens.

Empirical studies are currently under way to test the efficacy of cognitive therapy in suicidal, affectively disordered adolescents.

SELECTED READINGS

Asarnow JR, Carlson GA, Guthrie D: Coping strategies, self-perceptions, hopelessness, and perceived family environments in depressed and suicidal children. *Journal of Consulting and Clinical Psychology* 1987; 55:361–366.

Beck AT, Rush AJ, Shaw BF, Emery G: *Cognitive Therapy of Depression.* New York, Guilford Press, 1979.

Beck AT, Schuyler D, Herman J: Development of suicidal intent scales, in *The Prediction of Suicide.* Edited by Beck AT, Resnik HLP, Lettieri D. Bowie, MD, Charles Press, 1974.

Beck A, Steer R, Kovacs M, Garrison B: Hopelessness and eventual suicide: A 10-year prospective study of patients hospitalized with suicidal ideation. *American Journal of Psychiatry* 1985; 142:559–563.

Beck AT, Ward CH, Mendelson M, Mock J, Erbaugh J: An inventory for measuring depression. *Archives of General Psychiatry* 1961; 4:561–571.

Bedrosian RC, Epstein N: Cognitive therapy of depressed and suicidal adolescents, in *Suicide in the Young.* Edited by Sudak HS, Ford AB, Rushforth NB. John Wright, Boston, 1984.

Blackburn I, Bishop S, Glen A, Whalley LJ, Christie JE: The efficacy of cognitive therapy in depresion: A treatment trial using cognitive therapy and pharmacotherapy, each alone and in combination. *British Journal of Psychiatry* 1981; 139:181–189.

Boylan MB: *Feeling Better.* Pittsburgh, University of Pittsburgh, Western Psychiatric Institute and Clinic, unpublished manuscript, 1990.

Brent DA, Kalas R, Edelbrock C, Costello AJ, Dulcan MK, Conover N: Psychopathology and its relationship to suicidal ideation in childhood and adolescence. *Journal of the American Academy of Child and Adolescent Psychiatry* 1986; 25:666–673.

Brent DA, Kolko DJ: The assessment and treatment of children and adolescents at risk for suicide, in *Suicide over the Life Cycle: Risk Factors, Assessment, and Treatment of Suicidal Patients.* Edited by Blumenthal, SJ, Kupfer DJ. Washington, DC, American Psychiatric Press, 1990.

Brent DA, Kolko DJ, Goldstein CE, Allan MJ, Brown RV: Suicidality in affectively disordered adolescent inpatients. *Journal of the American Academy of Child and Adolescent Psychiatry* 1990b; 29:586–593.

Brent DA, Perper JA, Allman C: Alcohol, firearms, and suicide among youth: Temporal trends in Allegheny County, Pennsylvania, 1960–1983. *Journal of the American Medical Association* 1987; 257:3369–3372.

Brent DA, Perper JA, Goldstein CE, Kolko DJ, Allan MJ, Allman CJ, Zelenak JP: Risk factors for adolescent suicide: A comparison of adolescent suicide victims with suicidal inpatients. *Archives of General Psychiatry* 1988; 45:581–589.

Brent DA, Poling K, McKain B, Baugher M: A psychoeducational program for families of affectively ill children and adolescents. *Journal of the American Academy of Child and Adolescent Psychiatry* 1993; 32:770–774.

Brent DA, Zelenak JP, Bukstein O, Brown RV: Reliability and validity of the structured interview for personality disorders in adolescents. *Journal of the American Academy of Child and Adolescent Psychiatry* 1990a; 29:349–358.

Carlson G, Cantwell D: Suicidal behavior and depression in children and adolescents. *Journal of the American Academy of Child and Adolescent Psychiatry* 1982; 21:361–368.

Chambers WJ, Puig-Antich J, Hirsch M, Paez P, Ambrosini PJ, Tabrizi MA, Davies M: The assessment of affective disorders in children and adolescents by semi-structured interview. *Archives of General Psychiatry* 1985; 42:696–702.

Clum G, Patsiokas A, Luscomb R: Empirically based comprehensive treatment program for parasuicide. *Journal of Consulting and Clinical Psychology* 1979; 47:37–45.

D'Zurilla T, Goldfried M: Problem-solving and behavior modification. *Journal of Abnormal Psychology* 1971; 78:107–126.

Geller B, Cooper TB, Graham D: *Double-Blind Placebo Control Study of Nortriptyline in Depressed Adolescents.* Paper presented at the Annual NIMH NCDEU Meeting, Key Biscayne, FL, June 1, 1989.

Hawton K, Osborn M, O'Gray J, Cole D: Classification of adolescents who take overdoses. *British Journal of Psychiatry* 1982; 140:124–131.

Hibbard RA, Brack DJ, Rauchs, Rauch S, Orr DP: Abuse, feelings, and health behaviors in a student population. *American Journal of Diseases of Children* 1988; 142:326–330.

Hollon SD, Kendall PC: Cognitive self-statements in depression: Development of an automatic thoughts questionnaire. *Cognitive Therapy Research* 1980; 4:383–395.

Kapur S, Mann JJ: Antidepressant medications and the relative risk of suicide attempt and suicide. *Journal of the American Medical Association* 1992; 268:3441–3445.

Kazdin AE, French NHY, Unis AS, Esveldt-Dawson K, Sherick RB: Hopelessness, depression, and suicidal intent among psychiatrically disturbed inpatient children. *Journal of Consulting and Clinical Psychology* 1983; 51:504–510.

Kosky R, Silburn S, Zubrick S: Symptomatic depression and suicidal ideation: A comparative study with 628 children. *Journal of Nervous and Mental Diseases* 1986; 174:523–528.

Kovacs M, Rush AJ, Beck A, Beck AT, Hollon SD: Depressed outpatients treated with cognitive therapy or pharmacotherapy: A one year follow-up. *Archives of General Psychiatry* 1981; 38:33–39.

Kovacs M, Feinberg TL, Crouse-Novak M, Paulauskas SL, Finkelstein R: Depressive disorders in childhood: I. A longitudinal prospective study of characteristics and recovery. *Archives of General Psychiatry* 1984a; 41:229–237.

Kovacs M, Feinberg TL, Crouse-Novak M, Paulauskas SL, Pollock M, Finkelstein R: Depressive disorders in childhood: II. A longitudinal study of the risk for a subsequent major depression. *Archives of General Psychiatry* 1984b; 41:643–649.

Kramer A, Feiguine R: Clinical effects of amitriptyline in adolescent depression. *Journal of the American Academy of Child and Adolescent Psychiatry* 1981; 20:636–644.

Leitenberg H, Yost LW, Carroll-Wilson M: Negative cognitive errors in children: Questionnaire development, normative data, and comparisons between children with and without self-reported symptoms of depression, low self-esteem, and evaluation anxiety. *Journal of Consulting and Clinical Psychology* 1986; 54:528–536.

Lerner ML, Clum G: Treatment of suicide ideators: A problem-solving approach. *Behavior Therapy* 1990; 21:403–411.

Lewinsohn PM, Clarke GN: Cognitive-behavioral treatment for depressed adolescents. *Behavior Therapy* 1990; 21:385–401.

Linehan MM, Armstrong HE, Suarez A, Allmon D, Heard HL: Cognitive-behavioral treatment of chronically parasuicidal borderline patients. *Archives of General Psychiatry* 1991; 48:1060–1064.

Myers K, McCauley E, Calderon R, Mitchell MD, Burke P, Schloredt K: Risks for suicidality in major depressive disorder. *Journal of the American Academy of Child and Adolescent Psychiatry* 1991; 30:86–94.

Orvaschel H, Puig-Antich J, Chambers W, Tabrizi MA, Johnson R: Retrospective assessment of prepubertal major depressive episode with the K-SADS-E. *Journal of the American Academy of Child and Adolescent Psychiatry* 1982; 21:392–397.

Pfeffer CR, Newcord J, Kaplan G, Mizruchi MS, Plutchik R: Suicidal behavior in adolescent psychiatric inpatients. *Journal of the American Academy of Child and Adolescent Psychiatry* 1988; 27:357–361.

Poling K: *Living with Depression: A Survival Manual for Families.* Pittsburgh, University of Pittsburgh, Western Psychiatric Institute and Clinic, 1988.

Reynolds WM, Coates KI: Comparison of cognitive and behavioral therapy and relaxation training for treatment of depression in adolescents. *Journal of Consulting and Clinical Psychology* 1986; 54:653–660.

Robbins D, Alessi N: Depressive symptoms and suicidal behavior in adolescents. *American Journal of Psychiatry* 1985; 142:588–592.

Rotheram MJ: Evaluation of imminent danger for suicide among youth. *Journal of the American Orthopsychiatric Association* 1987; 57:102–110.

Rush AJ, Beck AT, Kovacs M, Hollon SD: Comparative efficacy of cognitive therapy and pharmacotherapy in the treatment of depressed outpatients. *Cognitive Therapy Research* 1977; 1:17–37.

Rush AJ, Beck AT, Kovacs M, Weissenburger J, Hollon SD: Comparison of the effects of cognitive therapy and pharmacotherapy on hopelessness and self-concept. *American Journal of Psychiatry* 1982; 139:862–866.

Ryan N: *A Controlled Study of Amitriptyline versus Placebo in Adolescent MDD.* Paper presented at the American Academy of Child and Adolescent Psychiatry, New York, NY, October 1989.

Ryan ND: Pharmacotherapy of adolescent major depression: Beyond TCA's. *Psychopharmacology Bulletin* 1990; 26:76–79.

Ryan ND, Puig-Antich J: Affective illness in adolescence, in *American Psychiatric Association Annual Review,* Vol. 5. Edited by Frances AJ, Hales RE. Washington, DC, American Psychiatric Press, 1986.

Ryan ND, Puig-Antich J, Ambrosini P, Rabinovich H, Robinson D, Nelson B, Iyengar S, Twomey J: The clinical picture of major depression in children and adolescents. *Archives of General Psychiatry* 1987; 44:854–861.

Schotte D, Clum G: Problem-solving skills in suicidal psychiatric patients. *Journal of Consulting and Clinical Psychology* 1987; 55:49–55.

Shaffer D: Suicide in childhood and early adolescence. *Journal of Child Psychology and Psychiatry* 1974; 15:275–291.

Shaffer D: The epidemiology of teen suicide: An examination of risk factors. *Journal of Clinical Psychiatry* 1988; 49 (Suppl. 9):36–41.

Shaffer D, Garland A, Gould M, Fisher P, Trautman P: Preventing teenage suicide: A critical review. *Journal of the American Academy of Child and Adolescent Psychiatry* 1988; 27:675–687.

Shafii M, Stelz-Lernarsky J, Derrick AM, Beckner C, Whittinghill JR: Comorbidity of mental disorders in the post-mortem diagnosis of completed suicide in children and adolescents. *Journal of Affective Disorders* 1988; 15:227–233.

Taylor EA, Stansfeld SA: Children who poison themselves. I: A clinical comparison with psychiatric controls. *British Journal of Psychiatry* 1984a; 145:127–132.

Taylor EA, Stansfeld SA: Children who poison themselves. II: Prediction of attendance for treatment. *British Journal of Psychiatry* 1984b; 145:132–135.

Topol P, Reznikoff M: Perceived peer and family relationships, hopelessness and locus of control as factors in adolescent suicide attempts. *Suicide and Life Threatening Behavior* 1982; 12:141–150.

Trautman PD, Rotherman-Borus, MJ: Cognitive-behavioral therapy with children and adolescents, in *American Psychiatric Association Annual Review,* Vol. 7. Edited by Frances AJ, Hales RE. Washington, DC, American Psychiatric Press, 1988.

Vallis TM, Shaw BF, Dobson KS: The cognitive therapy scale: Psychometric properties. *Journal of Consulting and Clinical Psychology* 1986; 54:381–385.

Velez CN, Cohen P: Suicidal behavior and ideation in a community sample of children: Maternal and youth reports. *Journal of the American Academy of Child and Adolescent Psychiatry* 1988; 27:349–356.

Weisman A, Worden W: Risk rescue rating in suicide assessment. *Archives of General Psychiatry* 1972; 26:553–560.

Wilkes TCR, Rush JR: Adaptations of cognitive therapy for depressed adolescents. *Journal of the American Academy of Child and Adolescent Psychiatry* 1988; 27:381–386.

PART V

Other Treatments for Depressed Adolescents

CHAPTER THIRTEEN

Cognitive Therapy with Hospitalized Adolescents

ANTHONY NOWELS

INTRODUCTION

Cognitive therapy can be used effectively with depressed patients who are hospitalized. The easiest methods employ the same understanding and strategies that one would use with any outpatient. To be truly effective, however, adjustments need to be made to compensate for the differences that are usually encountered with inpatient work, such as multiple therapists, "team" decisions, intensive three- or four-times weekly treatment, special program needs, and therapeutic strategies designed to resolve conflict.Cognitive therapy can be used as the "organizing philosophy" for an entire inpatient program, with all staff employing programmatic management and with treatment strategies evolving, in part, as extensions of individual strategies and interventions.

"TEAM" EFFECTS ON THE THERAPIST

The most obvious difference in providing inpatient psychotherapy arises from having to deal with a multidisciplinary treatment team, each member of which has his own views of the patient's problems and how they should be treated. Some members of the team may differ substantially from each other in their philosophies and therapeutic skills and strategies. Even where there is relatively good cooperation and mutual understanding, each of the caregivers frequently harbors the fantasy that his own particular interaction represents the "crucial" therapeutic intervention.When these views surface, and can be openly dealt with among professionals, the treatment team is usually more successful.

In some instances, the cognitive therapist may be the leader of the treatment team and, thus, be able to set the specific goals and adjust the strategies to his own liking. In other cases, the cognitive therapist must adapt to systems created by other members of the treatment team. It is also possible that other forms of psychotherapeutic intervention will be simultaneously applied to the same patient, with all of the complexities and potential conflicts such treatment can create.

STANDARDS FOR THE TREATMENT TEAM

For the inpatient therapy team to use cognitive approaches most effectively, the therapist should try to assure that a variety of standards are met so that:

1. Members of the treatment team mutually respect (if not understand) each other's approaches and do not undermine each other in an effort to be the "prime therapist."
2. A common language exists so that cognitive approaches can be discussed, understood, and implemented without conflict.
3. Therapists be of approximately equal skill and experience so that certain approaches are not relegated to "second-class" status by virtue of their being delivered by the new, inexperienced therapist.
4. Sufficient compulsory time for team meetings and other communication systems exists so that team members operate together as a "team," that the patient cannot "split" the therapists, and that conflicts with approaches and strategies can be identified and resolved. This is particularly crucial with cognitive therapy because of the logs, essays, and tasks that must be created, defined, and observed.
5. The team–patient interaction and communication systems (some teams have the patient as a team member) be constructed in such a way that the cognitive-behavioral approaches can be applied in an atmosphere of mutual cooperative interaction, an extension of one cotherapy approach.

Caroline's Case

Caroline was a 14-year-old admitted to the hospital when outpatient treatment failed to help failing school grades, constant arguments with parents at home, and refusal to follow the family rules for conduct. Her depression was largely defined by irritability, although her self-esteem was also very low. The new inpatient treatment team was trying to deal with Caroline's anger, rejection of help, refusal of sessions, and use of group session time to get her own personal needs met.

Caroline was skilled in inducing staff to disagree with each other, even over minor privilege issues, a behavior that was probably a replication of what occurred in the family. Individual cognitive therapy was still in its initial stages, even five sessions into the hospitalization. The therapist was trying to establish a cotherapy relationship, mutual goals, and civil behavioral ground-rules for the therapy sessions. The therapists working most closely with Caroline wanted to maintain her privileges at a relatively low level because of her noncompliance with therapy, whereas program staff insisted that she would not improve and that they could not help her self-esteem until she was allowed to participate in all aspects of the program with higher privilege levels.

Caroline came to the sixth session angry and demanding help in convincing other staff that she deserved an increase in privileges. This was the first time she had been so active and participatory, the first opportunity for a mutual goal. She explained that higher privileges would allow her to attend additional off-unit group therapies, the cafeteria, and a regular classroom—all excellent goals for her.

Caroline was pleased that her goal was supported, and she demanded that her therapist immediately call the other members of her treatment team. It was explained that this strategy was unlikely to work and that she needed something more convincing such as a written "petition." Caroline rejected the idea but at least listened while the details of such a document were suggested, including her own lists of reasons for moving to a higher level, with spaces for each staff member and therapist to comment and sign his or her name. It was suggested that she could add to the document each day as other reasons arose for staff to view her as being successful. She laughed and commented that the petition was like other "logs" and "essays" I had asked her to write during previous sessions.

The seventh session was similar to earlier meetings, and Caroline did not mention the petition until it was brought up toward the end. She reported that it was a stupid idea, that people had just said bad things about her, and, for the first time in a session, she began to cry. It turned out that she had solicited support not only from staff she believed would be supportive but also from peers. Their remarks about her self-centered and selfish behaviors had been painful but did serve to create the first self-observing Caroline had done. That the words were written down and had, in fact, been elicited by Caroline herself seemed to give them much more power. They also mirrored her own thoughts and fears. These events served to create a realistic discussion of Caroline's views of herself and to help her formulate new goals about her self-esteem and how others viewed her.

At the next treatment-team rounds, it was important to remind all the staff about Caroline's depression and low self-esteem. Her being a difficult patient created major countertransference feelings, and staff needed to identify those impulses when Caroline's "petition" was being completed. Her angry behavior needed to be translated into reactions based on assumptions she had about herself and how others would treat her. The treatment team needed to remind themselves of these issues when feeling angry with her.

The eighth session was the first one that Caroline attended eagerly, bringing a petition now grown to almost 15 pages, showing positive comments by peers, staff, and even her family. She had been writing the most negative things about herself, and she was surprised when this was pointed out to her. Logging and discussing these self-condemning thoughts consumed the major portions of the next two sessions. Caroline was asked to counter these ideas by not "hitting herself over the head"—by identifying the times she assumed negative thoughts about herself and trying to insert other ideas to replace them.

Session 11 showed a marked return toward anger, silence, and hostile recriminations. Caroline had *not* been granted the highest privilege level by the treatment team, and she was now deprecating the individual therapy and therapist as not having much influence or power. When it was finally pointed out that "some people were getting hit over the head" again, she laughed, said she knew that would be the response, and continued to be somewhat angry.

Caroline came to session 12 smiling, pleased that the treatment team had decided that she would be discharged at the end of the week to return to her previous therapist. She had drawn a picture of herself on her "petition log," showing her as a smiling stick figure hitting herself over the head. She reported that she knew when she was putting herself down. She also said her parents did not hit her over the head any longer.

The last session was used to say goodbye, to review her treatment petition, and to call her outpatient therapist on the speaker phone to explain what had happened at the hospital.

This example suggests some of the issues faced by a therapist conducting cognitive therapy in a hospital setting. The degree of resistance to therapy may be much more than usually seen, sessions may be much more frequent, and the goals and strategies must take into account the other members of the treatment team. Feedback from program staff can be very helpful, although some therapists may feel that their efforts are being "diluted" or "contaminated" by many other caregivers. An aftercare plan is usually developed to assure that therapy continues postdischarge, frequently with a different therapist. Patients are often admitted and discharged suddenly, with changes in therapists and treatment strategies, and with the inpatient therapist feeling in tenuous control or even discounted.Treatment team meetings become one forum for dealing with these issues.

PROGRAM ASSISTANCE IN IMPLEMENTING COGNITIVE THERAPY

One of the advantages of working in an inpatient setting, assuming that cooperation exists between the program and the cognitive therapist, is that the maintenance of logs and other written materials can be enforced through the program and can be richly supplemented by observations from the program staff. This situation creates an extremely productive environment for specific behavioral observations, as well as for initiating interventions that can be carried out consistently and powerfully through a variety of patient–staff systems.The therapist's influence can be multiplied and extended through the efforts of a cooperative, well-trained inpatient program staff.

Marcy's Case

Marcy was a white 17-year-old admitted for the first time because of worsening depression, suicidal ideation and behavior, severe unremitting bulimia, and cocaine abuse. She was an attractive blonde, who had been a high school cheerleader, but was now a drop-out, living at home and dating a much older man. Her mother strongly supported her chaotic lifestyle, living vicariously through it, whereas her stepfather (of 4 years) was trying to set some limits within the family. Multiple outpatient therapists had failed to be of help, and both she and the family felt that the situation was completely out of control.

During the first session, Marcy demonstrated her excellent verbal skills, extreme seductiveness, and intense feelings of humiliation at having to be hospitalized. She did not want to take medication and easily and quickly set high goals for herself: to get out of the hospital immediately, to cease needing therapy, and to go to college while having a modeling career on the side. She denied the risks of purging, which she used to control her weight, but agreed that she had to stop her cocaine use.

Marcy was "perfect" in the hospital, well liked by staff and peers, and quickly identified as a patient who would not need to remain in the hospital long. The utilization review nurse even started to question criteria for hospitalization.

The second and third sessions were similar to the first, with Marcy presenting well-written but unemotional logs. Marcy's only emotion surfaced when, in the fourth meeting, she detected that her logs and essays were not what I had expected. I expressed confusion that she had recently been depressed, bulimic, and suicidal; but now suddenly everything was fine. Several times she asked what I wanted her to do. I told her that she should stop writing and living what others wanted and instead talk about her true feelings. The fifth meeting was similar, so I asked her to write a detailed autobiography, imagining that she was much older, and describing her life, her friends, and how she felt about herself.

Marcy chose to send me her autobiography rather than present it at a session—she later explained her concern that I would not like the document. She had written about a sad and lonely woman who felt empty inside, never close to people, always seeming to make others happy, but never happy herself. She was afraid her mother had hated her; she had virtually no sexual feelings or relationships and just wanted to be a "good little girl." At the end of that meeting, she expressed feelings that she did not want to live if that was going to be her life. I asked her to create an inventory—reasons to live and reasons not to live.

She revealed her suicidal feelings in her next logs and was quickly put on suicide precautions by program staff, creating great chaos on the program and in her family sessions. Many staff did not want to see her as having problems and found it difficult to adapt to her new patient role. Her mother had to be specifically dissuaded from telling Marcy that she could not possibly have those feelings, with specific requests by the family therapist that "mind reading" in the family had to stop.

At the seventh, eighth, and ninth meetings, Marcy elaborated on her depressed, empty feelings and indicated how much she was now trying to be a "good patient" by providing all these symptoms. Angry feelings emerged as she attacked me for "not understanding" her and never feeling that she was "good enough." She demonstrated her inventory of reasons to live as being much longer than the reasons not to live and said she was surprised by this, but "no one else appreciated that."

Treatment-team rounds became a struggle as program staff tried to strike a balance between allowing Marcy to reveal her underlying despair and hopelessness while also letting her have some time off of suicidal precautions. Staff feelings of disappointment were pointed out as being similar to feelings that the parents described.

Session 11 was different in that Marcy talked about others in the program for the first time, describing another unhappy patient and how they had talked about their feelings. She was now off suicide precautions. For the first time, she agreed to antidepressant medication, talking about how she recognized the feelings as coming over her for parts of each day and saying she would never "make it" outside the hospital. Desipramine was begun immediately, in the hope that the drug would help with her bulimia and depression.

Sessions 12, 13, and 14 were classical "cognitive" meetings, now helping Marcy to uncover assumptions about herself, recognize negative self-statements, and reinterpret events from a more positive viewpoint. She become an "instructor" in her family meetings, teaching her mother, whom she described as being just like herself. She was described in progress notes as being far more "real" by all the staff. The treatment team set a discharge date 1 week away.

Marcy revealed in her last session (number 18) that she had had some return of bulimic symptoms and that she was afraid she would not be attractive to her friends outside the hospital, who would "never understand her" like her peers in the program had.

When asked how she was going to solve this problem, Marcy smiled and produced an inventory about herself, outlining what others would like and dislike. I suggested that she specifically record her bulimic symptoms as part of the inventory. She agreed to bring this to her first outpatient session the following week. She was also asked to create goals for her outpatient therapy and determine how long she would need to attend.

Marcy did well in weekly outpatient therapy for about 6 weeks. She continued on desipramine for 9 months after that, with monthly therapy sessions, after which she graduated from high school and went on to college.

In addition to presenting the classic problem of the "perfect patient," Marcy also demonstrated how the therapist initially had difficulty establishing an alliance, with so many competing relationships in the inpatient milieu. The pace of therapy was rapid, with 18 sessions in only 6 weeks. It was important to distinguish this patient's extreme cooperativeness in the service of being a "good little girl" from the desirable cotherapy process that is an important part of cognitive therapy.

The treatment team correctly wanted to protect Marcy from her suicidal impulses but was also in danger of discouraging her expression of feelings—always a difficult balance. Material in logs and essays must be used carefully in considering program management issues and then only as part of an overall treatment strategy. The therapist also had to guard against the treatment becoming just another "compliance" issue, with the patient learning to give just what the therapist "wanted." This was especially true at the end of hospitalization, where it was essential that the responsibility be turned over to the patient. Finally, even after the formal outpatient sessions stopped, the medication checks were utilized to serve as reinforcers of the process and to test for any signs of relapse.

COMPATIBLE PATIENT AND TEAM GOALS

The cognitive therapist operating within the inpatient or residential milieu must work with two "levels" of patient care—one directed at the patient in a traditional fashion, the other directed at the treatment team and program staff, who must be included as part of the "system" of cognitive therapy. The staff must be educated about cognitive therapy; they often become part of the treatment strategies and are "won over" to help implement logs, essays, and other tasks. The "group" of therapists need to understand each other's approaches, develop compatible goals, and establish strategies that can be implemented together or sequentially to achieve these goals. Flexibility becomes the most important asset. This complex system requires the cognitive therapist to be prepared to adapt constantly to the dynamic hospital environment by being willing to change goals and strategies, try new ideas, and blend cognitive approaches into the fabric of other philosophies and therapeutic techniques.

PROGRAMMATIC USE OF COGNITIVE THERAPY WITHIN HOSPITAL OR RESIDENTIAL ENVIRONMENTS

Cognitive therapy probably works best when the program, its staff, and the treatment team are receptive to its fundamental concepts and therapeutic techniques. One logical extension of this criterion is to use a cognitive paradigm as the basis for the inpatient treatment program. Logs, tasks, essays, cognitive reinterpretations, and petitions are just a few examples of how the usual cognitive approaches are particularly well suited to inpatient program operations. Even more important, the philosophy underlying cognitive therapy is especially compatible with inpatient adolescent programming. Although certainly not essential with hospitalized adolescents, a cognitive therapy program can greatly simplify and extend the treatment process.

COGNITIVE STRATEGIES FOR INPATIENT PROGRAMS

Inpatient cognitive therapy interventions offer the opportunity for a therapist not only to apply cognitive behavioral techniques to a patient who happens to be hospitalized (just as one would on an outpatient basis) but also to extend strategies and interventions to the entire program as it interacts with the patient hour by hour through each day. In this context, a variety of individuals, working closely with one another and communicating frequently, apply many of the same strategies that would be used in a one-to-one therapist–outpatient relationship and often with similar goals.

The power and appeal of such a technique is that it places the hospital caregivers in more of a "cotherapy" role, which is far more comfortable for both the staff and patients. It also reinforces the cognitive behavioral interventions through multiple contacts over the course of a day and frequently can be applied at times when patients are "behaving" or "feeling" the specific areas sought out for intervention.

Patients can also be helped to maintain detailed daily logs that describe events and the patients' emotional reactions to them, but where the inpatient staff is in fact *present* during the period being discussed in the logs. This validation opportunity allows for more meaningful and accurate use of cognitive methods.

All program interventions, from the nurse who might feel a PRN (as-needed medication) is indicated to a group therapist encouraging the expression of feelings, can take advantage of the overall treatment team's goals and cognitive strategies. "Time-outs" can be replaced or supplemented with written "essays" intended to have the patient self-observe and report his reactions during particular events. In adolescent settings, the teachers and family members are also important members of the team and can assist greatly in the successful adaptation of cognitive strategies.

The program can establish a series of tasks whereby each patient must describe and write about certain ideas in his own words. This written component becomes a step in the process of moving up a privilege level or perhaps toward discharge. Thus, the patient can become "interwoven" into the fabric of therapy and the goal-creation process. It is especially important to understand how the patient views the goals and the underlying assumptions motivating his interaction with the treatment team. With many patients, particularly adolescents, this system recapitulates the underlying family dynamics.

The treatment team can also establish other, more specific written or behavioral tasks that the patient must understand and report. A process of having the patient "teach" other patients about issues related to his success and the achievement of some of these goals can be an important step in the process of the patient's therapy. This technique allows the adolescent to apply the cognitive learning process to everyday experience and, at the same time, to experience self-esteem and support through success and praise from peers. This exercise becomes a true cotherapy experience.

Inpatient care of teenagers is directed at several separate levels and implemented by different staff, as shown in Table 13.1. Hospital or facility policies and procedures usually dictate levels I to III whereas treatment plan/treatment team supervises levels IV and V.

Employing cognitive techniques becomes gradually more difficult as one moves from level V downward. Most well-trained therapy staff can easily become familiar with cognitive therapy, and most readily accept the specificity of tasks and concrete goals. However, most current patient management systems employ "police"-type attitudes and see

TABLE 13.1. Workers Involved in Various Levels of Care

Levels of care	Workers
I. Basic services—food, shelter	Hospital departments and child-care workers
II. Safe environment through supervision	Nursing and child-care workers
III. School, activities—creation of typical adolescent experience	Teachers, activity therapists
IV. Programmatic therapy groups and interventions	Nursing, social work, child-care workers, other master's-level therapists
V. Individual, family, medication	Psychiatry, psychology, social work, nursing staff

their role as doing something *to* a patient. It takes time and practice to substitute more cognitive interventions, and some nursing and child-care staff initially experience feelings of loss of authority. Only later do some staff enjoy the sense of being "more therapeutic."

In bringing cognitive strategies into the inpatient program, some of the most important changes include helping staff view their interventions as a "cotherapy" experience with the patient—to use essays, contracts, and petitions to deal with behavior problems. It is also useful to have staff feel comfortable "going public" with their own problem-solving skills—serving as a model for teenagers to develop systems for corrective internal self-statements. In employing this technique, the staff must become comfortable describing their own thought processes, including initial mistakes or poor ideas and then comfortable explaining how thinking about one's thoughts can lead to a solution.

Teachers can be particularly helpful by using planned essays, classroom teaching experiences, and even direct psychoeducational approaches to help implement cognitive strategies within the classroom. Some of the newest teaching techniques employ meta-cognitive strategies to teach students new internalized self-statements to augment problem solving—a direct analogue of cognitive therapy.

The written documentation of how the patient completed these assignments and tasks becomes an additional log of the patient's therapeutic process, opening opportunities for the individual therapist to explore these issues and for the patient to reconstruct events through different viewpoints based on staff feedback. The entire medical record can become a living, useful document, with the patient's own material playing an important role.

Although these issues may at first seem complex or difficult, programmatic use of cognitive therapy appears to work well with depressed teenagers. Its use should be expanded and eventually interwoven with the variety of other successful change techniques.

SELECTED READINGS

Baum JC, Clark HB, McCarthy W, Sandler J, Carpenter R: An analysis of the requisition and generalization of social skills in troubled youths: Combining social skills training, cognitive self talk, and relaxation procedures. *Child and Family Behavior Therapy* 1986; 8:1–27.

Feindler EL: *Training Childcare Workers in Anger Reduction Methods to Reduce Aggressive Incidents in Delinquents.* New York, Association for Advancement of Behavior Therapy, 1980.

Feindler EL: *Adolescent Anger Control: Cognitive Behavioral Techniques.* New York, Pergamon Press, 1986.

Hansen D, St. Lawrence JS, Christoff KA: Conversations skills of inpatient conduct disordered youths: Social validation of component behaviors and implications for skills training. *Behavior Modification* 1988; 12:424–444.

Kendall PC, Braswell L: *Cognitive-Behavioral Therapy for Impulsive Children,* second edition. New York, Guilford Press, 1993.

Kettlewell PW, Kausch DF: The generalization of the efforts of a cognitive behavioral treatment program for aggressive children. *Journal of Abnormal Child Psychology* 1983; 11:101–114.

Lochman JE, Lampron LB: Cognitive behavior interventions for aggressive boys: 7-month followup effects. *Journal of Child and Adolescent Psychology* 1988; 5:15–23.

Meichenbaum D: *Cognitive Behavior Modification.* New York, Plenum Press, 1977.

CHAPTER FOURTEEN

General Management and Psychopharmacological Treatment of Depression in Adolescents

GRAHAM J. EMSLIE
A. JOHN RUSH
WARREN A. WEINBERG

INTRODUCTION

This chapter briefly reviews the general management of depression in adolescents, psychopharmacological treatment alone and in combination with cognitive therapy, and special considerations in treating the depressed, learning-disabled, adolescent. Because cognitive therapy often is not or cannot be used alone to treat a youngster with depression, it is important for the therapist to understand other treatment options and the patient's potential therapeutic needs.

NONMEDICATION MANAGEMENT

Depression in adolescents is best understood and managed using a biopsychosocial model (Engel, 1977). A multimodal approach to therapy (Petti, 1978; Weinberg and Emslie, 1988), including the concomitant management of the adolescent, the environment (home and school), and the patient's biological imbalance, is recommended. The adolescent, parents, and others in the environment need to work together in treatment. Table 14.1 summarizes a general approach to treatment manage-

TABLE 14.1. General Approach to Treatment Management

1. Remove inappropriate stressors: Bypass strategies; demands and tasks in keeping with the adolescent's facilities.
2. Inform: Emphasis on genetics, biology, and maturation with potential cycles.
3. Educate: Emphasize what is known and not known; avoid rationalization and misinformation.
4. Support: Be a positive advocate.
5. Reassure: A treatable and self-limiting condition with anticipation of long periods of wellness.
6. Assist with order and planning: Toward school, work, play, and pursuit of assets and talents.
7. Assist with decision making: "Continue usual pursuits"/"do not drop out."
8. Cognitive coaching on a "mini" daily basis: "Learn to think positive—act positive; come to know that actions should dictate feelings; intelligence should overrule emotions."

ment. The emphasis is on cognitive training on a "mini" daily basis with support, reassurance, continued and reiterative education about depression, and assistance in planning school, work, and play. Cognitive training in this context is the understanding that actions must dictate feelings: "It is not how you feel but how you act." Intelligence must overrule emotions. Continuation of usual pursuits and avoidance of "dropping out" are mandatory during depressed cycles. Rationalization and misinformation from the patient, parents, or teachers are discouraged; and all parties are educated about what is known and not known about the causes of depression. Daily attendance at school, pursuit of extrascholastic activities, and comforting, nonconfronting, but well-disciplined home, school, and play environments are expected. Specific instructions are offered, and implementation is continuously encouraged. The preliminary aim of treatment is to shorten the period of depression and to decrease the negative consequences of a depressive episode.

It is common during an episode of depression that the family, adolescent, or school will seek to understand the behavior in the form of some external cause; for example, the school blames the parents or adolescents, or the parents or adolescents blame the school. Such attribution occurs more frequently when the depressed adolescent expresses the depression more in one environment than in another. For example, if the adolescent is more depressed in school, the parents will change schools, blaming the school environment for the patient's problems. For these reasons, depressed adolescents and their families are encouraged not to make major life changes during a depressive episode. More rational decisions can be made when the depression has remitted.

The behavioral management of a depressed adolescent can pose a particular challenge to parents. The common consequences of progressive "groundings," with some adolescents being grounded for months, does nothing to help the situation and worsens the depressed adolescent's social withdrawal and loss of interest. However, not setting any limits is equally destructive. A more reasonable approach is to make consequences for actions time-limited but consistent, with the family taking one day at a time. This approach, combined with the adolescent's continued involvement in positive activities, can be helpful. It is also important for the adolescent and the family to realize that little is achieved in terms of compromise once a negative situation has developed. Time is needed to cool off before attempts are made to address specific problems. It is common to see depressed adolescents and their families engaged in prolonged arguing and nagging, which activities are highly unproductive on both sides.

In adolescence, substance abuse is commonly a presenting symptom of depression and may be a primary disorder. In this situation, treatment of the substance abuse is initially the primary concern: the adolescent must be free of substances for the therapist to determine whether the depression requires treatment. This necessity, however, does not mean that all adolescents using drugs require specialized inpatient drug treatment. The drug problem and its treatment need to be appropriately assessed and resolved.

Thirty to fifty percent of depressed adolescents will have a parent who is affectively ill at the time of the initial visit or during the treatment period. The parent's problem will require concomitant recognition and treatment. Beardslee and Podorefsky (1988) have identified several factors they feel help adolescents remain resilient to their parents' affective disorders, independent of whether they themselves have depression. These include self-understanding, a problem-solving orientation, the availability of additional supportive figures, and the ability to separate their own feelings from those of their depressed parents and not feel responsible for them. The majority of depressed children and adolescents can be successfully treated as outpatients. Short-term hospitalization (3–8 weeks) is required for those who are acutely suicidal, homicidal, out of control, abusing drugs, or for whom the home is either in need of respite from the patient or too unstable to offer appropriate care.

In addition to the management principles discussed above, several studies have suggested that cognitive or cognitive-behavioral therapy may be specifically helpful in the treatment of depression (Wilkes and Rush, 1988). These treatment approaches stem largely from two major theoretical perspectives. The first, proposed and studied by Beck (1967,

1976) and colleagues, is that faulty beliefs and cognitions (cognitive errors) are associated with the depressive syndrome. The second is that of attributional style (Abramson et al., 1978) or learned helplessness, whereby a depressed individual believes that negative events are internally mediated (internal), long-lasting (stable), and applicable to broad-based situations (global). These theories have been supported by empirical research in adults (Coyne and Gotlib, 1983) and children (Lewinsohn et al., 1981; Asarnow and Bates, 1988; McCauley et al., 1988). In a recent, well-designed study, Tems (1989) found that inpatient children and adolescents meeting DSM-III criteria for major depressive disorder evidenced more self-reported depressive symptoms, more cognitive errors, and lower self-esteem than nondepressed psychiatric inpatients. When compared to nondepressed control subjects, they differed on the above variables and also had a more internal–stable–global attributional style. Over the course of treatment, the patients' depressive symptoms, cognitive errors, low self-esteem, and attributional style improved, suggesting that these symptoms are "state dependent." As yet, no controlled studies of cognitive-behavioral therapy in this age group have been done. However, this approach is an exciting development in child and adolescent clinical psychology and psychiatry.

MEDICATION MANAGEMENT

Some general issues regarding the medication management of depressed adolescents are as follows:

1. Medical evaluation
2. Developmental issues in diagnosis
3. Normal versus pathological processes
4. Ethical issues
5. Psychological meaning of medication
6. Systemic rating (subjective, objective)
7. Risk–benefit ratio

Clearly important initially is a comprehensive diagnostic and medical evaluation, as delineated in Chapter 3, to rule out medical problems, assess developmental issues, and determine whether the adolescent suffers from a diagnosed disorder. The ethical issues in treating adolescents primarily center around who is the patient. If a school insists that an adolescent is disruptive and needs medication or the parents say the child is depressed and needs medication, but in both situations the adolescent disagrees, the therapist must ask whether the adolescent should be treated. Although there are no definitive answers, such questions should always be asked, particularly in the context of understanding what treatment is appropriate given the patient's developmental phase. It is probably also not appropriate that an immature 13-year-old make the treatment decision autonomously. Generally, the therapist is able to get consent from the parents and assent from the adolescent. Even the more resistant adolescent will often agree to a "trial" of treatment.

The psychological meaning of medication may be influenced by whether the adolescent's primary mode of coping is one of external or internal locus of control (Petti and Law, 1982). Adolescents with a more internal locus of control will have more trouble accepting an outside source or possible solution to their problems. Young adolescents also may retain some of the child's magical thinking about medication. Placebo response rates appear to be higher in children and adolescents, a fact that should be remembered when the therapist sees an excellent response to treatment.

Finally, it is important to assess change systematically, using self- and observer reports of symptoms. Some symptoms can improve while others worsen; without a systematic review, these variations will be missed. The risk–benefit ratio is always assessed.

ANTIDEPRESSANT MEDICATION

The efficacy of tricyclic antidepressants (TCAs) for major depressive disorder in adults is well established. Currently, only four placebo-controlled studies of TCAs in children (Kashani et al., 1984; Puig-Antich et al., 1987; Preskorn et al., 1987; Geller et al., 1989) have been undertaken. These used amitriptyline (Kashani, et al., 1984), imipramine (Puig-Antich et al., 1987; Preskorn et al., 1987), and nortriptyline (Geller et al., 1989). Only Preskorn's study with imipramine showed a difference between depressed children and controls. It has been suggested that a more serotonergic antidepressant may be more effective (Geller et al., 1989). Nortriptyline has been extensively studied in children and adolescents with regard to its pharmacokinetics, steady-state plasma levels, safety, and efficacy (Geller et al., 1984, 1985a, 1985b). Data on the use of TCAs in adolescents are even more meager. Kramer and Feiguire (1981) studied 20 adolescent inpatients in a randomly assigned, placebo-controlled, double-blind study of 200 mg of amitriptyline per day. The investigators found no difference between active medication and placebo, with significant improvement occurring in both groups (80% and 70%, respectively). In an open protocol assessing plasma level and response to imipramine in 34 outpatient adolescents, 44% were clinical responders (Ryan et al., 1986). Ryan (1988) has also reported on the efficacy of monoamine oxidase inhibitors (MAOIs) in TCA treatment nonresponders. He reported that 74% achieved a good or fair response, although concerns were raised about adolescents' following the dietary restrictions mandated by MAOI therapy. A recent open study (Ambrosini, 1989) suggested that adolescents may take longer to respond to pharmacotherapy than the usual 6 weeks.

In summary, no controlled experimental evidence is yet available to show that any pharmacological treatment is effective for treating major depressive disorder in adolescents. However, in general, controlled treatment studies in this age group, be they pharmacological or psychosocial, are limited. Given this limited information, the combination of cognitive therapy and medication in treating depressed adolescents should be approached with caution but may be a reasonable option in some cases.

COMBINING COGNITIVE THERAPY AND PHARMACOTHERAPY IN DEPRESSION

The overall objectives of both pharmacotherapy and short-term psychotherapies are to reduce or remove symptoms of depression, prevent relapse, prevent recurrence, and/or reduce the secondary consequences of the disorder. In addition, psychotherapy may be useful in achieving medication adherence. When to combine psychotherapy and pharmacotherapy is unclear—especially in child or adolescent depressives given the dearth of available data. For which patients or for which disorders are both treatments indicated? Does each treatment accomplish a different goal? Do these two treatments produce an effect that is greater than either alone? Are certain types of psychotherapy compatible with pharmacotherapy while others are not? Is the course of the mood disorder relevant to predicting whether psychotherapy, pharmacotherapy, or the combination is the optimal treatment(s)? These questions remain untested in controlled clinical research.

The effects of pharmacotherapy depend on a variety of factors, including the chemical effects of the agent, the dose, the length of time the drug is prescribed, patient adherence to the regime, and the disorder under treatment. Similarly, if "psychotherapy" has specific therapeutic effects, it would be logical to expect these effects also to depend on the specific psychological effects of the treatment, the length (i.e., frequency of sessions) of the treatment, the patient's participation in therapy, and the disorder being treated. Only recently have the these speculations been empirically tested.

Cognitive therapy has been most thoroughly assessed in nonpsychotic, nonbipolar depressed adult outpatients. Data from a recent review of randomized controlled trials of cognitive, behavioral, and other psychotherapies (Jarrett, 1990) indicate that (1) cognitive therapy exceeded the efficacy of wait-list control conditions, (2) cognitive therapy largely equaled the efficacy of the psychotherapy contrast condition, and (3) cognitive therapy largely equaled the efficacy of the medication contrast.

The question of when and whether to combine antidepressant medication with psychotherapy remains unanswered, although three reports have evaluated such a combination. Rush and Watkins (1981), in a small study, found no difference between individual cognitive therapy alone and the combination of cognitive therapy plus antidepressant medications in outpatients. However, the limited sample size may have precluded detection of significant differences. Beck and colleagues (1985) found that the addition of amitriptyline to cognitive therapy did not increase its efficacy. Other evidence (Blackburn et al., 1981) indicates that, with depressed outpatients treated in general practice, cognitive therapy alone is equivalent to the combination treatment; with psychiatric clinic outpatients, however, the combination treatment exceeded cognitive therapy alone. This study suggests that patient source may influence the probability of response to combination treatment. Murphy and colleagues (1984) did not find the combination treatment to exceed the effects obtained with either cognitive therapy alone or with medication alone in depressed patients. Apparently some, but clearly not all, patients were uniquely benefited by the combination treatment. Other patients, however, may benefit from cognitive therapy without medication.

All of these data relate to adult patients. Given the dearth of findings regarding the use of both medication and cognitive therapy in adolescents, the combination may be tried as a relatively "last resort" option. However, the patient should be monitored carefully because of the untested status of the treatment.

MANAGEMENT OF THE DEPRESSED AND LEARNING-DISABLED CHILD

The management of the depressed and learning-disabled child is a particular challenge. The brain has a great capacity to remove itself from unhealthy environments if allowed to do so. It stands to reason that children and adolescents with depression and specific learning disabilities will require appropriate management of their learning disability in order to remove inappropriate stress that might be inducing or worsening the depression (Weinberg and Emslie, 1988; Brumback and Weinberg, 1990).

Education about learning disabilities for both the children and their parents is an important intervention in the management of depression in children. Symbolic, verbal, and nonverbal communication skills are presented as genetically determined higher cortical functions that probably have their own rate of development (Weinberg et al., 1971; Weinberg and McLean, 1986; Weinberg and Emslie, 1988). Families are advised that the development of these skills may not depend on drill, reiteration, or excessive "time on task" but will develop with aging and rather informal exposure.

Bypass/compensatory strategies for the youngster are strongly recommended to avoid inappropriate stress and to maximize the possibility of success in school (Silberberg et al., 1973; Silberberg and Silberberg, 1969a, 1969b; Mosby, 1979; Weinberg, 1975; Weinberg and McLean 1986; Weinberg et al., 1988, 1989a, 1989b, 1989c). Adolescents, in comparison to prepubertal children, have some insight into their deficits and will begin to implement (and request) bypass strategies on their own volition. For those children and adolescents with alphabetic language problems (reading, spelling, and writing), input can be of the multimedia (lectures, tapes, and "talking books") variety. The youngsters can limit their reading to abstracts, synopses, well-prepared teacher handouts, and "fact sheets" and make sure they know what they must learn prior to listening and/or reading. Such children should not be penalized for poor spelling, and spelling tests should be by multiple-choice technique. Writing in the form of assisted outlines using memo style and assessment for content rather than quantity, syntax, or grammar are encouraged. Some children can learn to dictate, type, or use a word processor. A "poor speller" dictionary is also helpful. If the child is defective in numeric language, he can use a calculator and "mini" computer and be tested in multiple-choice format. Multiple-choice untimed tests, either written or oral, that avoid "recall" and "naming" are advised for those having difficulty with nominal recall, specific word finding, and word-to-word definitions.

Assistance with order and planning, the one-task-at-a-time approach, pictorial systems for self-reminding, and reminders offered by others in a positive and supportive manner are helpful. Avoiding overload is important to prevent willful neglect and excessive anxiety, with resultant worsening in immediate recall and less output of known material.

Cognitive approaches, such as identifying irrational thoughts, correcting cognitive errors, and offering support, should be used daily by parents and teachers. The emphasis is on awareness, self-control, and planned methods for expression when the child is "frustrated" in the group setting of school. Extrascholastic activities that use the child's assets, talents, and creativities should be encouraged; deprivation of such activities should not be used to punish the youngster for a "failed" test or course.

CONCLUSION

Developing a specific plan of treatment for an adolescent with depression requires a multidimensional assessment and usually a multidimensional intervention. Areas to be covered include the individual adolescent's strengths and weaknesses, family and social environment, and school functioning. It is not uncommon for the treatment needs in one area to conflict with those in another or for different environments to have different goals. For example, an adolescent may need to function more autonomously and take more individual responsibility; yet, the depressive illness may require the adolescent to be more dependent on the family.

Research in psychopharmacological treatment of depression in this age group lags far behind clinical practice. It is important to remember that, of more than 200 studies in adults, one-fifth had negative results. Whether adolescent depression is more resistant to psychopharmacological treatment than adult depression is still to be determined. Depression in adolescents remains a disorder with attendant morbidity and mortality that is in need of extensive further research.

SELECTED READINGS

Abramson LY, Seligman MEP, Teasdale JD: Learned helplessness in humans: Critique and reformulation. *Journal of Abnormal Psychology* 1978; 87:49–74.
Ambrosini P: *Open Nortriptyline Treatment over 10 Weeks in Depressed Adolescent Outpatients.* Paper presented at the Annual Meeting of American Academy of Child and Adolescent Psychiatry, 1989
Asarnow JR, Bates S: Depression in child psychiatric inpatients: Cognitive and

attributional patterns. *Journal of Abnormal Child Psychology* 1988; 16:601–615.

Beardslee WR, Podorefsky D: Resilient adolescents whose parents have serious affective and other psychiatric disorders: Importance of self-understanding and relationships. *American Journal of Psychiatry 1988*; 145:63–69.

Beck AT: *Depression: Causes and Treatment.* Philadelphia, University of Pennsylvania Press, 1967.

Beck AT: *Cognitive Therapy and the Emotional Disorders.* New York, International Universities Press, 1976.

Beck AT, Hollon DS, Young JE, Bedrosian RC, Budnez D: Treatment of depression with cognitive therapy and amitriptyline. *Archives of General Psychiatry* 1985; 42:142–148.

Blackburn IM, Bishop S, Glen AM, Whalley LJ, Christie JE: The efficacy of cognitive therapy in depression: A treatment trial using cognitive therapy and pharmacotherapy, each alone and in combination. *British Journal of Psychiatry* 1981; 139:181–189.

Brumback RA, Weinberg WA: Pediatric behavioral neurology: An update on the neurological aspects of depression, hyperactivity, and learning disabilities. *Neurology Clinics* 1990; 8:677–703.

Coyne JC, Gotlib IH: The role of cognition in depression: A critical appraisal. *Psychology Bulletin* 1983; 94:472–505.

Engel GL: The need for a new medical model: A challenge for biomedicine. *Science* 1977; 196:129–136.

Geller B, Cooper TB, Chestnut E, Abel AS, Anker JA: Nortriptyline pharmacokinetic parameters in depressed children and adolescents: Preliminary data. *Journal of Clinical Psychopharmacology* 1984; 4:265–269.

Geller B, Cooper TB, Chestnut EC, Anker JA, Price DT, Yates E: Child and adolescent nortriptyline single dose kinetics predict steady state plasma levels and suggested dose: preliminary data. *Journal of Clinical Psychopharmacology* 1985a; 5:154–158.

Geller B, Cooper TB, McCombs HG, Graham D, Wells J: Double-blind placebo-controlled study of nortriptyline in depressed children using a "fixed plasma level" design. *Psychopharmacology Bulletin* 1989; 25:101–108.

Geller B, Farooki ZQ, Cooper TB, Chestnut EC, Abel AS: Serial ECG to measurements at controlled plasma levels of nortriptyline in depressed children. *American Journal of Psychiatry* 1985b; 142:1095–1097.

Jarrett RB: Psychosocial aspects of depression and the role of psychotherapy. *Journal of Clinical Psychiatry* 1990; 51(Suppl. 6):26–35.

Kashani J, Shekin WO, Reid JC: Amitriptyline in children with major depressive disorder: A double-blind crossover pilot study. *Journal of the American Academy of Child Psychiatry* 1984; 23:348–351.

Kramer AD, Feiguire BA: Clinical effects of amitriptyline in adolescent depression. *Journal of the American Academy of Child Psychiatry* 1981; 20:636–644.

Lewinsohn PM, Steinmetz JL, Larson DW, Franklin J: Depression-related cognitions: Antecedent or consequence? *Journal of Abnormal Psychology* 1981; 90:213–219.

McCauley E, Mitchell JR, Burke P, Moss S: Cognitive attributes of depression in children and adolescents. *Journal of Consulting and Clinical Psychology* 1988; 56:903–908.

Mosby RJ: A bypass program of supportive instruction for secondary students with learning disabilities. *Journal of Learning Disabilities* 1979; 12:187–190.

Murphy GE, Simons AD, Wetzel RD, Lustman PJ: Cognitive therapy and pharmacotherapy. *Archives of General Psychiatry* 1984; 41:33–41.

Petti TA: Depression in hospitalized child psychiatry patients: Approaches to measuring depression. *Journal of the American Academy of Child Psychiatry* 1978; 17:49–59.

Petti TA, Law W: Imipramine treatment of depressed children: A double-blind pilot study. *Journal of Clinical Psychopharmacology* 1982; 2:107–110.

Puig-Antich J, Perel JM, Lupatkin W, Chambers WJ, Tabrizi MA, King J, Goetz R, Davies M, Stiller RL: Imipramine in prepubertal major deprssive disorders. *Archives of General Psychiatry* 1987; 44:81–89.

Preskorn SH, Weller EB, Hughes CW, Weller RA, Bolte K: Depression in prepubertal children: Dexamethasone nonsuppression predicts differential response to imipramine vs. placebo. *Psychopharmacology Bulletin* 1987; 23:128–133.

Rush AJ, Watkins JT: Group versus individual cognitive therapy: A pilot study. *Cognitive Therapy and Research* 1981; 5:95–103.

Ryan ND, Puig-Antich J, Cooper T, Rabinorich H, Ambrosini P, Davies M, King J, Torres D, Fried J: Imipramine in adolescent major depression: Plasma level and clinical response. *Acta Psychiatrica Scandinavica* 1986; 73:275–288.

Ryan ND, Puig-Antich J, Rabinovich H, Fried J, Ambrosini P, Meyer V, Torres D, Dachille S, Mazzie D: MAO's in adolescent major depression unresponsive to tricyclic antidepressants. *Journal of the American Academy of Child and Adolescent Psychiatry* 1988; 27:755–758.

Silberberg NE, Iversen IA, Goins JT: Which remedial method works best? *Journal of Learning Disabilities* 1973; 6:547–556.

Silberberg NE, Silberberg MC. Myths in remedial education. *Journal of Learning Disabilities* 1969a; 2:34–42.

Silberberg NE, Silberberg MC: The bookless curriculum: An education alternative. *Journal of Learning Disabilities* 1969b; 2:302–307.

Tems CLC: *Cognitive Patterns in Depressed and Nondepressed Children and Adolescents.* Doctoral dissertation, University of Texas Southwestern Medical Center at Dallas, 1989.

Weinberg WA: Delayed symbol language skills and their relationship to school performance: diagnosis and management, in *The Practice of Pediatric Neurology.* Edited by Swaiman KF, Wright FS. St. Louis, Mosby, 1975.

Weinberg WA, Emslie GJ: Adolescents and school problems: Depression, suicide and learning disorders. *Advances in Adolescent Mental Health* 1988; 3:181–205.

Weinberg WA, McLean A: A diagnostic approach to developmental specific learning disorders. *Journal of Child Neurology* 1986; 1:158–172.

Weinberg WA, McLean A, Brumback RA: Comparison of reading and listening techniques for administration of PIAT reading comprehension subtest: Justification for the bypass approach. *Perceptual and Motor Skills* 1988; 66:672–674.

Weinberg WA, McLean A, Snider RL, Nuckols AS, Rintelmann JW, Erwin PR, Brumback RA: Depression, learning, disability, and school behavior problems. *Psychological Reports* 1989a; 64:275–283.

Weinberg WA, McLean A, Snider RL, Rintelmann JW, Brumback RA: Comparison of nominal recall (standard) and multiple-choice methods for administration of WISC-R information subtest: A preliminary study indicating a learning effect of multiple choice testing. *Psychological Reports* 1989b; 64:659–665.

Weinberg WA, McLean A, Snider RL, Rintelmann JW, Brumback RA: Comparison of reading and listening–reading techniques for administration of SAT reading comprehension subtest: Justification for the bypass approach. *Perceptual and Motor Skills* 1989c; 68:1015–1018.

Weinberg WA, Penick E, Hammerman M, Jackoway M: An evaluation of a summer reading program: A preliminary report on the development of reading. *American Journal of Diseases of Children* 1971; 122:494–498.

Wilkes TCR, Rush AJ: Adaptations of cognitive therapy for depressed adolescents. Journal of the American Academy of Child and Adolescent Psychiatry 1988; 27:381–386.

PART VI

Further Considerations

CHAPTER FIFTEEN

Treatment Failures, Obstacles, and Options

T. C. R. WILKES

A. JOHN RUSH

GAYLE BELSHER

INTRODUCTION

In the first section of this chapter, we examine some reasons for apparent therapy failures. The second section of the chapter uses a question-and-answer format to review many of the obstacles therapists face in attempting to conduct cognitive therapy with depressed adolescents. Finally, the third section highlights the 10 recommendations most frequently given to novice cognitive therapists. Our goal in listing recommendations is to provide a "checklist" of things to consider when one is evaluating the effectiveness of cognitive therapy with depressed adolescents.

CAUSES OF FAILURE WITH COGNITIVE THERAPY

Treatment failures are perhaps the most instructive of all experiences for psychotherapists. Some types of depression or some adolescents may be unresponsive to psychotherapy. Thus, the lessons gleaned from each failure have implications for improved patient selection, refinement and innovation of psychotherapeutic techniques, differential diagnosis of the disorders themselves, improved strategies for enhancing compliance with homework, improved strategies to deal with countertherapeutic forces in the social system, and the identification of patients who may have only short-term as opposed to long-term gains. Treatment failures may be attributed to a variety of factors, each of which is discussed below.

Lack of Patient Motivation

Perhaps the rationale most commonly offered for treatment failures is that the patient was not motivated. However, this "explanation" is both logically untenable and obfuscating. By definition, the syndrome of depression involves a reduction in energy and motivation. Thus, all depressed patients are less motivated than nondepressed patients to undertake most activities, including psychotherapy. Depressed cognitive therapy patients, all of whom are somewhat unmotivated, are required both to attend the sessions and to complete various homework assignments in order to obtain a therapeutic effect. Although "lack of motivation" may be used in an attempt to explain therapy failures, the therapist must realize that those patients who do respond were also "unmotivated" at the outset of therapy. Thus, lack of motivation is associated with both successes and failures in therapy and, therefore, explains little.

Engagement Problems

Some patients are more difficult to engage in the treatment process than others. We believe this initial difficulty stems from two major sources: the patient's negative anticipations, and difficulty with trust. Each of these issues should be reframed in cognitive terms and addressed early in treatment.

Negative Anticipations

Cognitive therapy for adolescent depression is one of many potential treatment modalities. Indeed, many adolescents become involved in school counseling on an ad hoc basis. Others may be receiving individual or family counseling through a host of private practitioners. Often hospital-based programs or mental health clinics are not consulted until other psychosocial interventions have been unsuccessful. Thus, cognitive therapists sometimes feel that treatment failures are related to the negative anticipations of adolescents that have arisen because of previous, failed attempts at intervention. However, negative expectations can be elicited by the therapist and corrected with information, logical discussion, and experimental tasks. Furthermore, unlike previous caregivers, cognitive therapists who are part of a large mental health team or an established institution may benefit from the "edifice complex" fostered by the treatment setting. In other words, the hospital or clinic itself may help to promote high expectations for a positive treatment outcome, thus compensating a little for the therapist's disadvantaged position of being "yet another" person consulted about the adolescent's problems.

Lack of Trust

Trust issues may be indicated by beliefs such as "If I really tell you [the therapist] how I think, you won't like me." Expectations of rejection or failure often underlie reluctance to engage fully in treatment. Patients who lack trust will often begin to work in therapy but later reduce adherence and voice hopeless or helpless ideas. Sometimes these patients denigrate the therapist or the therapy process itself. Adolescents are more likely than adults to exhibit this kind of behavior because it protects them from developing an emotional, personal relationship with the therapist and, consequently, helps them to avoid the anticipated disappointment of therapy termination. These fears should be identified, framed into "if–then" statements (e.g., "If I put my hopes into this treatment or therapist and don't get better, then I'll be shattered, or it means I'm incurable"), and discussed logically.

The more severe the depression, the more likely are problems regarding trust and negative anticipation. As such, the engagement of severely depressed patients is both critical and difficult. However, the therapist can usually engage such patients by identifying behavioral patterns that appear to represent these maladaptive assumptions, raising the assumptions in the form of questions early in treatment, and addressing them repeatedly throughout treatment.

Adversarial Social System

Forces within the patient's family or social system may also pose problems for the efficacy of therapy. Significant others may unwittingly conceptualize the depressed patient as a helpless, negative, hostile person from whom nothing better can be anticipated, particularly if the depression has been present for a long period of time or if the patient has chronic interpersonal difficulties independent of the depression. Thus, positive behavioral or attitudinal changes made by the patient may inadvertently be minimized because of the rigid views of the patient held by significant others. And since many depressed patients will overvalue the opinions and views of others, the efficacy of therapy may be even further challenged. Potentially countertherapeutic social forces exist for all adolescents, so it is imperative that family members be engaged in the adolescent's therapy. When family members themselves have lost hope of seeing meaningful change in the adolescent, behaviors or attitudes generated by the depression may be erroneously attributed to the adolescent's character. Specific techniques for addressing these issues are discussed in Chapter 6 and throughout the chapters in Part III.

Inadequate Initial Assessment of Biopsychosocial Factors

If the cognitive therapist has not seen some improvement in the adolescent's depressive symptomatology after about six sessions, reassessment may be required. The adolescent may be struggling with significant comorbidity, such as an early schizophrenic process, attention-deficit hyperactivity disorder, posttraumatic stress disorder, substance abuse, an eating disorder, or a major personality disturbance. Additionally, the family situation may be so unhealthy for the adolescent, because of neglect or abuse, that relocating to foster care or a child-welfare residence is the only alternative. The therapist must be able to identify three separate but interwoven threads in the matrix of the adolescent's phenomenology: (1) signs and symptoms associated with the primary diagnosis or associated comorbid diagnoses; (2) the contribution of the adolescent's temperament or personality to the current phenomenological picture; and (3) the process of adolescence itself, which can give rise to dysphoria, anxiety, and difficulties coping with authority figures or self-regulation of impulses. Consistent with the biopsychosocial model of mental illness, the primary diagnosis, temperament or personality, and phase of adolescence all interact to give rise to the composite clinical picture. Failure to progress in cognitive therapy may be a result of underestimating the relative contribution of the different factors involved.

Poor "Fit" of the Adolescent and Therapy

If no obvious reason for treatment failure is evident after further reassessment, the therapist must consider the goodness of "fit" between the adolescent and therapy before deciding that treatment should be abandoned. Treatment failures can develop because the therapist and patient have not matched psychological deficits or needs with specific interventions. At first, it is wise to remember the theoretical basis of cognitive therapy. The traditional view is that faulty beliefs, a biased attributional style, or cognitive errors are associated with the depressive syndrome. Furthermore, cognitive theory of depression emphasizes the role of impaired self-monitoring, impaired self-evaluation, and impaired self-reinforcement. Impaired self-monitoring refers to the proclivity of depressed individuals to focus on negative events, selecting only data that are consistent with their negative schemas. Such individuals often focus on immediate rather than delayed gratification. Impaired self-evaluation refers to the stringent and often highly unrealistic standards that depressed individuals impose on themselves. Finally, impaired self-reinforcement refers to insufficient engagement in pleasant, rewarding activities and a tendency to elevate the rate of self-punishment. When progress in therapy is elusive, the therapist should consider these factors and attempt to identify those most suitable for intervention (see Kendall and Hollon, 1981).

Consider the following two patients who demonstrate the importance of choosing the appropriate type of intervention. The first case involves a depressed adolescent with the associated problems of attention-deficit hyperactivity disorder, learning disorders, and oppositional defiant disorder. The therapist will need to focus on techniques for solving problems, monitoring negative consequences of behavior, delaying gratification, and engaging in more reflective thought. The goal would be to help the adolescent set higher standards of personal conduct that are in keeping with social values. Here, emphasis is on the acquisition of social arbitrary knowledge (in contrast to physical and logical mathematical knowledge, the other traditional Piagetian division of knowledge), which includes values, ethics, observation of social rules, and affective regulation. In Piagetian theory, cognitive development places constraints on affect and judgment, so in order to facilitate better integration of the adolescent's cognitive domains of self, world, and future, his homework assignments would be arranged to provide opportunities to gain experience in appropriate social interactions.

By way of contrast, consider a second case that involves a depressed adolescent who pays excessive attention to negative events, holds very high expectations, and demonstrates little ability to play or to reward himself. Emphasis now would be less on the acquisition of social arbitrary knowledge and more on challenging the adolescent's logical mathematical knowledge and egocentrism. This therapeutic focus would facilitate transformation of the adolescent's idealistic perception of his world and self to a more logical and realistic view. Homework would again focus on social interactions but also on the identification of cognitive errors in order to help the adolescent acquire alternative views of his problems. The therapist would also emphasize achieving immediate rewards and altering the adolescent's depressogenic attributional style. This approach would be in direct contrast to that used with the former patient, with whom the therapist would work to establish a greater sense of personal responsibility and accountability.

Inadequate Therapeutic Alliance

A more fundamental problem when therapy seems to have failed may be the relationship between therapist and patient, or lack of a therapeutic alliance. Perhaps the adolescent and therapist have not found a common language or frame of reference. Perhaps the therapist is perceived as an agent of coercion employed by the adolescent's parents. It should be remembered that the use of narrative is important in establishing a therapeutic alliance. Psychoanalysis, hermeneutics, and family therapy have long used the personal narrative as a way of gaining access to an individual's inner world and its organizing properties. Cognitive therapy achieves this goal through its emphasis on constructivist structuralism, the view that knowledge is represented as internalized constructs, schemas, or models, which are refined by ongoing experiences, thus producing new models or schemas. This paradigm readily lends itself to examination of the individual's personal narrative. By asking an adolescent, "What is your story up to now?" the therapist creates a new opportunity for developing a therapeutic alliance. People change their stories according to their cognitive development and their social orientation. They may perceive themselves as "victims" at one stage in the narrative and as "survivors" at another. In other words, therapy with a depressed adolescent may be "stuck" because the therapist has failed to appreciate the adolescent's story. How does the adolescent see himself in his world? What is his story now? What stage has he reached in the story? What ending is he expecting? We know that a person's self-narrative gives a sense of continuity and purpose; however, there are often gaps that offer opportunities for therapeutic change (see Popper and Eccles, 1977).

Therapeutic relationships with adolescents need to be flexible, avoiding futile power struggles. The therapist must show a willingness to engage in play, humor, paradox, and irony. If an adolescent does not complete homework, it does not mean cognitive therapy stops. Rather, cognitive therapy should be viewed as an approach, an orientation, a therapeutic stance. It uses experience to foster cognitive restructuring in a depressed individual. The reader is reminded of Piaget's emphasis on the importance of experience, social interaction, maturation, and equilibrium (freedom from cognitive conflict) in cognitive development.

Lack of Intelligence

We do not feel that general intelligence is a critical factor in dictating the success or failure of therapy. However, impairments in memory or concentration may make treatment more demanding of some patients. The therapist would be advised to remember that some patients may present with depressions that are the consequence of underlying medical disorders, or medications.

QUESTIONS THERAPISTS ASK

During the course of learning cognitive therapy for the first time or learning to adapt the adult model for application with an adolescent population, therapists often ask important questions that can lead to greater theoretical understanding and better model adherence. The questions that appear below are those therapists have posed during their training in cognitive therapy for depressed adolescents. Questions and their answers have been grouped into one of four content categories: those that relate to the cognitive therapy model itself, those regarding application of the model with the adolescent's family, those reflecting problems that arise during implementation of the model, and those concerning case management more generally. Although a much lengthier response to each question could have been provided, we have opted for greater brevity in order to address as broad a range of queries as possible. Where appropriate, reference is made to specific chapters in this volume that contain relevant additional information or instruction.

Questions about the Cognitive Therapy Model

Q. Since I am already familiar with cognitive therapy for depressed adults, what major adjustments will be necessary for application with an adolescent population?

A. Because of adolescents' emotional dependency and the significance of attachment issues in this stage of development, it will be important to include the adolescent's family members in the therapy process. Since "adolescence" spans an age range of 7 years and represents the passage from childhood to adulthood, normative development and the stage of adolescence should be considered. The issues of younger adolescents usually will be different from the issues of older patients. Adolescents' characteristic egocentricity will be a significant factor influencing the nature of your therapeutic interactions. Awareness of the adolescent's cognitive development will be essential; in particular, you will want to guard against incorrectly assuming that the adolescent has developed formal thinking skills. Perhaps most importantly, progress in therapy will depend largely on your flexibility in every aspect of your work with the adolescent. Remember that a cooperative, hard-working patient one week can become a sullen, angry, or reluctant patient the next week. In general, you should be prepared to be more concrete and persistent and to use more exaggeration to communicate therapeutic messages. Chapter 2 includes several references to the difference between cognitive therapy with adults and adolescents. Also, the three chapters in Part II (Chapters 4–6) of the manual discuss the special issues that arise when cognitive therapy is undertaken with an adolescent population.

Q. How should I respond when adolescents or their parents seem to favor a biological explanation of the depression and postulate a "chemical imbalance" or "family heredity" as the primary causal factor?

A. Discuss the "biopsychosocial" perspective of emotional disorders, acknowledging brain chemistry and genetic predisposition as relevant biological factors. Then discuss the role of psychological factors in depression, explaining the relationship between cognitions and depression. Indicate that the therapy sessions you conduct with the adolescent will focus primarily on this "psychological" part of the larger model. Because the family has an important influence on the development of the adolescent's belief system and provides important social experiences for him, you should indicate that family members' participation in therapy will be required. It will be important to communicate that a strictly biological view of the depression may result in the adoption of a passive rather than an active role with respect to the disorder, a reluctant "acceptance" of problems rather than an aggressive "attack" on them. A more active stance acknowledges the significance of choice in the adolescent's life; for example, he might schedule pleasant activities even though he does not feel like it. In the presence of choice, feelings of helplessness and hopelessness fade. Hope, in turn, can have a profound effect on increasing tolerance of pain or decreasing anxiety about the emotional disorder.

Q. Referrals to therapy usually involve complaints about behaviors and requests to "fix" problems. How do I frame these concerns in a cognitive model?

A. Begin by eliciting the family's views about which problems are most likely to be related to the "normal" struggles of adolescence (e.g., separation–individuation) and which are probably a manifestation of the depression. The former can be addressed by exploring family beliefs and expectations about adolescence. Intervene to change maladaptive cognitions about this stage of development, and "normalize" the difficulties when appropriate. Problems that arise in the context of depression are the primary targets for intervention using cognitive therapy techniques. However, it will be important to remember that your role as a cognitive therapist is not to "fix" problems, because the adoption of such a role may encourage the perception that you are the "expert," precipitating a dependent or helpless stance on the part of the adolescent and his family. Rather, it would be more appropriate to emphasize that your role is to help the family develop its own skills for problem resolution by teaching its members how to examine the relationship between the problems they present and the cognitions normally associated with depression. When the adolescent does make positive behavioral changes, draw the family's attention to the choice the adolescent has made, exploring the relationship between the adolescent's choices and his views about himself, his circumstances, and his future. Remember that problem-solving in the absence of interventions to address maladaptive cognitions will be appropriate in relatively few situations (refer to the introductory discussion in Chapter 8).

Q. How do I engage in "short-term" cognitive therapy involving a contracted number of sessions without feeling pressure to be overly directive, thereby threatening collaboration?

A. The anxiety associated with a limited-term psychotherapy contract can be a positive stimulus for both you and the adolescent, helping to focus your attention on amelioration of the depressive symptoms and resolution of the functional problems. As a cognitive therapist, you will provide explicit direction only about how to approach problems (the cognitive therapy model), not about what should be done to solve them. Since families will have been socialized into the cognitive therapy model during the initial phase of therapy (refer to Chapter 7), you need not feel apologetic about being directive in this regard.

Q. How do I focus on the "present" and address issues in the "here and now" when current problems seem to have historical antecedents, suggesting that the adolescent's past life and experiences need to be explored?

A. Your desires both to focus on current problems and to explore the adolescent's past experiences are neither mutually exclusive nor unrelated. In fact, you would be advised to explore the way in which past life experiences have helped to shape the adolescent's belief system because certain of these beliefs may be contributing to current emotional distress. Exploring the role that past experience has played in the formation of beliefs can be a liberating experience for the adolescent and/or his family because they may come to realize for the first time that beliefs previously developed can now be reformulated. The fact that they have some choice in what to believe means that change is possible.

Q. How can patients with strong religious affiliations be expected to reconcile the cognitive therapy model with a religious model that may prescribe a rigid belief system, perhaps one that holds that members of the faith "must always" remain true to religious tenets?

A. If your adolescent patient or his family members indicate that they will not tolerate any examination of their religious beliefs, then it may be impossible to establish a therapeutic contract. Consideration of some other method of intervention may be necessary. If you do embark on a course of cognitive therapy, you should realize that this group of patients is at greater risk of attrition in the event that strongly held religious beliefs are identified as the ones most closely associated with the depression because evaluating or challenging these beliefs will be disallowed. However, as a cognitive therapist, you should remember that several beliefs may be contributing to the adolescent's depression, and many of these beliefs may bear no direct relationship to the family's religious faith. If this were the case, then these maladaptive cognitions would become the focus of cognitive therapy interventions.

Questions Regarding Cognitive Therapy in Family Sessions

Q. What would a cognitive therapist do in a family session that would be notably different from what a systemic family therapist would do?

A. Generally speaking, the cognitive therapist would provide a more detailed explanation of the theoretical model underlying therapy. A concerted effort to impart an understanding of the model to family members would be made so that they would be better able to collaborate with the therapist as "experts" on identifying relevant family beliefs. To the greatest extent possible, parents or other family members would be encouraged to become "cotherapists" in helping the adolescent to overcome his depression. The cognitive therapist usually would be less directive in "prescribing" homework; the adolescent and his family should be active participants in this endeavor after they have assisted in the identification of maladaptive cognitions. The cognitive therapist would not employ interventions that reframed a symptom as "helpful" to the family system. Neither would the cognitive therapist prescribe more of the symptom in the hope of activating the family's defenses against it. Although the cognitive therapist might employ various techniques with the intent of changing family members' beliefs or behaviors, the primary purpose of such interventions always would be relief of the adolescent's depression. At all times, the adolescent patient, rather than the family in general, would remain the focus of therapy. As a result, any problems in marital or family functioning would be explored only to the extent that they had relevance for the adolescent in question.

Q. How do I explain depression in cognitive terms to the family?

A. By using examples relevant to the adolescent's life, describe how your patient's views of himself, his "world," and his future are related to the depression. In so doing, include mention of both the emotional and the behavioral manifestations of the depression. Indicate that the adolescent's cognitions (or "ideas") in these three domains will be the focus of the therapy and that the family will be an invaluable asset in helping you to develop an accurate and comprehensive understanding of the adolescent's cognitive domains. In addition, indicate the role the family can play in helping the adolescent to develop more adaptive ways of thinking or behaving.

Q. How do I initiate a discussion about family beliefs in a family session?

A. Begin by eliciting family members' views on relevant issues. Engage parents in a discussion of their own adolescence and families of origin and explore with them how beliefs held by their parents were the same as or different from their own views of adolescence. Throughout such a discussion, your goal will be to show parents that just as their families influenced their experiences of adolescence, so their children (and the adolescent patient in question) are affected by the prevailing nuclear family beliefs. And just as they, as adults, may have chosen to adopt views different from those of their parents, so may their children choose to challenge the family's "party line." By introducing the concept of choice in what an individual believes, you will be introducing the possibility of change, which usually will be a harbinger of hope for both the adolescent and the parents.

Q. When and how often should I invite the family to therapy sessions?

A. The parents or guardians of the adolescent should always participate in the initial assessment. From that point forward, the extent of family involvement in the adolescent's therapy will depend to some extent on the contract established. In general, family members should be included in therapy sessions more often when the adolescent is younger because his cognitive skills will be more limited. Greater family involvement is also indicated when the adolescent has the comorbid diagnoses of attention-deficit hyperactivity disorder, learning disabilities, or a personality disorder. More specifically, you should schedule a family session whenever the adolescent raises significant issues that implicate other family members during individual sessions (e.g., a specific problem with one of his parents). Furthermore, you would be advised to plan a family session as a "reality check" any time the adolescent denies that there are issues that need to be addressed in therapy and whenever you wish to assess the extent to which gains in specific domains are generalizing to other situations. It will be especially important to include family members when you feel that therapeutic progress is insufficient because the family's participation may reveal additional factors that would help to explain the adolescent's continuing depression.

Q. What is the best response when only some of the family members come to family sessions even though all were asked to attend?

A. If only one session is unavoidably missed, the absent individual can be informed about the session as part of the review process that would occur at the beginning of the next family session. Alternatively, missing family members could be sent a letter summarizing the main points of the family session. If an individual's absence is consistent, you might phone that person, asking for his "help" in treating the adolescent by attending the next family session. Generally, the absence of a family member is most critical when it is one of the parents who consistently refuses to attend. A parental absence may indicate significant marital distress or the parent's own psychopathology, which, if persistent, usually will be negative indicators for the adolescent's progress in therapy. If you feel this is the case, you might attempt to meet with the marital dyad alone or discuss the importance of appropriate intervention with the parent who does attend the family sessions.

Q. How do I maintain a neutral stance to avoid alienating either the adolescent or his parents when they are presenting different stories about the problem or various individual's roles in it?

A. You should use the disagreement to your advantage by indicating "confusion" about the conflicting stories. Adopt the "Columbo" technique of innocently asking for further explanation to help you understand the different points of view. Clarify for the entire family that you want to understand the differences in opinions and that opinions are not facts. Unlike correct or incorrect facts, opinions are not "right" or "wrong." As opinions or beliefs about an issue are revealed, emphasize that your goal is to help the adolescent and his family evaluate which are more and less helpful. Thereafter, apply cognitive therapy techniques to evaluate and change beliefs, whenever appropriate. In exploring the controversial issue, convey a willingness to listen equally to each "side" by directing questions and apportioning time for explanations equally. You also will be able to indicate your neutrality as a therapist by stating overtly that your goal is to keep in mind the best interests of the adolescent patient. Sometimes his best interests will require that you make statements that either the adolescent or his parents would rather not hear. However, by indicating your concern for the adolescent as your primary motivation, both parties to the disagreement will be more likely to accept your views, whatever they are, as neutral ones.

Q. How should I interpret and react to the extreme emotional volatility that some adolescents display during family sessions?

A. Welcome the display of affect as an opportunity to learn more about the adolescent's cognitions. Acknowledge the affect openly and explore it. Label the adolescent's extreme emotionality to the family as an indication of the adolescent's strong beliefs about something important. By so doing, you will be challenging the perceptions of many parents that their adolescent is "out of control" or a "bad kid" in general. Parental views such as these will tend to diminish their feelings of competence and augment the family's general sense of hopelessness. By observing your response to the adolescent's emotional outburst, parents may learn how to "contain" the adolescent's emotion, "contain" their own emotional and behavioral reactions, avoid a judgmental stance, and seek an understanding of the cognitions that underlie the adolescent's emotion by probing it instead of rushing to calm or disallow it. In effect, the adolescent who displays extreme emotional volatility during a family session provides you with a prime opportunity to model an appropriate response for the family members. It will be important for you and the parents to consider the emotional outburst in the context of the adolescent's cognitive development. If an older adolescent displays behaviors more like those you would expect of a much younger child, it may be appropriate to respond as if he were much younger. For example, if a 17-year-old who was accustomed to using the family car began having temper tantrums that included destruction of property, then it would be appropriate to withdraw privileges (such as driving the car) that normally would be reserved for more age-appropriate responses to frustration or anger.

Q. When there appear to be marital or parenting issues, how can I address them with the adolescent present in the session?

A. Even if the adolescent does not know the details of disputes involving his parents, he will usually be aware that friction exists. Inquire about what the adolescent does know and about his interpretation of the situation. Remember that the adolescent is your patient, so you can think of discussions about marital or parenting issues as pursuits of issues that may affect his depression. In practice, more leverage usually is gained with parents if their problems are addressed indirectly, in the service of treating the adolescent, because they did not seek therapy for their own problems.

Q. When there are comorbid diagnoses such as attention-deficit hyperactivity disorder, learning disabilities, or schizoid personality disorder, how can I discuss the adolescent's limitations without giving him an excuse for continuing nonperformance or behavioral problems?

A. Adolescents will best be able to use cognitive or personality limitations as excuses only when parents are unsure about the implications of the comorbid diagnoses. Therefore, clarification of reasonable expectations in light of the comorbid diagnoses will allow parents to set standards and uphold expectations appropriately. Cognitive therapy will emphasize the choice that the adolescent has between giving in to his limitations or accepting some "ownership" and "responsibility" for them. If he chooses the former, then he must be prepared for the consequences. You should also remember that failure to discuss the adolescent's limitations with parents has at least two serious potential repercussions. First, parental expectations may be too high, predisposing the adolescent to failure and the parents themselves to grave disappointment. Second, the adolescent who wishes to meet his parents' expectations may become overwhelmed with anxiety or guilt about his abilities to achieve or perform.

Questions about the Implementation of Cognitive Therapy Strategies

Q. Should I attempt to identify maladaptive cognitions in the assessment and include them in setting goals and contracting for therapy?

A. No, in the assessment you should be concerned with the symptoms of depression and the manifestations of them in the day-to-day life of the adolescent. In contracting for therapy, you normally will want to target the areas of functional impairment, for example, school failure. Maladaptive cognitions become the focus of attention in the middle phase of therapy. Specifically, steps two and three in the therapeutic process involve elicitation of automatic thoughts and identification of beliefs. Refer to Chapter 8, which discusses the process and techniques of the "working" phase of therapy.

Q. The adolescent appears to have so many problems that need to be addressed. Where do I begin?

A. Ask the patient and his parents to prioritize the problems. If one thing could be improved, what would they choose it to be? In addition, consult your initial formulation, which will suggest important domains for therapeutic intervention. Your own question about where to begin should be answered by considering two kinds of information: (1) the emotional, cognitive, or behavioral problems most distressing to the adolescent, and (2) the likelihood of successful intervention in a particular area.

Q. How do I proceed to use cognitive therapy techniques when the adolescent appears to have no specific problem or complaint other than a global, amorphous depression?

A. When utilization of techniques such as a mood chart fails to reveal any consistent relationship between particular situations, emotions, and thoughts, it may be more useful to explore the adolescent's general views about himself, his circumstances, and his future. Attempt to elicit beliefs rather than automatic thoughts using techniques such as down arrow questioning or others discussed in Chapter 8. The adolescent's depression could, for example, be related to an active perfectionistic schema.

Q. How do I engage younger adolescents or learning-disabled patients who deny or minimize problems?

A. Involve the family in therapy to determine whether they hold a different perspective. If they do, use the discrepancy to engage the adolescent in a discussion. During therapy sessions, pay particular attention to the adolescent's behaviors, which may demonstrate what he is unable to state verbally. With these patients, cognitive deficits (limitations) often will play a bigger role in the depression than cognitive distortions. Thus, your emphasis should be on providing concrete examples, modeling, and using exaggeration to convey a message.

Q. How should I respond when patients say they will do the homework but do not, or do it but forget to bring it to the session?

A. If the adolescent decided not to do the homework, inquire about his rationale, expressing concern that he did not view it as potentially helpful. In your own mind, review the appropriateness of the homework in light of your initial formulation. If the adolescent attempted to do the homework but abandoned his attempt, explore the reasons for his difficulty so that similar problems are avoided in the future. If motivation was a problem, consider using techniques such as the pro–con analysis, antiprocrastination, or activity scheduling applied to the task of therapy homework, specifically. In the future, take an active role in anticipating potential problems and solve them, with the adolescent's help, in advance. When feasible, engage family members in helping the adolescent to complete the homework. It is critical that you explore the adolescent's cognitions about the homework, both those contributing to and resulting from its noncompletion. If the adolescent simply forgot to bring the homework to the session, discuss what the adolescent remembers about its content.

Q. When patients collect empirical data (e.g., homework) that appear to verify their depressogenic views, how should I respond?

A. Remember that cognitive distortions can exert their influence in various domains, including the reporting of information as part of a homework exercise. The presentation of empirical data that consistently appear to verify negative views as realistic may be an indication that the adolescent is selectively attending to negative information, for example. Involve the adolescent's family members in therapy as soon as possible to determine whether the patient's reporting is accurate. Naturally, this strategy must be employed with sensitivity so as not to offend the adolescent by giving him the message that you do not believe him. If the patient's report was accurate, the existence of empirical data verifying a problematic situation often indicates the need to consider the (optional) sixth step in the therapeutic process, problem-solving. Refer to Chapter 8 for more discussion of the circumstances under which the therapist's focus would shift from changing cognitions to changing some aspect of the adolescent's environment.

Q. When therapy appears to be progressing well, how do I know that an active "approval schema" is not operating to enhance the adolescent's compliance with homework or his reporting of improvement that will not be sustained?

A. Since it is developmentally appropriate for adolescents to explore "identification" with various heroes, self-images, behaviors, interpersonal styles, or philosophies, the identification that occurs with the cognitive model of depression might be regarded as quite normal. To the extent that this identification with the model results in the successful completion of homework and enhances internalization of the cognitive therapy concepts, its effects probably will be more lasting than temporary. Furthermore, even if "approval seeking" initially motivated the adoption of new behaviors or ways of thinking, these changes usually will result in benefits to the adolescent that will reinforce continued utilization of the new cognitive or behavioral repertoire. If the adolescent has developed formal thinking skills, you might discuss the issue with him directly, for example, by asking, "How does people pleasing affect you and me?"

Q. How can I respond when a patient who understands the model "parrots" adaptive responses to maladaptive cognitions in a mocking way with obvious sarcasm, superficially telling me what he thinks I want to hear?

A. In a nonjudgmental way, comment on the tone of his voice or his apparent disbelief in the cognitive therapy techniques you have been discussing. Ask whether the adolescent thinks his style of working with you will be helpful to him in the long run. Since he apparently has not adopted the cognitive model as one that applies to himself, ask about his alternative explanations for the depression. Include his ideas or suggestions in future therapy. By discussing his apparent rejection of the therapy technique you employed, you probably will elicit cognitions about therapy that can themselves be subjected to empirical analysis.

Q. After using various techniques such as logical analysis or examining empirical data to challenge the maladaptive cognitions of an adolescent, he states that he agrees with the logic but does not feel any differently. What do I try next?

A. Acknowledge that changes of the "heart" often lag behind those of the "head" when adapting to a new situation. As such, improvement in the adolescent's feelings of depression may require a little more time than he expected. Also, remind the adolescent that his mood depends on a variety of things in his life about which he may have maladaptive cognitions; indicate that you would like to address other issues that may be maintaining his depression. The adolescent's report that logical argument has failed to make him feel emotionally better may be an indication that he is using dichotomous categories to classify his emotions. In other words, since he does not feel "completely happy," he may have concluded that he is still "completely depressed." Chapter 2 discusses the importance of challenging the adolescent's binary motif, and Chapter 8 reviews various suggestions for emphasizing a cognitive continuum rather than dichotomous categorization. In addition to the black-and-white thinking style, other cognitive errors may be acting to distort the adolescent's view of his emotional gains in therapy. Inquire about the possibility of minimization or predicting the future, for example.

Q. I am working hard to convey the cognitive therapy model to the adolescent but am concerned that he is not internalizing anything. How can I proceed?

A. Encourage application of cognitive therapy concepts to the adolescent's life outside of therapy sessions by presenting hypothetical but realistic situations and asking him what he has learned in cognitive therapy that would help him cope with the situation. Attempt to involve family members in the adolescent's homework, putting them in the role of "cotherapists" so that cognitive therapy has advocates who go home with the adolescent. If possible, relate cognitive therapy concepts to real-life "heroes" or fictional characters whom the adolescent admires because these characters have already been internalized. Finally, remember that repetition will be important for all adolescents, particularly for those who have limited cognitive skills because of their young age or comorbid diagnoses.

Q. What can I do when I feel discouraged about the progress a patient is making or feel "stuck" about what to try next?

A. Consult your original assessment report to see if there are some significant factors you had forgotten about while you pursue other issues in weekly therapy sessions (e.g., historical or family issues). Also consult your original written formulation to see if therapy with the adolescent has addressed your original hypotheses about cognitive factors and the depression. Family sessions will be essential in order to provide additional information about the adolescent's progress or continuing problems. Exploration of family beliefs on relevant issues is critical because the family system could inadvertently be working against your efforts in therapy. Consider the possible role of personality factors or cognitive limitations. Finally, examine your own role with the patient and family to see if you have become so "helpful" that they have been placed in a dependent "helpless" position and have delegated the adolescent's emotional well-being to your continued care.

Questions Related to Case Management

Q. When a patient repeatedly cancels or misses sessions, should I pursue him? If so, how soon, how often, and by what method?

A. Yes, you should pursue contact with the adolescent and his parents because the patient may be missing sessions without the knowledge of his parents who assume that therapy is continuing as usual. It will be important to gain an understanding of the reasons for cancelations or absences because you may be able to correct the problem easily. The family should normally be contacted within a day or two every time the adolescent misses a session. Phone contact is preferable to a letter because you will ensure that your message is received and will have an opportunity to gain an immediate understanding of the adolescent's attendance problems. Acknowledge how hard it is for the adolescent to come to therapy. Discuss his ambivalence and listen for the associated automatic thoughts, beliefs, or cognitive distortions that may be expressed. A family session will usually be required in order to explore the ways in which therapy could be more helpful to the adolescent. At such times, parents may reveal their own role in the adolescent's absences, for example, by refusing to provide transportation. Remember that adolescents may have difficulty terminating relationships and may be using the cancellations or absences to indicate that they feel termination is appropriate. If this is the case, review the various styles of termination outlined in Chapter 9.

Q. How can I respond when parents indicate that they can no longer afford the time or the money to pay for therapy?

A. In most cases, you can preclude the possibility of this problem arising by discussing relevant issues during the initial phase of therapy when contracting is done. Parents should understand the time and financial implications before you embark on a course of cognitive therapy. Even though initially supportive, parents may be most inclined to withdraw their support if they are doubtful about the benefits of therapy and if they feel estranged from the process of therapeutic change. Remember that it will be important to include parents in periodic family sessions and to use them as "cotherapists" between sessions. Listen for parents' maladaptive cognitions about their adolescent's therapy, and address them using appropriate cognitive therapy techniques. You should be vigilant for marital or family problems that the parents may be attempting to avoid by withdrawing from therapy. Address any concerns you have directly by engaging parents in a discussion of the consequences of their choices for the adolescent. The technique of time projection may be particularly useful, for example, inquiring about the long-term future prospects for the adolescent if therapy does not address the depression and/or behavioral problems now.

Q. Under what circumstances should I refer the adolescent to other types of therapy or other therapists?

A. Remember that patients sometimes present for treatment of depression with significant hidden agendas (refer to Chapter 6). If you become aware of hidden agendas, you may wish to consider referral to more appropriate agencies. If the adolescent has significant skill deficits, he may require more attention to skill development than is appropriate for your therapy sessions, in which case referral should be considered. Consider the possibility that significant personality factors, such as schizoid personality disorder, may be better treated in longer-term group therapies. Also, primary substance abuse/dependence may be better treated in a "dual-diagnosis" clinic. If sexual abuse is a significant factor in the formulation for an adolescent, carefully consider your relationship with the patient, as referral may be indicated. Refer to Chapter 11 for discussion of the issues in treating depressed adolescents who have been the victims of sexual abuse. If the depression worsens significantly or suicidal risk becomes extreme, you may wish to consider hospitalization. If the adolescent indicates no improvement within six or eight sessions in spite of your attempts to involve the family and observe the other cognitive therapy principles (refer to Chapter 2), antidepressant medication may be indicated, if not already in place.

NOVICE COGNITIVE THERAPISTS: A CHECKLIST OF 10 RECOMMENDATIONS FOR IMPROVED THERAPY

During the process of teaching cognitive therapy and supervising the first cases of therapists within the "new" paradigm, we observed that some aspects of the therapy were harder to learn or easier to forget than others. Although there were individual differences, depending on the therapist's prior experience and previous theoretical background, it became apparent that the same recommendations for improvement were often repeated. The 10 most frequent suggestions offered to therapists are summarized below and may serve as a guide to others who are learning or beginning to practice cognitive therapy with depressed adolescents. Of course, it is assumed that, prior to anticipating the application of cognitive therapy with depressed adolescents, therapists will have acquired a comprehensive understanding of the cognitive theory of depression and will have digested several relevant publications about the treatment of depression using a cognitive therapy model (e.g., Beck et al., 1979; Burns, 1980). Given that this knowledge is an essential prerequisite, the discussions that follow make no attempt to provide basic instruction in the theory or general practice of cognitive therapy. Rather, the 10 recommendations might best be viewed as a checklist for therapists wishing to improve their skills.

1. Prepare a Written Cognitive Formulation

Each depressed adolsecent will present with a unique array of symptomatology and functional difficulties in day-to-day living. The purpose of a formulation is to interpret the presenting problems using the theoretical concepts that are central to cognitive therapy. The act of preparing a written formulation assists the therapist in his own thought process, thereby encouraging greater systematic review of the "facts" as presented by the patient and the relationship between them and the theoretical model that is the basis of cognitive therapy. If a conscious effort is not made to incorporate all of the adolescent's emotional and behavioral manifestations of depression in a written formulation, therapists risk embarking on a course of therapy that will be disjointed and characterized by weekly shifts in focus from one issue to another seemingly unrelated one. Although discussions from session to session may indeed reflect different "surface content," the formulation provides an overview of them all and allows the therapist to adopt a "metaposition" from which different problems can be viewed as examples of the same theme. The ability to identify this theme and communicate it to the patient is central to therapy because a theme is like a superordinate category that helps adolescents to organize their experiences. Rather than feeling overwhelmed by their inability to cope with a myriad of problems, depressed adolescents gain a sense of perspective and hope if a host of emotional and behavioral difficulties can be reduced to only one or two central issues.

When novice cognitive therapists are asked about their case formulation for a particular adolescent, one problem that arises is that they tend to respond by repeating the "facts" as presented by the adolescent, mentioning only a superficial relationship between them and theoretical concepts. For example, an adolescent's failing school grades, conflict with friends or family, and social withdrawal may be summarily dismissed as bearing some relationship to "low self-esteem." But this is not an adequate formulation of the case. The failing school grades and interpersonal conflict may be contributors to low self-esteem, whereas the social withdrawal may be a result of it. Furthermore, although an unrealistically negative view of "self" is one part of the cognitive triad central to cognitive theory, the therapist may neglect to consider the other two components of the triad: the adolescent's view of his current "world" or circumstances and his future. By disciplining himself to write a formulation, the therapist enhances the likelihood that he will carefully consider all aspects of the adolescent's phenomenological field and all aspects of the cognitive therapy model.

A second problem that arises in the absence of a written case formulation is the tendency of therapists to offer an explanation of the causal relationships between "facts" or events in the adolescent's life in stimulus–response behavioral terms without accounting for the role of cognition. For example, the therapist may explain that an adolescent's uncontrolled angry behavior (the presenting problem) is the result of unresolved conflict with parents, which is the result of failing school grades, which are the result of disorganized study habits, which are in turn the result of learning difficulties caused by attention-deficit hyperactivity disorder. Although the therapist's speculations about this cause-and-effect sequence may be quite reasonable, this explanation of the presenting problem excludes hypotheses about the adolescent's views of himself (e.g., "I am stupid and a bad person"), his current life circumstances (e.g., "Nobody understands or cares about me"), and his future (e.g., "There's no point in trying since I'll just fail anyway"). But the central premise of cognitive therapy is that the individual's maladaptive automatic thoughts or underlying beliefs can exacerbate or maintain the depressive symptomatology, so a cognitive therapist must seek to intervene in the patient's maladaptive cognitive process and will be critically hampered in so doing if the case formulation fails to take account of the role of cognition. The preparation of a written formulation will decrease the likelihood that cognitive factors are omitted from the explanatory hypothesis.

A third problem that often occurs in the absence of a written case formulation is the therapist's failure to incorporate relevant information derived from family members. Remember that an adolescent is largely dependent on his family system and will be heavily influenced by its prevailing beliefs. Thus, failure to include significant family views in the formulation will result in an inability to speculate about the impact of its members on the adolescent's views of himself, his circumstances, or his future. For example, a depressed adolescent may present with complaints about his inability to achieve the academic performance to which he aspires. As a result, he may report automatic thoughts such as "I should have done better on that exam," and hold beliefs such as "I'm not good enough," or "I'll never amount to anything." A formulation that took these cognitions into account might lead to therapeutic interventions directed at altering the adolescent's perception of his abilities and future, or at adjusting the high expectations he places on himself. However, such a formulation would be incomplete and therapeutic interventions could be relatively ineffective if the therapist neglected to consider the fact that both parents were high-achieving professionals who upheld perfectionistic standards for themselves and their children, or the fact that the adolescent's older siblings were intellectually gifted individuals who were apparently successful in following their parents' covert directives with respect to achievement, career endeavors, and financial success. A comprehensive formulation would, of necessity, incorporate the family's beliefs about personal worth and valued endeavor. A comprehensive treatment plan would examine the adaptiveness of this family schema for the adolescent in question.

In some cases, the apparent reluctance of therapists to develop a written case formulation or their oversight in so doing may be related to their assumption that an initial formulation is the same thing as a definitive explanation. Laboring under this misconception, therapists might claim to feel more comfortable writing a formulation at the conclusion of therapy rather than at the beginning. But such an orientation fails to credit the formulation with its dynamic properties of change and development over time. Initial formulations can and should be amended as greater understanding is gained about the adolescent's depression, environmental influences, personality, and cognitive development.

2. Maintain a Metaposition

A *metaposition* refers to the mental activity of the therapist that is directed at processing the ongoing therapist–patient interaction as it relates to cognitive theory and the adolescent's case formulation. In essence, the cognitive therapist must learn to split his attention between the observable activity in a session (e.g., semantic content, grammatical syntax, pace of interaction, application of particular interventions and techniques) and his own nonobservable mental activity in a session (e.g., forming hypotheses, amending the formulation, assessing the purpose of ongoing interaction).

Failure to maintain a metaposition is manifested in various ways. Perhaps the most obvious indication is the therapist's oversight in relating the content of the current session to previous sessions. Repetition across therapy sessions may occur with respect to the nature of problematic situations experienced, the emotional or behavioral patterns displayed, the schemas represented by various automatic thoughts, or the type of cognitive errors evidenced in the adolescent's thought processes. Inadequate maintenance of a metaposition also may be indicated by the therapist's premature utilization of a specific therapy technique without enough consideration of its purpose. For example, the techniques appropriate for eliciting automatic thoughts (step II in the middle phase of therapy) are usually not appropriate for identifying beliefs (step III in the therapeutic process). And attempts to evaluate maladaptive cognitions (step IV) will appear somewhat pointless unless the adolescent has first developed an adequate awareness of the relationship between precipitating situations and his emotional reactions to them (the first step in the "working" phase of therapy) as well as an awareness of the relationship between his emotions and his thoughts or beliefs (steps II and III). Finally, a therapist committed to treating an adolescent's depression usually works hard to ameliorate the extreme negative emotion that precipitated the request for therapy. Since most therapists are predisposed to helping their adolescent patients feel better emotionally, they may exhibit premature attempts to "rescue" a patient who displays strong negative affect during a session, for example, by shifting the focus of discussion to something less emotionally provocative. But rushing to the adolescent's aid in such a manner may indicate that the therapist has abandoned his metaposition, which would suggest that the most appropriate course of action is pursuit of the adolescent's thoughts and beliefs associated with strong affective displays, rather than withdrawal from them.

Sometimes it appears as if therapists have adopted an adequate metaposition because they relate part of the cognitive model to the content of a session. For example, a therapist may skillfully elicit an adolescent's automatic thoughts associated with a particular situation but neglect to show the patient the relationship between these particular thoughts and his depressed mood or maladaptive behavior in the situation being examined. Or a therapist may succeed in helping the adolescent to identify and evaluate his beliefs but fail to assist the adolescent in the formation of new, more adaptive beliefs to replace the old ones.

The skill of dividing one's attention between the adolescent present in the room and the theoretical model underlying therapy is one that is developed over time. Maintenance of a metaposition will be particularly challenging during family sessions when the therapist's attention will be drawn to several people at once. However, the therapist's ability to divide his attention effectively will be enhanced greatly if the therapist attempts to review critically his own videotaped sessions or discusses them with knowledgeable observers. The sooner a metaposition can be maintained, the faster a therapist's skill will develop because cognitive therapy is founded in theory, not in technique.

3. Adjust Your Own Negative Bias

By definition, mental health professionals expect their referrals to be patients who have emotional and/or behavioral problems. By the nature of the disorder, depression is usually characterized by unrealistic negative cognition. Thus, therapists treating depressed adolescents usually enter the therapeutic relationship with the expectation that the primary focus of therapy will be identifying, evaluating, and changing the patient's unrealistic negative cognition. Although the therapist's bias to attend to distressing affect, undesirable life experiences, problematic behavior, and negative cognition may be a reasonable one in the initial stages of therapy, it usually becomes increasingly less appropriate as therapy progresses.

The inappropriateness of noticing primarily "the negative" has several serious repercussions. First, therapists who are in the habit of attending to the negative aspects of an adolescent's experience may inadvertently neglect to reinforce the adolescent for his successes in changing dysfunctional negative cognitions or problematic behavior. If relatively little attention is paid to these accomplishments, the unspoken message that may be communicated to the adolescent is that his progress is insignificant or unimportant. As a result, the adolescent may become discouraged and suffer a loss of self-efficacy. Second, since therapists are always in the role of modeling behaviors and cognitive styles for adolescents, cognitive errors made by therapists communicate a covert message about how the patient's accomplishments should be evaluated. The therapist who neglects to notice small positive accomplishments demonstrates his own cognitive error by minimizing the adolescent's success. In addition, the therapist demonstrates a tendency to selectively attend to only part of the adolescent's life experience. This may be quite confusing for the adolescent who simultaneously receives two conflicting directives. On the one hand, the adolescent hears the therapist overtly stressing the importance of avoiding the "mental filter" or the "binocular vision" cognitive style. On the other hand, the adolescent experiences the therapist demonstrating the opposite in his own behavior by apportioning little time and attention to content with a positive rather than negative valence. Third, therapists who listen almost exclusively for negative emotion or cognition will often miss opportunities to correct depressogenic attributions for positive life events because the positive event or experience is dismissed as something not requiring exploration. Important questions about the adolescent's attributions for the positive event may never be asked, thus precluding the opportunity to discover depressogenic external, unstable, or specific attributions for it. Fourth, the therapist who is primed to investigate only negative content in the adolescent's verbalizations will likely fail to investigate unrealistically positive views the adolescent may hold. Although some researchers have argued that most nondepressed people hold unrealistically positive views to some degree, if the extent of discrepancy between "reality" and the adolescent's overly positive perception of it becomes too great, he will eventually experience severe disappointment and will be at risk for relapse into more severe depression. Furthermore, the adolescent who presents unrealistically positive points of view after being in therapy for some time may, in fact, be demonstrating dichotomous thinking with his radical switch from an "all negative" to an "all positive" perspective.

Obviously, the therapist's inclination to attend to negative emotion, behavior, and thought will serve him well in terms of maximizing therapeutic "sensitivity" to maladaptive negative cognition. But, as tends to be the case with all screening procedures, excessive sensitivity will exact a price in terms of "specificity," this being the exploration of only appropriate negative aspects of the adolescent's experience. Thus, one important requirement for the maintenance of an adequate metaposition will be the therapist's careful assessment of his own bias to attend to the negative.

4. Seek a Comprehensive Understanding of the Adolescent's World View

A "comprehensive" understanding of the adolescent's world view cannot be achieved unless the therapist becomes an active, inquisitive participant in conversation about the adolescent's weekly life experiences. Novice therapists sometimes make the mistake of assuming they know what a patient means when complaining about common adolescent issues such as "school" or "rules." By accepting the adolescent's vague reference to problems, the therapist forgoes the opportunity to discover potentially maladaptive cognitions and, as such, compromises the therapeutic process greatly. For example, it would not be uncommon for a depressed adolescent to claim, "It's hard to deal with the pressures of school." A therapist who was aware of parental concerns about the adolescent's declining academic performance might mistakenly conclude that the adolescent's reference to "pressures of school" meant trouble completing homework or passing exams when, in fact, the adolescent might have been referring to social pressures from peers to engage in dishonest or illegal activities. Alternatively, a therapist who was aware of a history of learning disabilities might mistakenly assume that the adolescent's "difficulty dealing" with the pressures of school meant trouble concentrating or expressing himself verbally when, in fact, the patient might have been referring to his dilemma in choosing between a group of athletically oriented friends and a group of party-oriented friends who were both competing for his allegiance. Only by inquiring about the precise meaning of the adolescent's words "dealing with pressures" could the therapist hope to achieve a comprehensive understanding of the adolescent's world view.

With many adolescents it will not be sufficient to probe with statements like "Tell me the meaning of your words 'dealing with school pressures.'" Greater understanding will be achieved by posing questions such as "What particular part of school is hardest?" or "How do you try to deal with school?" or "Who else does/doesn't have the same pressures?" or "When have you been somewhat successful?" or "If you were in another school, would the pressures be fewer/greater/the same?" Of course, everything the adolescent says cannot be explored in such detail. The therapist must be selective, paying particular attention to the intensity of emotion attached to various topics. Remember that affect is the "radar beam" that will most readily lead to maladaptive cognition.

As greater comprehension of the adolescent's world view is gained, this information should be used to amend the initial formulation. Since the formulation is an evolving explanation of the adolescent's depression, it will serve to guide both the content and process of therapy.

5. Employ Questions Rather Than Statements Whenever Possible

The use of Socratic dialogue is central to cognitive therapy because a series of questions leading the patient to verbalize a conclusion is more powerful than the same conclusion stated by the therapist. The therapeutic impact of carefully formulated questions derives from at least four sources. First, questions posed by the therapist usually imply a request for a response from the patient. As such, adolescents are more likely to become engaged in an active thought process focusing on some issue than would be the case if they were only passively listening to the therapist's declarations. Second, the developmental stage of adolescence is characterized by egocentricity, a quest for independence, and caution in trusting adults. Here, the Socratic dialogue fosters a guided discovery of the adolescent's beliefs and invites him into a metaposition as well. As a result, the adolescent patient is likely to give more credence to the observations he verbalizes himself than to those offered by the therapist. Third, many adolescents will have experienced lengthy "lectures" delivered by their parents or other adults and will be relatively unfamiliar with the role of voicing their own opinions. Therefore, the use of questions may indicate to the adolescent that his relationship with the therapist is notably different from that with many other adults, and this difference will most often be interpreted as a positive one. Fourth, questions indicate respect on the part of the interviewer for the respondent. As such, the therapist's frequent use of questions helps to convey interest, open-mindedness, and a willingness to consider the adolescent's point of view, which will enhance the therapeutic alliance.

Sometimes novice cognitive therapists may resort to statements because they feel uncertain about their ability to pose a series of questions which will lead the adolescent to the "right" or "desired" conclusion. However, this fear arises only in the presence of the therapist's assumption that there are, in fact, "correct" or "better" answers to questions. In fact, any response offered by the adolescent is useful information. Sometimes novice cognitive therapists may hesitate to examine an issue using a series of questions because they feel that they will retain greater control over the direction of conversation if they make statements designed to "teach" or make some point. Ironically, this strategy may result in less control because the adolescent may "tune out" yet another "lecture." The opposite may also occur with overuse of statements relative to questions. In the case where the therapist's statements are regarded as the "absolute truth," the adolescent may become overly dependent on the therapist for guidance, resulting in the false appearance of increased helpfulness on the part of the therapist but greater helplessness on the part of the patient.

6. Prioritize the Issues to Be Addressed

Adolescents often present with many functional problems in addition to the symptoms of depression. Common complaints of parents are that the adolescent is performing poorly in school, exhibiting destructive behavior when angry, fighting with friends and siblings, secluding himself in his bedroom, refusing to perform regular household tasks, or even making suicidal threats and gestures. Discussion with the adolescent usually results in further elaboration of specific problems such as dislike of a certain school teacher, a recent fight with his best friend, refusal by his father to provide money for some desired purchase, the expectations of his mother regarding his music lessons, or virtually endless other possibilities. In addition, the adolescent may identify chronic difficulties such as feeling guilty about participating in an illegal activity a few months previously or feeling inadequate relative to his siblings who he has always believed are the "favorites" of his parents. Faced with so many varied issues, the therapist may wonder where to begin. If prioritization of the problems has not been accomplished during the initial phase of therapy, the therapist may attempt to address everything in a rather haphazard fashion. The result will usually be frequent changes in focus and topic without adequate resolution of any one issue.

In deciding where to begin, the therapist may be tempted to address the "biggest" problem first, assuming that resolution of it will provide the greatest relief to the adolescent. For example, a depressed girl who has the comorbid diagnosis of post traumatic stress disorder may identify recurrent nightmares, experiences of dissociation, and guilt about an incident of past sexual abuse as the problems most disturbing to her. Less serious from her perspective may be her feelings of inadequacy relative to her sisters, her sense of worthlessness among her circle of friends, and her guilt because she appears unable to ensure her mother's happiness at all times. Common themes throughout discussions with this adolescent may be her belief that she should be able to control other people's behaviors or emotions and that it is her fault because she has been unable to do so. The therapist might hypothesize that two factors are central to the adolescent's depression: (1) her inability to meet the perfectionistic standards she has set for herself, and (2) her depressogenic attributions for negative life events.

Rather than address the adolescent's maladaptive cognitions in the context of discussion about the incident of sexual abuse (the biggest problem from the patient's point of view), the therapist might be advised to begin by focusing on the girl's ongoing life experiences with her sisters, mother, and friends (lesser problems from the patient's point of view). The major advantage of this strategy is that examination of current experiences will afford the opportunity to collect relevant empirical data during the time between sessions. As the adolescent learns to relax her perfectionistic standards, change her depressogenic attributional style, and correct her "should-y" thinking errors related to her sisters, her friends, and her mother, these cognitive changes can be expected to transfer to the issues of responsibility and guilt the girl felt in relation to the sexual abuse. Typically, the symptoms associated with this traumatic experience will decrease, even though they were not addressed directly as the first course of action. Naturally, the therapist would want to assess the adolescent's symptoms and cognitions regarding the sexual trauma before terminating therapy.

The important point to abstract from the example above is that cognitive change made in relation to one issue will reap benefits in relation to other issues. Furthermore, in setting priorities for therapy, the therapist should carefully consider both the importance of the issues in the overall picture and the likelihood of achieving cognitive change in relation to them. Preparation of a case formulation and maintenance of a metaposition will be invaluable aids to the process of setting appropriate priorities.

7. Watch for Subtle Behavioral Cues

Novice cognitive therapists often report that they feel mentally very "busy" during a therapy session. Attention must be devoted to the therapeutic alliance, time management, the content of discussion, the formulation of their own comments or questions, and the memory of details from previous sessions, while simultaneously a metaposition must be maintained that requires consideration of cognitive theory, the case formulation, depressive symptomatology, functional problems, developmental stage, personality factors, family factors, the stages of therapy, and therapeutic techniques. Given the significant demands on their attention, therapists sometimes miss subtle behavioral cues provided by the adolescent. However, many adolescents will be unable to communicate certain information orally either because they lack the verbal skills or because they lack an immediate awareness of the issue. In such cases, the adolescent's actions will speak louder than words and successful communication of the message will depend on the therapist's ability to notice and correctly interpret the patient's behaviors.

The importance of attending to subtle behavioral cues most often will arise in relation to depressed adolescents who have comorbid problems with attention, learning disabilities, and personality style. Diagnoses such as attention-deficit hyperactivity disorder, specific learning disabilities (Axis II), or schizoid personalty disorder may not have been made at the time of initial assessment; and, even if they were, the therapist may forget to watch for behavioral indications of the adolescent's confusion or inattention.

When novice cognitive therapists become frustrated with the rate of progress in therapy, most seem inclined to attribute the difficulty to their own skill deficits. Consequently, they may redouble their efforts to use a greater variety of intervention techniques. But if the major impediment to progress in therapy is actually the adolescent's cognitive limitation or personality style, the therapist's misattribution of problems to himself will only result in further frustration. Reviewing a difficult case with questions such as the following may help the therapist to make more appropriate attributions for the apparent lack of progress. Does the adolescent decrease his verbal participation at some point in the session? Do responses to questions become increasingly brief, vague, or evasive? Does the adolescent show clear cognitive deficits with sequential reasoning or with auditory processing as compared to visual processing of information? Does eye contact decrease, fidgeting increase, or posture become more distanced? Does the therapist find himself repeating ideas more frequently because the adolescent misses the point? Does the adolescent indicate an exaggerated preference for discussing fantasy, science fiction, or his own imaginal characters? Are the "heroes" with whom the adolescent identifies bizarre or unusual (e.g., the android on *Star Trek*)? Do the adolescent's gestures or general presentation in the session exceed even the range that would include "eccentric"? Because a therapist who is accustomed to working with adolescents comes to expect and tolerate more extreme behaviors, he may be predisposed to ignore or misinterpret subtle cues such as those identified above. He would be advised to reset his threshold for them accordingly. In so doing, the therapist will better be able to recognize significant comorbidity such as pervasive developmental disorder, schizoid personality disorder, or attention-deficit hyperactivity disorder with severe learning problems.

8. Develop Your Skills for Setting an Agenda

Almost invariably, novice cognitive therapists will begin a session by asking, "What should we put on our agenda?" or "What's important for us to discuss today?" Although the therapist's intentions are admirable, his execution of them is less than adequate. The attempt to set an agenda by posing questions such as these is a rather formal beginning to a therapy session and, as such, does not "fit" well with the general tendency of adolescent therapy to be somewhat informal, spontaneous, or even "playful" in nature. Furthermore, a direct request for agenda items implies that the adolescent should be able to state the issues of concern to him in a succinct and clear manner. For many adolescents, this will be a skill beyond their abilities. A direct request for agenda items may also be experienced as threatening to adolescents, who may feel an obligation to state the "right" things for inclusion on the list. Finally, if the adolescent says there is nothing important to discuss, proceeding to develop an agenda based on the therapist's own perspective might be interpreted by the adolescent as evidence that he is inadequate in some way, or worse, as a confrontational gesture by the therapist.

A more natural and appropriate way of establishing an agenda is for the therapist to ask about the adolescent's general well-being or various life spheres that are known to be of relevance. For example, the therapist might inquire about the current status of some aspect of the adolescent's depressive symptomatology, such as a significant sleep disturbance. Or the therapist might ask if there have been any significant developments in the areas of school, friends, activities, or home life. If appropriate, the therapist will want to inquire about the adolescent's homework from the previous session. By taking a quick "survey" in this manner, the therapist will cue the adolescent about what topics are of potential importance for the current session and may help jog the adolescent's memory about issues he meant to highlight but had forgotten.

Throughout the somewhat superficial exploration of the adolescent's life in the opening minutes of the session, the therapist should be noting any topics he feels are appropriate to address in the remainder of the session. Those identified as potential agenda items should be identified for the adolescent, who may then assist with prioritization of them. While developing an agenda for the session, it will be important for the therapist to use his professional judgment about the number of issues to be addressed, truncating the list if necessary, in a collaborative manner. Too many agenda items can leave both the adolescent and the therapist feeling overwhelmed and can impose a sense of urgency to finish one topic so that the next can be addressed. Both problems will be counterproductive.

Skill and practice are required in order to survey various spheres of the adolescent's life without becoming engaged in substantive discussion while attempting to set the agenda. When the therapist probes an area of particular relevance to an adolescent, the patient may launch into a lengthy and detailed account of some experience. However, most adolescents are quite tolerant of the therapist's gentle interruption suggesting that they defer further discussion to later in the session, after development of the agenda. Of course it will be important to return to the deferred topic or else the adolescent may conclude that setting an agenda is a rather pointless exercise, thereby becoming less inclined to participate in the process in future sessions. As each session nears its conclusion, if the therapist discovers that the agenda was overly ambitious, deferring some topics to the next session is an acceptable strategy. The important thing is that agenda items are not merely "dropped."

When verbalizing agenda items, the therapist is advised to watch for opportunities to use cognitive therapy concepts with which the adolescent is familiar. For example, instead of listing "Anger about exam mark" as an agenda item, the therapist might relabel exactly the same issue as "Perfectionistic standards and self-expectations." In this way, agendas may display some continuity from session to session even though the specific content of the real-life difficulties may change.

9. Develop Your Skills for Designing Homework

In therapy sessions conducted by novice cognitive therapists, homework assignments are often given hurriedly in the last few minutes of the session. Pressured by time constraints, the therapist may quickly state, for example, "I'd like you to keep track of your feelings and some of your automatic thoughts in the coming week." But if homework is introduced to adolescents in this vague and hurried way, they will be unlikely to understand or comply with the suggestion. Like other aspects of cognitive therapy, homework should be a collaborative endeavor, with the adolescent participating in a discussion about the rationale and the requirements of a particular homework exercise. To the extent that the adolescent is involved in such a discussion, he likely will feel that the homework is not a directive imposed by the therapist but, rather, an activity that he himself decided to pursue. The advantage of this perspective is that the adolescent will be more inclined to remember and complete the homework exercise.

Although the discussion of homework often occurs in the latter part of a session, it need not be relegated to the closing few minutes. Periodically throughout each session, the therapist would be advised to summarize the point of discussion. For example, sometime during the middle of a session the therapist might ask, "What's the important thing we have just learned about you during our discussion of [your fear about changing schools]?" If the adolescent were to respond by stating something like "I jump to conclusions about what other people are thinking and predict the worst about things in the future," then the therapist could use this insight to introduce a discussion of homework that would help the patient to correct these cognitive errors. For example, the therapist might ask, "Since you've discovered this about yourself, do you think it would be helpful for us to figure out a way of breaking your habit?" Assuming that the adolescent responded in the affirmative, a collaborative discussion of homework could follow. Perhaps the therapist could suggest that the adolescent become more aware of how often and in what situations he tended to jump to conclusions. For example, the therapist might explain the triple-column technique, suggesting that the adolescent review each day in the coming week and record each instance of mood disturbance (e.g., anxiety, depression, anger), the situation that engendered it, the thoughts that occurred when the adolescent was feeling particularly upset, and more adaptive responses to each maladaptive thought.

Various options regarding the format of the homework could be offered as well, with the adolescent choosing the one he thought would be most helpful to him. For example, younger adolescents might prefer to indicate the height of "mercury" in an emotional thermometer and write the precipitating situation and their automatic thoughts beside it. Alternatively, younger adolescents might prefer to keep a frequency record of the occurrence of "typical" automatic thoughts that had been listed during the session, noting the occurrence of each thought on the list with checkmarks and the dates and situations when each occurred. Older adolescents might like to keep notes in a personal diary or in a "daytimer" that they already use to record appointments or school assignments. By raising the issue of homework at any appropriate point in the session, the therapist will have more time to engage in a collaborative discussion of it, and the adolescent will understand better the direct relationship between issues discussed during the session and the homework exercise. Both factors will enhance the likelihood of homework being completed.

Regardless of when in the session homework is discussed, it will be important for the therapist to inquire about the adolescent's understanding of the rationale for it at the end of the session. For example, the therapist may wish to state, "Earlier today, we talked about some observations you were going to make on yourself this week. How do you think that is going to help you with your depression?" If the adolescent has difficulty explaining the rationale for the homework, the therapist will have an opportunity to ensure that it is understood.

When adolescents fail to complete homework assignments, it is often because they were unsure about what to do. Although it may have seemed clear to them during discussion in the session, later in the week at home they may be more uncertain. Rather than risk doing it the "wrong way," the adolescent often will not attempt the exercise at all. Verbal instructions provided during the session will seldom suffice when it comes time for the adolescent to do the homework later in the week. Therefore, it is advisable for the therapist to write something specific on a paper for the adolescent to take home. These instructions should be demonstrative to the greatest extent possible. For instance, providing an "empty" mood chart, complete with allocated space for each day and a written example of a mood rating and corresponding situation will help to remind the adolescent what is to be recorded during the week. Alternatively, the therapist could provide a blank form indicating the five-column format for the dysfunctional thoughts daily record, complete with an example relevant to the adolescent's life written in by the therapist. The therapist might attempt to preempt the adolescent's frustration or neglect of the homework by inviting him to phone the therapist if he encounters any problems remembering what to do in the coming week.

The technique of cognitive rehearsal can be particularly useful when applied to issues of homework. The therapist might inquire about when the adolescent anticipates doing the homework each day, or how he will remember to do it. For example, it is often useful to ask questions such as "How will you remember to do this exercise each day?" or "Where will you put the [mood chart] so that you see it and remember to fill in the information?" or "Do you think it would be best for you to write some things down when you get home from school or just before you go to bed at night? How will you remember to do it on the weekends?" To check the adolescent's understanding of the homework, it is often useful to provide a hypothetical example and ask the adolescent what information he would record. Of course, the therapist should inquire about any potential problems the adolescent anticipates could arise in attempting to complete the homework. In sum, the therapist will want to ensure that the adolescent understands clearly the rationale for doing homework, what and when it is to be done, and how he should cope with any difficulties encountered while attempting the exercise.

10. Remember to Summarize the Session

One of the most common omissions from therapy sessions conducted by novice cognitive therapists is a summary of what has been discussed. This oversight occurs most frequently when the therapist suddenly realizes that the time allocated for a session has nearly expired and rushes to address a few more issues such as the assignment of homework, renewal of prescriptions for medication, and scheduling the next appointment. The risk in terminating a session without a summary is that the adolescent will leave feeling somewhat overwhelmed by the extent of discussion, unsure about which part of it deserves particular attention. Under such circumstances, the adolescent's internalization of therapeutic concepts will be severely compromised.

　　In its most extreme form, the inappropriate termination of a session will be characterized by statements such as "We have to stop for today, but we can continue this discussion next time." In effect, the adolescent is left in limbo, uncertain of what to think or do differently during the interim between sessions. This kind of termination leaves issues unfinished and, as such, can even exacerbate the adolescent's emotional distress. To avoid the confusion and discomfort that may arise from overly rapid terminations of sessions, the therapist must use his metaposition to maintain a perspective on time and the pacing of activities in a session.

Just as the discussion of homework need not be deferred to the closing minutes of a session, summaries need not occur only at the termination of the therapeutic hour. In fact, it is advisable for therapists to inquire about the adolescent's understanding of what is being discussed periodically throughout the session. By so doing, the therapist invites the adolescent to adopt his own metaposition and to consider the relevance of the discussion for his depression, forming hypotheses about his affect and maladaptive cognitions or behaviors. If the points to be extracted from discussion are identified periodically during therapy, the summary at the end of the session can make reference to them, leaving the adolescent with a sense of continuity and completion.

Some novice cognitive therapists will attempt to summarize a session by referring to the specific content of various topics addressed. For example, the therapist might state, "Today we have discussed your trouble studying for exams and the fights you are having with your mom." While this may be true at one level of abstraction, a summary that identifies only specific content issues in the adolescent's life will fail in its attempt to aid internalization of the therapy process. Instead, the therapist who had discussed inadequate study habits or conflict with a parent would be better advised to summarize the session by referring to cognitive theory and the concepts that had been imparted to the adolescent during the session. For example, the therapist might state, "While discussing your trouble with exams and the fights with your mother, we learned that your problems often stem from a tendency to procrastinate, which occurs because you sometimes magnify the size of the task to be done. Is that right?" By summarizing the session with reference to cognitive therapy concepts, the therapist models and reinforces the importance of adopting a metaposition from which to view problems. In addition, the therapist provides the adolescent with a generalized statement of problems or solutions that will be applicable across a variety of situations with different specific content.

The summarization of a session, like all other endeavors in cognitive therapy, should be a collaborative exercise. The therapist can encourage the adolescent to participate in summarizing important concepts by asking questions rather than making statements. For example, the therapist might ask, "What have we learned about the connection between your depression and the way you view yourself?" or "Did we discover anything about your thinking style that will help you to fight the depression?" The therapist usually will want to inquire about what part of the session was most useful to the adolescent or what part of the discussion the adolescent will be most likely to remember through the coming week. In this way, the therapist gains feedback about what information is being attended to and internalized by the adolescent. Finally, the therapist should ask if there was any part of the session which the adolescent did not understand or felt was not particularly helpful so that clarification can be offered and future sessions can be designed to better meet the adolescent's needs.

NEED FOR ALTERNATE INTERVENTIONS

Cognitive therapy is clearly most helpful in cases where the onset of adolescence, with its associated tasks of increasing autonomy, self-regulation, and self-actualization, has activated dysfunctional depressogenic schemas. Although the original schemas may have served the adolescent quite well initially, a changing social context may challenge him and overwhelm personal resources, resulting in depression. Cognitive therapy can then focus on helping the adolescent to adapt to a new biopsychosocial matrix. However, cognitive therapy may not be enough. If it is not, medication, hospitalization, and relocation to the child-welfare system or the legal system are some options available to the patient and therapist. These options need to be discussed actively with the adolescent and his family, who may offer their own solutions as alternatives. Of course, second opinions and referral to a different therapist with a different theoretical orientation may also be in order. Finally, no treatment modality is 100% successful. A "tincture" of time is often the greatest intervention of all.

SELECTED READINGS

Beck AT, Rush AJ, Shaw BF, Emery G: *Cognitive Therapy of Depression*. New York, Guilford Press, 1979.

Burns DD: *Feeling Good*. New York, William Morrow, 1980.

Kendall PC, Hollon SD (eds): *Assessment Strategies for Cognitive-Behavioral Interventions*. New York, Academic Press, 1981.

Popper KR, Eccles JC: *The Self and Its Brain*. New York, Springer International, 1977.

Index